Current Topics in SARS-CoV-2/COVID-19 - Two Years After

Edited by Alfonso J. Rodriguez-Morales

Published in London, United Kingdom

Current Topics in SARS-CoV-2/COVID-19 - Two Years After
http://dx.doi.org/10.5772/intechopen.100818
Edited by Alfonso J. Rodriguez-Morales

Contributors
Lesley Burgess, Matthew Wilson, Jurie Johannes Jordaan, Alfonso J. Rodriguez-Morales, D. Katterine Bonilla-Aldana, Josphert N. Kimatu, Huseyin Tombuloglu, Galyah Alhamid, Marco Pellegrini, Cesare Saccani, Alessandro Guzzini, Arbind Kumar, Sanjay Kumar, Narendra Vijay Tirpude, Yogendra Padwad, Aashish Sharma, Shaifali Sharma, Yong Yang, Yanyan Li, Tahereh Alinejad, Danial Zareh, Cheng-shui Chen, Zuo Hao, Tengfei Zhou, Chang-qing Xu, Andres Escobar, Adekunle Sanyaolu, Aleksandra Marinkovic, Stephanie Prakash, Chuku Okorie, Abdul Jan, Priyank Desai, Abu Fahad Abbasi, Jasmine Mangat, Zaheeda Ansaara Hosein, Kareem Hamdy, Nafees Haider, Nasar Khan, Rochelle Annan, Olanrewaju Badaru, Ricardo Izurieta, Stella Smith, Črtomir Podlipnik, Radostina Alexandrova, Marko Jukič, Sebastian Pleško, Urban Bren, Bahadır Ertürk, Zamir Kemal Ertürk, Ericka Matus, Lorena Matus, Carmen Cristina Diaconu, Ioana Madalina Pitica, Mihaela Chivu-Economescu, Laura Georgiana Necula, Anca Botezatu, Iulia Virginia Iancu, Ana Iulia Neagu, Elena L. Radu, Lilia Matei, Simona Maria Ruta, Coralia Bleotu, Marco Bassanello, Ugo Coli, Antonio Tegon, Matteo Geretto, Maurizio D'Aquino, Maria Teresa Pasqualini, Aldo Farencena, Sadia Sana, Naheed Akhter, Muhammad Adnan Ahsan, Abu Huraira, Zafaar Siddique, Somara Sana, Gonzalo Moratorio, Mercedes Paz, Pilar Moreno, Balram Ji Ji Omar, Ankur Kumar, Manju O. Pai, Gaurav Badoni, Arpana Singh, Ankit Agarwal

First published in London, United Kingdom, 2023 by IntechOpen
IntechOpen is the global imprint of INTECHOPEN LIMITED, registered in England and Wales, registration number: 11086078, 5 Princes Gate Court, London, SW7 2QJ, United Kingdom
Printed in Croatia

British Library Cataloguing-in-Publication Data
A catalogue record for this book is available from the British Library

Additional hard and PDF copies can be obtained from orders@intechopen.com

Current Topics in SARS-CoV-2/COVID-19 - Two Years After
Edited by Alfonso J. Rodriguez-Morales
p. cm.

This title is part of the Infectious Diseases Book Series, Volume 18
Topic: Viral Infectious Diseases
Series Editor: Alfonso J. Rodriguez-Morales
Topic Editor: Shailendra K. Saxena

Print ISBN 978-1-80356-233-9
Online ISBN 978-1-80356-234-6
eBook (PDF) ISBN 978-1-80356-235-3
ISSN 2631-6188

An electronic version of this book is freely available, thanks to the partial funding support of libraries working with Knowledge Unlatched. KU is a collaborative initiative designed to make high quality books Open Access for the public good. More information about the initiative and links to the Open Access version can be found at www.knowledgeunlatched.org

For EU product safety concerns:
IN TECH d.o.o., Prolaz Marije Krucifikse Kozulić 3, 51000 Rijeka, Croatia,
info@intechopen.com or visit our website at intechopen.com.

IntechOpen Book Series
Infectious Diseases
Volume 18

Aims and Scope of the Series

This series will provide a comprehensive overview of recent research trends in various Infectious Diseases (as per the most recent Baltimore classification). Topics will include general overviews of infections, immunopathology, diagnosis, treatment, epidemiology, etiology, and current clinical recommendations for managing infectious diseases. Ongoing issues, recent advances, and future diagnostic approaches and therapeutic strategies will also be discussed. This book series will focus on various aspects and properties of infectious diseases whose deep understanding is essential for safeguarding the human race from losing resources and economies due to pathogens.

Meet the Series and Volume Editor

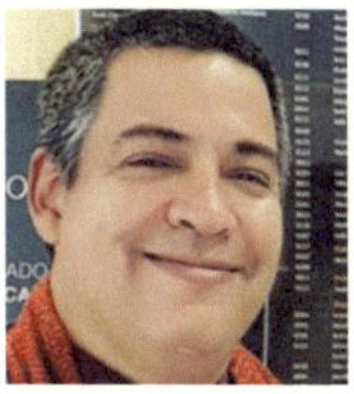

Dr. Rodriguez-Morales is an expert in tropical and emerging diseases, particularly zoonotic and vector-borne diseases (notably arboviral diseases), and more recently COVID-19 and Monkeypox. He is the president of the Publications and Research Committee of the Pan-American Infectious Diseases Association (API), as well as the president of the Colombian Association of Infectious Diseases (ACIN). He is a member of the Committee on Tropical Medicine, Zoonoses, and Travel Medicine of ACIN. Dr. Rodriguez-Morales is a vice-president of the Latin American Society for Travel Medicine (SLAMVI) and a member of the Council of the International Society for Infectious Diseases (ISID). Since 2014, he has been recognized as a senior researcher at the Ministry of Science of Colombia. He is a professor at the Faculty of Medicine of the Fundacion Universitaria Autonoma de las Americas, in Pereira, Risaralda, Colombia, and a professor, Master in Clinical Epidemiology and Biostatistics, at Universidad Científica del Sur, Lima, Peru. He is also a non-resident adjunct faculty member at the Gilbert and Rose-Marie Chagoury School of Medicine, Lebanese American University, Beirut, Lebanon, and an external professor, Master in Research on Tropical Medicine and International Health, at Universitat de Barcelona, Spain. Additionally, an invited professor, Master in Biomedicine, at Universidad Internacional SEK, Quito, Ecuador, and a visiting professor, Master Program of Epidemiology, at Diponegoro University, Indonesia. In 2021 he was awarded the "Raul Isturiz Award" Medal of the API and, the same year, the "Jose Felix Patiño" Asclepius Staff Medal of the Colombian Medical College due to his scientific contributions to the topic of COVID-19 during the pandemic. He is currently the Editor in Chief of the journal Travel Medicine and Infectious Diseases. His Scopus H index is 55 (Google Scholar H index 77) with a total of 725 publications indexed in Scopus.

Contents

Preface

The Severe Acute Respiratory Syndrome Coronavirus 2 (SARS-CoV-2) has probably been the most important disease to emerge in the 21st century. The COVID-19 pandemic was declared a Public Health Emergency of International Concern (PHEIC). This viral zoonotic disease has been a significant cause of morbidity and mortality worldwide, but with a higher impact in low- and middle-income countries of Africa, Asia, and Latin America. As with other emerging diseases, this condition is strongly associated with social conditions, along with other factors whose improvement leads to better control of the disease and pathogen transmission. Research has been of the utmost importance in solutions to the COVID-19 crisis: a great deal of knowledge was gathered between December 2019 and December 2022 [1–17]. Up to December 4, 2022, more than 645,195,564 cases had been reported globally, with 6,640,845 deaths. Appropriate evidence-based management and the development of safe and effective vaccines have been key to controlling the virus [18–25], and more than 13,054,668,703 doses of a vaccine had been given by December 2022.

This book presents a selection of the learning from research and clinical practice during the last two years regarding SARS-CoV-2/COVID-19. The 18 chapters are organized into four major sections: “Overview and Epidemiology”, “Diagnosis and Treatment”, “Genomics, Bioinformatics and Immunology” and “Trials and Studies”.

Among the reasons for the commissioning of this book by IntechOpen is my long commitment to tropical and emerging disease research, especially vector-borne, zoonotic, and neglected tropical diseases. I am a Council Member of the International Society for Infectious Diseases (ISID), and President of the Colombian Association of Infectious Diseases (Asociación Colombiana de Infectología, ACIN), as well as of the Committee on Tropical Medicine, Zoonoses and Travel Medicine of the ACIN. In 2020 I founded the Latin American Network of Research on COVID-19 (LANCOVID).

Following the same philosophy that was used for my eleven previous books with IntechOpen [26–36], this book is not intended to be an exhaustive compilation. Research in SARS-CoV-29/COVID-19 has become highly dynamic and requires the most recent available evidence to be consulted for appropriate diagnostic and specialty decisions.

I am grateful to IntechOpen for the opportunity to edit this interesting and important book. I would especially like to thank Author Service Managers Josip Knapić and Marica Novakovic and Commissioning Editor Lucija Tomicic Dromgool for their constant support.

This book is dedicated to my family in Venezuela, Chile, and Colombia (Aurora, Alfonso José, Alejandro, and Andrea, the neurologist), and to my beloved wife Katterine, who makes every day special and cares for me in every aspect of my life.

I would also like to thank my friends and my undergraduate and postgraduate students in Colombia, Venezuela, and Latin America. In 2019, I began work at the Fundación Universitaria Autónoma de las Américas, Pereira, Risaralda, Colombia, a new "home" that has given me support and trust in my research and teaching endeavors. Special thanks are due to Dr. Maria Monica Murillo, Dean at the Faculty of Medicine, and former School of Medicine Director Dr. Jaime Cardona-Ospina, a long-time friend and colleague. I would like to acknowledge the significant support given by Dr. Jose Antonio Suárez, "Tony" (Venezuela/Panama), and my friend Dr. Alberto Paniz-Mondolfi (Venezuela/USA).

I hope that readers will enjoy this publication as much as I enjoyed putting it together with my talented and knowledgeable collaborators.

Alfonso J. Rodriguez-Morales
MD, MSc, DTM&H, DipEd, FRSTMH(Lon), FFTM RCPS(Glasg),
FACE, FISAC, HonDSc
Professor,
Senior Researcher,
Grupo de Investigación Biomedicina,
Faculty of Medicine,
Fundación Universitaria Autónoma de las Américas – Institución Universitaria
Visión de las Américas,
Pereira, Risaralda, Colombia

Lecturer,
Universidad Científica del Sur,
Lima, Peru

Research Adjunct Faculty,
Gilbert and Rose-Marie Chagoury School of Medicine,
Lebanese American University,
Beirut, Lebanon

President,
Colombian Association of Infectious Diseases (ACIN)

Member of the Committee on Tropical Medicine,
Zoonoses and Travel Medicine,
ACIN

President,
Committee on Research and Publications,
Pan-American Association of Infectious Diseases

References

[1] Ahmad T, Khan M, Haroon, Musa TH, Nasir S, Hui J, et al. COVID-19: Zoonotic aspects. Travel Medicine and Infectious Disease. 2020;**36**:101607.

[2] Bastola A, Sah R, Rodriguez-Morales AJ, Lal BK, Jha R, Ojha HC, et al. The first 2019 novel coronavirus case in Nepal. The Lancet Infectious Diseases. 2020;**20**:279-280.

[3] Benites-Zapata VA, Herrera-Añazco P, Benites-Meza JK, Bonilla-Aguilar K, Urrunaga-Pastor D, Bendezu-Quispe G, et al. Prevalence of parents' non-intention to vaccinate their children and adolescents against COVID-19: A comparative analysis in Colombia and Peru. Vaccine: X. 2022;**12**:100198.

[4] Biscayart C, Angeleri P, Lloveras S, Chaves T, Schlagenhauf P, Rodríguez-Morales AJ. The next big threat to global health? 2019 novel coronavirus (2019-nCoV): What advice can we give to travellers? - Interim recommendations January 2020, from the Latin-American society for travel medicine (SLAMVI). Travel Medicine and Infectious Disease. 2020;**33**:101567.

[5] Dhama K, Patel SK, Sharun K, Pathak M, Tiwari R, Yatoo MI, et al. SARS-CoV-2 jumping the species barrier: Zoonotic lessons from SARS, MERS and recent advances to combat this pandemic virus. Travel Medicine and Infectious Disease. 2020;**37**:101830.

[6] Iqbal Yatoo M, Hamid Z, Parray OR, Wani AH, Ul Haq A, Saxena A, et al. COVID-19 - Recent advancements in identifying novel vaccine candidates and current status of upcoming SARS-CoV-2 vaccines. Human Vaccines & Immunotherapeutics. 2020;**16**:2891-2904.

[7] León-Figueroa DA, Abanto-Urbano S, Olarte-Durand M, Nuñez-Lupaca JN, Barboza JJ, Bonilla-Aldana DK, et al. COVID-19 and dengue coinfection in Latin America: A systematic review. New Microbes and New Infections. 2022;**49**:101041.

[8] Panduro-Correa V, Arteaga-Livias K, Rodríguez-Morales AJ. Coronavirus disease 2019 (COVID-19) and surgical recommendations in Latin America. The American Surgeon. 2020;**86**:596-598.

[9] Park SH, Hong SH, Kim K, Lee SW, Yon DK, Jung SJ, et al. Non-pharmaceutical interventions reduce the incidence, and mortality of COVID-19: A study based on the survey from the international COVID-19 research network (ICRN). Journal of Medical Virology. 2022.

[10] Patel SK, Singh R, Rana J, Tiwari R, Natesan S, Harapan H, et al. The kidney and COVID-19 patients - Important considerations. Travel Medicine and Infectious Disease. 2020;**37**:101831.

[11] Rodriguez-Morales AJ, Bonilla-Aldana DK, Balbin-Ramon GJ, Rabaan AA, Sah R, Paniz-Mondolfi A, et al. History is repeating itself: Probable zoonotic spillover as the cause of the 2019 novel coronavirus epidemic. Le Infezioni in Medicina. 2020;**28**:3-5.

[12] Rodríguez-Morales AJ, MacGregor K, Kanagarajah S, Patel D, Schlagenhauf P. Going global - Travel and the 2019 novel coronavirus. Travel Medicine and Infectious Disease. 2020;**33**:101578.

[13] Romaní L, León-Figueroa DA, Rafael-Navarro D, Barboza JJ, Rodriguez-Morales AJ. Association between the use of antibiotics and the development of

acute renal injury in patients hospitalized for COVID-19 in a hospital in the Peruvian amazon. Journal of Clinical Medicine. 2022;**11**.

[14] Solante R, Alvarez-Moreno C, Burhan E, Chariyalertsak S, Chiu NC, Chuenkitmongkol S, et al. Further implications on the global real-world vaccine effectiveness against SARS-CoV-2. Expert Review of Vaccines. 2022;**21**:1355-1357.

[15] Solante R, Alvarez-Moreno C, Burhan E, Chariyalertsak S, Chiu NC, Chuenkitmongkol S, et al. Expert review of global real-world data on COVID-19 vaccine booster effectiveness and safety during the omicron-dominant phase of the pandemic. Expert Review of Vaccines. 2022:1-16.

[16] Toro-Huamanchumo CJ, Hilario-Gomez MM, Pinedo-Castillo L, Zumarán-Nuñez CJ, Espinoza-Gonzales F, Caballero-Alvarado J, et al. Clinical and epidemiological features of patients with COVID-19 reinfection: A systematic review. New Microbes and New Infections. 2022;**48**:101021.

[17] Vasquez-Bonilla WO, Orozco R, Argueta V, Sierra M, Zambrano LI, Muñoz-Lara F, et al. A review of the main histopathological findings in coronavirus disease 2019. Human Pathology. 2020;**105**:74-83.18.

[18] Cardona-Ospina JA, Rojas-Gallardo DM, Garzón-Castaño SC, Jiménez-Posada EV, Rodríguez-Morales AJ. Phylodynamic analysis in the understanding of the current COVID-19 pandemic and its utility in vaccine and antiviral design and assessment. Human Vaccines & Immunotherapeutics. 2021;**17**:2437-2444.

[19] Dhama K, Singh Malik Y, Rabaan AA, Rodriguez-Morales AJ. Special focus 'SARS-CoV-2 / COVID-19: advances in developing vaccines and immunotherapeutics'. Human Vaccines & Immunotherapeutics. 2020;**16**:2888-2890.

[20] Patel SK, Pathak M, Tiwari R, Yatoo MI, Malik YS, Sah R, et al. A vaccine is not too far for COVID-19. Journal of Infection in Developing Countries. 2020;**14**:450-453.

[21] Petersen E, Lucey D, Blumberg L, Kramer LD, Al-Abri S, Lee SS, et al. COVID-19 vaccines under the International Health Regulations - We must use the WHO International Certificate of Vaccination or Prophylaxis. International Journal of Infectious Diseases. 2021;**104**:175-177.

[22] Rabaan AA, Al-Ahmed SH, Sah R, Al-Tawfiq JA, Al-Qaaneh AM, Al-Jamea LH, et al. Recent advances in vaccine and immunotherapy for COVID-19. Human Vaccines & Immunotherapeutics. 2020;**16**:3011-3022.

[23] Rabaan AA, Al-Ahmed SH, Sah R, Tiwari R, Yatoo MI, Patel SK, et al. SARS-CoV-2/COVID-19 and advances in developing potential therapeutics and vaccines to counter this emerging pandemic. Annals of Clinical Microbiology and Antimicrobials. 2020;**19**:40.

[24] Shrestha S, Khatri J, Shakya S, Danekhu K, Khatiwada AP, Sah R, et al. Adverse events related to COVID-19 vaccines: The need to strengthen pharmacovigilance monitoring systems. Drugs & Therapy Perspectives. 2021;**37**:376-382.

[25] Urrunaga-Pastor D, Bendezu-Quispe G, Herrera-Añazco P, Uyen-Cateriano A, Toro-Huamanchumo CJ, Rodriguez-Morales AJ, et al. Cross-sectional analysis of COVID-19 vaccine intention,

perceptions and hesitancy across Latin America and the Caribbean. Travel Medicine and Infectious Disease. 2021;**41**:102059.

[26] Rodriguez-Morales AJ, Editor. Current Topics in Tropical Medicine. Croatia: InTech. March 2012. ISBN 978-953-51-0274-8. Available from: http://www.intechopen.com/books/current-topics-in-tropical-medicine

[27] Rodriguez-Morales AJ, Editor. Current Topics in Public Health. Croatia: InTech. May 2013. ISBN 978-953-51-1121-4. Available from: http://www.intechopen.com/books/current-topics-in-public-health

[28] Rodriguez-Morales AJ, Editor. Current Topics in Echinococcosis. Croatia: InTech. September 2015. ISBN 978-953-51-2159-6. Available from: http://www.intechopen.com/books/current-topics-in-echinococcosis

[29] Rodriguez-Morales AJ, Editor. Current Topics in Chikungunya. Croatia: InTech. August 2016. ISBN 978-953-51-2595-2. Available from: http://www.intechopen.com/books/current-topics-in-chikungunya

[30] Rodriguez-Morales AJ, Editor. Current Topics in Malaria. Croatia: InTech. November 2016. ISBN 978-953-51-2790-1. Available from: http://www.intechopen.com/books/current-topics-in-malaria

[31] Rodriguez-Morales AJ, Editor. Current Topics in Giardiasis. Croatia: InTech. December 2017. ISBN 978-953-51-5260-6. Available from: http://www.intechopen.com/books/current-topics-in-giardiasis

[32] Rodriguez-Morales AJ, Editor. Current Topics in Zika. United Kingdom: InTech. June 2018. ISBN 978-1-78923-271-4. Available from: https://www.intechopen.com/books/current-topics-in-zika

[33] Rodriguez-Morales AJ, Editor. Current Topics in Tropical Emerging Diseases and Travel Medicine. United Kingdom: InTech. December 2018. ISBN 978-1-78984-824-3. Available from: https://www.intechopen.com/books/current-topics-in-tropical-emerging-diseases-and-travel-medicine

[34] Rodriguez-Morales AJ, Editor. Current Topics in Neglected Tropical Diseases. United Kingdom: InTech. December 2019. ISBN 978-1-78923-890-7. Available from: https://www.intechopen.com/books/current-topics-in-neglected-tropical-diseases

[35] Rodriguez-Morales AJ, Editor. Current Concepts in Zika Research. United Kingdom: InTech. February 2021. ISBN 978-1-83880-876-1. Available from: https://www.intechopen.com/books/current-concepts-in-zika-research

[36] Rodriguez-Morales AJ, Editor. Current Topics and Emerging Issues in Malaria Elimination. United Kingdom: InTech. July 2021. ISBN 978-1-83968-484-5. Available from: https://www.intechopen.com/books/9528

Section 1

Overview and Epidemiology

Chapter 1

Introductory Chapter: Lessons from SARS-CoV-2/COVID-19 after Two Years of Pandemic

Alfonso J. Rodriguez-Morales and D. Katterine Bonilla-Aldana

1. Introduction

In December 2019, the apparent emergence of a new disease, the Coronavirus Disease 2019 (COVID-19), in Wuhan, Hubei, China, caused by a new coronavirus, the Severe Acute Respiratory Syndrome Coronavirus 2 (SARS-CoV-2), occurred [1–4]. This viral emerging zoonotic disease was initially linked to a fresh seafood market in Wuhan city, with the secondary human-to-human transmission, initially considered by droplets and later confirmed in an aerosolized way, among other potential and alternate routes of transmission [5–11], even including transmission from human-to-animals, particularly to dogs, different felines (cats, lions, and tigers) and minks, among others [12, 13]. Initially affecting China [14–16], the SARS-CoV-2 spread rapidly in a few days to other countries in Asia, as well as later to Europe [17–20], North America [21–23], Africa, and Latin America [9, 24–27]. On January 30, 2020, after the assessments of the Emergency Committee, under the International Health Regulations (IHR), the World Health Organization (WHO) Director General declared that the SARS-CoV-2 outbreak constitutes a Public Health Emergency of International Concern (PHEIC). On March 11, 2020, the WHO declared the SARS-CoV-2 outbreak as a pandemic. Two years later, the pandemic continues, summarizing a total of 628,184,448 cases up to October 25, 2022, with 6,580,107 deaths (**Figure 1**).

Over this time, the initial impact of the outbreak lead globally to generalized lockdowns and quarantine [28–30], a collapse of the health systems, especially in low- and middle-income countries [31], as well as devastating impacts on travel, tourism, economy, education, and multiple other societal sectors [32, 33]. Fortunately, only a low proportion of infected individuals develop mild or severe diseases that required hospitalization and admittance to an intensive care unit, but still, given the magnitude of the pandemic, imply a collapse in countries with limited resources and facilities. During 2020, no effective treatments and vaccines were available, only non-pharmacological interventions (NPI), including the massive use of face masks (including personal protection equipments [PPE], such as N95 filters, especially for healthcare workers), and after December 2021, some treatments, including the use dexamethasone [34–38], and RNA and viral vector vaccines, such as BNT162b2 vaccine (Pfizer/BioNTech®), the ChAdOx1 nCoV-19 vaccine (AstraZeneca/Oxford®), mRNA-1273 (Moderna®), among others, were available and widely used [39–45].

One of the major issues after 2021 was the emergence of the mutations of the SARS-CoV-2 leading to variants of different nature, particularly the variants of

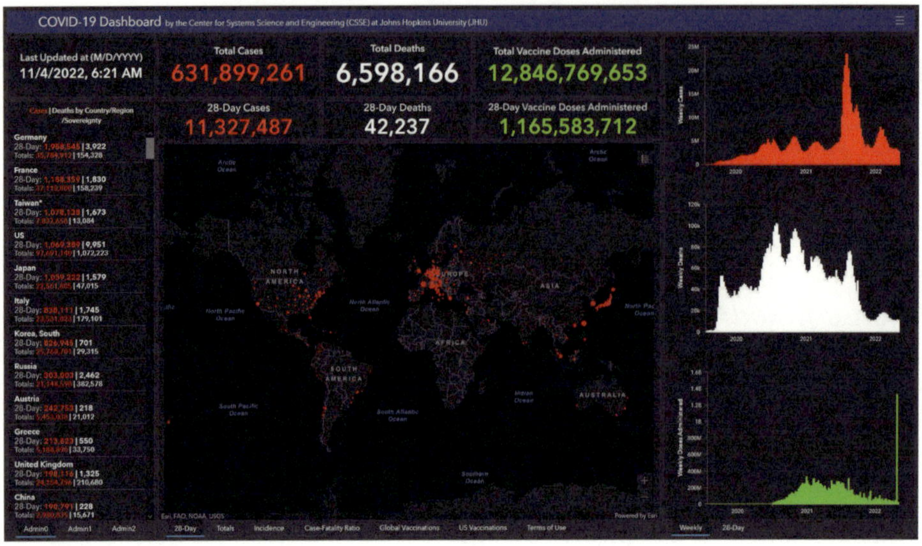
COVID-19 Dashboard by the Center for Systems Science and Engineering (CSSE) at Johns Hopkins University (JHU)
Last Updated at (M/D/YYYY)
11/4/2022, 6:21 AM
Total Cases
631,899,261
Total Deaths
6,598,166
Total Vaccine Doses Administered
12,846,769,653
28-Day Cases
11,327,487
28-Day Deaths
42,237
28-Day Vaccine Doses Administered
1,165,583,712
Germany
France
Taiwan*
US
Japan
Italy
Korea, South
Russia
Austria
Greece
United Kingdom
China
NORTH AMERICA
SOUTH AMERICA
EUROPE
AFRICA
ASIA
AUSTRALIA
2020
2021
2022
Admin0
Admin1
Admin2
28-Day
Totals
Incidence
Case-Fatality Ratio
Global Vaccinations
US Vaccinations
Terms of Use
Weekly
28-Day

Figure 1.
COVID-19 dashboard showing the cumulated incidence, mortality, and vaccination, as well as their total during the last 28 days, evolution since 2020, and the top of countries in such indicators; up to October 25, 2022. (https://gisanddata.maps.arcgis.com/apps/dashboards/bda7594740fd40299423467b48e9ecf6).

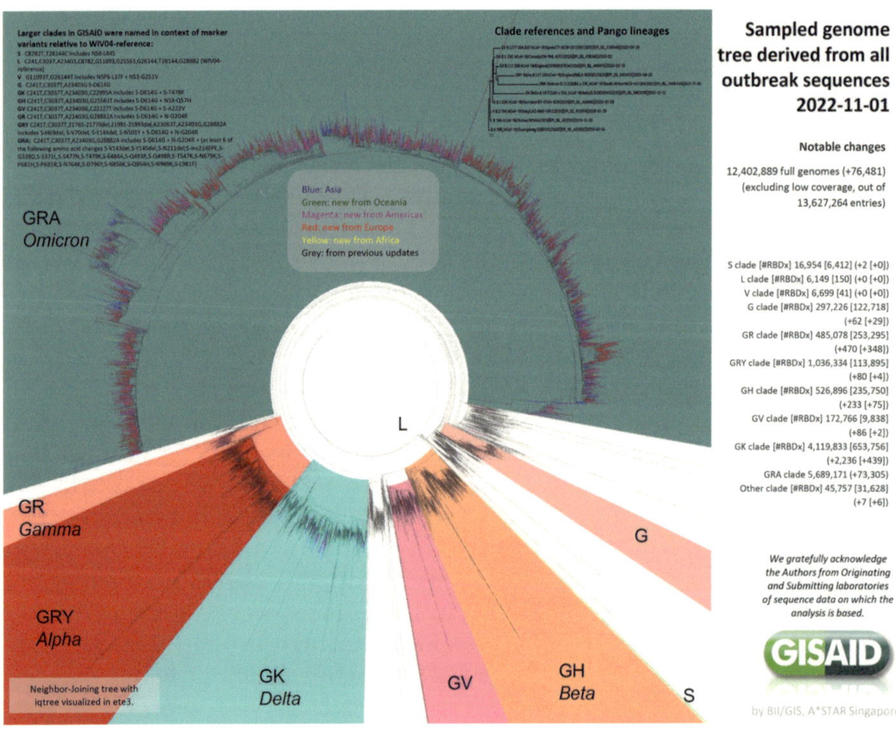

Figure 2.
SARS-CoV-2 variants and genomes were sequenced and collected at the GISAID database up to October 25, 2022. (https://www.gisaid.org/).

interest (VOI), and the variants of concern (VOC), which decrease the protection capacity of used vaccines [40, 44, 46, 47]. The emergence of the VOCs, Alpha, Beta, Gamma, Delta, and Omicron (**Figure 2**), as well as the Omicron's sublineage during those months, have been a real challenge for prevention and control of the pandemic.

2. Vaccines impact on the course of pandemic

Despite all the issues and difficulties, the humankind succeeds enough against the SARS-CoV-2/COVID-19, returning to a new "normal" life, after a successfully deployed and globally aggressive plan of vaccination against SARS-CoV-2/COVID-19 with multiple vaccine types. Up to October 25, 2022, a total of 12,822,482,039 vaccine doses have been administered in the world, representing the largest historical effort in vaccination [44, 47–49]. Over these months, multiple studies on vaccine impacts, pre-clinical, phase 1, phase 2, phase 3 (efficacy), and phase 4 (effectiveness, real-world impact), as well as their corresponding side effects assessment, have been developed showing the high efficacy, effectiveness, and safety of the used anti-COVID-19 vaccines (**Figure 3**) [41, 50–53].

Using vaccines with 50% of efficacy, or more, some of them above 75–80%, together with other measures, transmission was affected, but particularly mortality. Additionally to the published studies (**Figure 3**), multiple countries (e.g., the United States of America) monitor data regarding incidence and mortality among non-vaccinated and vaccinated people.

Case fatality rate among those not-vaccinated according to some analyses in the United States of America reached up to 12 times higher than compared with

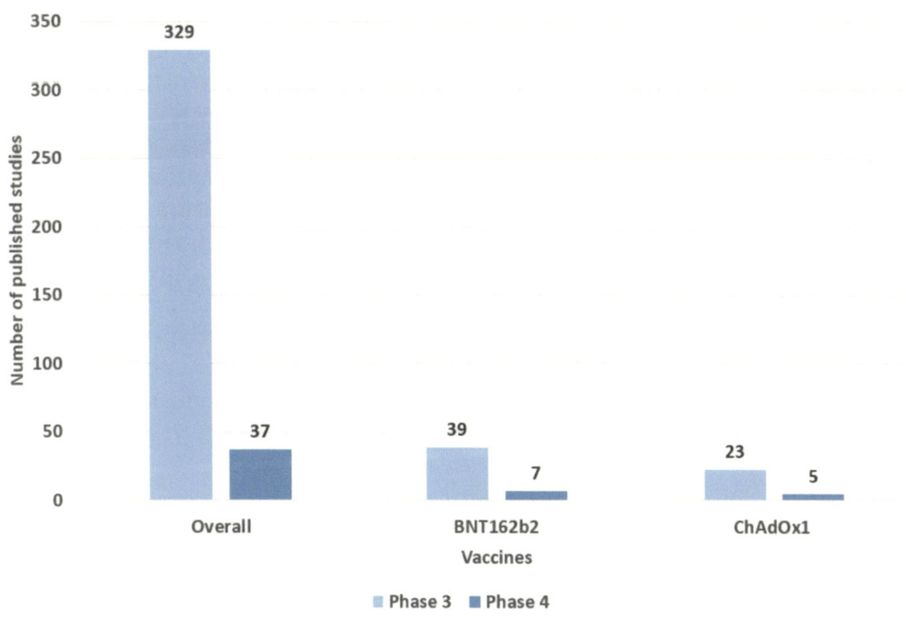

Figure 3.
Phase 3 and phase 4 COVID-19 vaccine studies published in PubMed-indexed journals up to October 25, 2022.

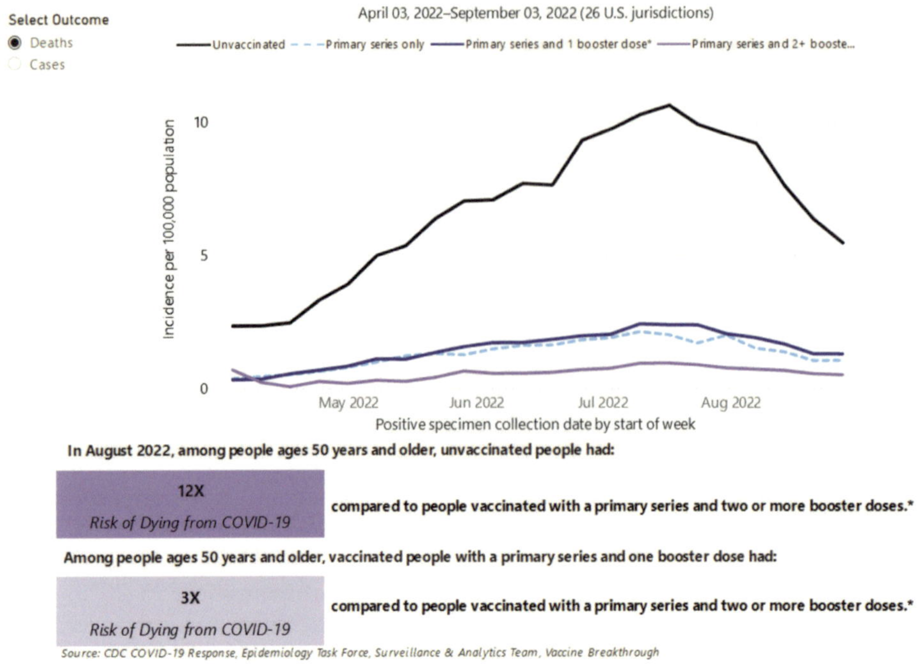

Figure 4.
Rates of COVID-19 deaths by vaccination status and two or more (2+) booster doses in ages 50+ years. (https://covid.cdc.gov/covid-data-tracker/#rates-by-vaccine-status).*

people with boosters, especially in elderly people (**Figure 4**). Anti-COVID-19 vaccines save lives.

For October 2022, multiple countries have applied a fourth dose or second booster in their populations. Obviously, the coverage at primary and booster schemes is highly variable among countries. Prioritizing vaccination coverage must remain as one of the key factors driving vaccine uptake [54]. Also, vaccine hesitancy is important and should be prevented with comprehensive population education [55].

It is now clear that none of the available COVID-19 vaccines provides robust, lasting protection against infection, particularly in the Omicron era, and likely due to inadequate and/or short-lived mucosal immunity [56, 57]. However, booster doses of all widely used vaccines offer very high levels of protection against severe outcomes [54]. With this consistency of protection against severe disease across different variants, the case for developing variant-specific vaccines becomes less urgent, particularly if heterologous schedules can potentially circumvent some of the challenges homologous schedules may encounter in the face of new variants [58–60].

3. Conclusions

COVID-19 pandemic has not been over. Although the evolution during the last months, especially in 2022, has been significantly positive, still SARS-CoV-2 and its variants, particularly the sublineages of Omicron (**Figure 5**), continue changing and circulating. That means preparedness, vaccination, assessment, and research, considering this evolving scenario, should be considered and continuously applied.

DOI: http://dx.doi.org/10.5772/intechopen.108769

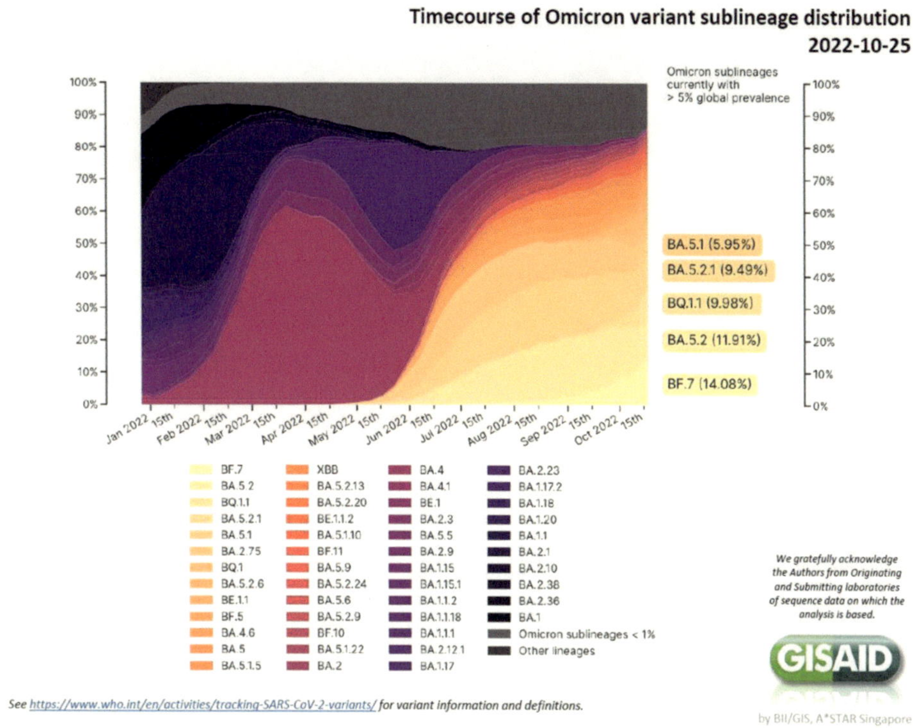

Figure 5.
Omicron sublineages over time, up to October 25, 2022. (https://www.gisaid.org/).

Prevention is key in general, continued education, surveillance, and monitoring, has been essential, and still will be up to the time SARS-CoV-2 became endemic or disappear. Many lessons have been learnt at differential levels [61, 62], but is essential to be highly, and even, better prepared for the next pandemic, to be caused by a coronavirus, another zoonotic virus making a spillover [3, 62] (e.g., zoonotic Influenza or monkey pox) [63, 64], or in general by another emerging or remerging pathogen. In the future outbreaks, we cannot fall into some of the mistakes done during the COVID-19 pandemic [65]. We have to work on the impacts of COVID-19 on other infectious diseases, such as the decrease of vaccine coverages against other vaccine-preventable diseases [66], as well as to deal with long-COVID-19 syndrome [67], among others.

We need to be better prepared for viral threats, monitor risks, and increase our preparedness and effective responsiveness against outbreaks, epidemics, and pandemics, to promote a safer and healthier world.

Author details

Alfonso J. Rodriguez-Morales[1,2,3,4,5]* and D. Katterine Bonilla-Aldana[3,4]

1 Faculty of Medicine, Grupo de Investigación Biomedicina, Fundación Universitaria Autónoma de las Américas, Pereira, Colombia

2 Universidad Cientifica del Sur, Lima, Peru

3 Latin American Network on COVID-19 Research (LANCOVID), Pereira, Colombia

4 Research Unit, Universidad Continental, Huancayo, Peru

5 Gilbert and Rose-Marie Chagoury School of Medicine, Lebanese American University, Beirut, Lebanon

*Address all correspondence to: alfonso.rodriguez@uam.edu.co; arodriguezmo@cientifica.edu.pe

References

[1] Biscayart C, Angeleri P, Lloveras S, Chaves T, Schlagenhauf P, Rodriguez-Morales AJ. The next big threat to global health? 2019 novel coronavirus (2019-nCoV): What advice can we give to travellers? - interim recommendations January 2020, from the Latin-American society for travel medicine (SLAMVI). Travel Medicine and Infectious Disease. 2020;**33**:101567

[2] Millan-Oñate J, Rodríguez-Morales AJ, Camacho-MorenoG,Mendoza-RamírezH, Rodríguez-SabogalIA,Álvarez-MorenoC. A new emerging zoonotic virus of concern: The 2019 novel coronavirus (COVID-19). Infection. 2020;**24**(3): 187-192

[3] Rodriguez-Morales AJ, Bonilla-Aldana DK, Balbin-Ramon GJ, Paniz-Mondolfi A, Rabaan A, Sah R, et al. History is repeating itself, a probable zoonotic spillover as a cause of an epidemic: The case of 2019 novel coronavirus. Le Infezioni in Medicina. 2020;**28**(1):3-5

[4] Rodriguez-Morales AJ, MacGregor K, Kanagarajah S, Patel D, Schlagenhauf P. Going global - travel and the 2019 novel coronavirus. Travel Medicine and Infectious Disease. 2020;**33**:101578

[5] Ahmad T, Haroon DK, Sharun K, Khan FM, Ahmed I, et al. Biosafety and biosecurity approaches to restrain/contain and counter SARS-CoV-2/COVID-19 pandemic: A rapid-review. Turk. Journal of Biology. 2020;**44**(Special issue 1):132-145

[6] Al-Tawfiq JA, Rodriguez-Morales AJ. Super-spreading events and contribution to transmission of MERS, SARS, and SARS-CoV-2 (COVID-19). The Journal of Hospital Infection. 2020;**105**(2):111-112

[7] Diaz-Guio DA, Diaz-Guio Y, Pinzon-Rodas V, Diaz-Gomez AS, Guarin-Medina JA, Chaparro-Zuniga Y, et al. COVID-19: Biosafety in the intensive care unit. Current Tropical Medicine Reports. 2020;**7**(4):104-111

[8] Malik YS, Kumar N, Sircar S, Kaushik R, Bhat S, Dhama K, et al. Coronavirus disease pandemic (COVID-19): Challenges and a global perspective. Pathogens. 2020;**9**(7):519

[9] Rodriguez-Morales AJ, Gallego V, Escalera-Antezana JP, Mendez CA, Zambrano LI, Franco-Paredes C, et al. COVID-19 in Latin America: The implications of the first confirmed case in Brazil. Travel Medicine and Infectious Disease. 2020;**35**:101613

[10] Rodriguez-Morales AJ, Katterine Bonilla-Aldana D, Tiwari R, Sah R, Rabaan AA, Dhama K. Covid-19, an emerging coronavirus infection: Current scenario and recent developments - an overview. Journal of Pure and Applied Microbiology. 2020;**14**(1):5-12

[11] Sawano T, Ozaki A, Rodriguez-Morales AJ, Tanimoto T, Sah R. Limiting spread of COVID-19 from cruise ships: Lessons to be learnt from Japan. QJM. 2020;**113**(5):309-310

[12] Tiwari R, Dhama K, Sharun K, Iqbal Yatoo M, Malik YS, Singh R, et al. COVID-19: Animals, veterinary and zoonotic links. The Veterinary Quarterly. 2020;**40**(1):169-182

[13] Bonilla-Aldana DK, García-Barco A, Jimenez-Diaz SD, Bonilla-Aldana JL, Cardona-Trujillo MC, Muñoz-Lara F, et al. SARS-CoV-2 natural infection in animals: A systematic review of

studies and case reports and series. The Veterinary Quarterly. 2021;**41**(1):250-267

[14] Li Q, Guan X, Wu P, Wang X, Zhou L, Tong Y, et al. Early transmission dynamics in Wuhan, China, of novel coronavirus-infected pneumonia. The New England Journal of Medicine. 2020;**382**(13):1199-1207

[15] Munster VJ, Koopmans M, van Doremalen N, van Riel D, de Wit E. A novel coronavirus emerging in China - key questions for impact assessment. The New England Journal of Medicine. 2020;**382**(8):692-694

[16] Zhu N, Zhang D, Wang W, Li X, Yang B, Song J, et al. A novel coronavirus from patients with pneumonia in China, 2019. The New England Journal of Medicine. 2020;**382**(8):727-733

[17] Martellucci CA, Sah R, Rabaan AA, Dhama K, Casalone C, Arteaga-Livias K, et al. Changes in the spatial distribution of COVID-19 incidence in Italy using GIS-based maps. Annals of Clinical Microbiology and Antimicrobials. 2020;**19**(1):30

[18] Day M. Covid-19: Surge in cases in Italy and South Korea makes pandemic look more likely. BMJ. 2020;**368**:m751

[19] Giovanetti M, Benvenuto D, Angeletti S, Ciccozzi M. The first two cases of 2019-nCoV in Italy: Where they come from? Journal of Medical Virology. 2020;**92**(5):518-521

[20] Livingston E, Bucher K. Coronavirus disease 2019 (COVID-19) in Italy. Journal of the American Medical Association. 2020;**323**(14):1335

[21] Holshue ML, DeBolt C, Lindquist S, Lofy KH, Wiesman J, Bruce H, et al. First case of 2019 novel coronavirus in the United States. The New England Journal of Medicine. 2020;**382**(10):929-936

[22] Team C-I. Clinical and virologic characteristics of the first 12 patients with coronavirus disease 2019 (COVID-19) in the United States. Nature Medicine. 2020;**26**(6):861-868

[23] Mollalo A, Vahedi B, Rivera KM. GIS-based spatial modeling of COVID-19 incidence rate in the continental United States. Science of the Total Environment. 2020;**728**:138884

[24] Sanchez-Duque JA, Arce-Villalobos LR, Rodriguez-Morales AJ. Coronavirus disease 2019 (COVID-19) in Latin America: Role of primary care in preparedness and response. Atencion Primaria. 2020;**52**(6):369-372

[25] Cimerman S, Chebabo A, Cunha CAD, Rodriguez-Morales AJ. Deep impact of COVID-19 in the healthcare of Latin America: The case of Brazil. The Brazilian Journal of Infectious Diseases. 2020;**24**(2):93-95

[26] Bonilla-Aldana DK, Holguin-Rivera Y, Perez-Vargas S, Trejos-Mendoza AE, Balbin-Ramon GJ, Dhama K, et al. Importance of the one health approach to study the SARS-CoV-2 in Latin America. One Health. 2020;**10**:100147

[27] Rodriguez-Morales AJ, Sah R, Paniz-Mondolfi A. Should the holy week 2020 be cancelled in Latin America due to the COVID-19 pandemic? Travel Medicine and Infectious Disease. 2020:101633

[28] Liyanage P, Rocklöv J, Tissera HA. The impact of COVID-19 lockdown on dengue transmission in Sri Lanka; a natural experiment for understanding the influence of human mobility.

PLoS Neglected Tropical Diseases. 2021;**15**(6):e0009420

[29] Ruiz-Arrondo I, Portillo A, Palomar AM, Santibáñez S, Santibáñez P, Cervera C, et al. Detection of SARS-CoV-2 in pets living with COVID-19 owners diagnosed during the COVID-19 lockdown in Spain: A case of an asymptomatic cat with SARS-CoV-2 in Europe. Transboundary and Emerging Diseases. 2021;**68**(2):973-976

[30] Lombardi A, Bozzi G, Mangioni D, Muscatello A, Peri AM, Taramasso L, et al. Duration of quarantine in hospitalized patients with severe acute respiratory syndrome coronavirus 2 (SARS-CoV-2) infection: A question needing an answer. The Journal of Hospital Infection. 2020;**105**(3):404-405

[31] Diaz-Guio DA, Villamil-Gomez WE, Dajud L, Perez-Diaz CE, Bonilla-Aldana DK, Mondragon-Cardona A, et al. Will the Colombian intensive care units collapse due to the COVID-19 pandemic? Travel Medicine and Infectious Disease. 2020;**38**:101746

[32] Ayittey FK, Ayittey MK, Chiwero NB, Kamasah JS, Dzuvor C. Economic impacts of Wuhan 2019-nCoV on China and the world. Journal of Medical Virology. 2020;**92**(5):473-475

[33] Baettig SJ, Parini A, Cardona I, Morand GB. Case series of coronavirus (SARS-CoV-2) in a military recruit school: Clinical, sanitary and logistical implications. BMJ Mil Health. 2021;**167**(4):251-254

[34] Dellapiana G, Naqvi M, Leggett C, Tholemeier L, Burwick RM. Preferential use of dexamethasone for fetal lung maturation in severe COVID-19. American Journal of Obstetrics & Gynecology MFM. 2020;**2**(4):100218

[35] Mahase E. Covid-19: Demand for dexamethasone surges as RECOVERY trial publishes preprint. BMJ. 2020;**369**:m2512

[36] Group RC, Horby P, Lim WS, Emberson JR, Mafham M, Bell JL, et al. Dexamethasone in hospitalized patients with Covid-19. The New England Journal of Medicine. 2021;**384**(8):693-704

[37] Ahmed MH, Hassan A. Dexamethasone for the treatment of coronavirus disease (COVID-19): A review. SN Compr Clinical Medicine. 2020;**2**(12):2637-2646

[38] Patel SK, Saikumar G, Rana J, Dhama J, Yatoo MI, Tiwari R, et al. Dexamethasone: A boon for critically ill COVID-19 patients? Travel Medicine and Infectious Disease. 2020:101844

[39] Rabaan AA, Al-Ahmed SH, Sah R, Tiwari R, Yatoo MI, Patel SK, et al. SARS-CoV-2/COVID-19 and advances in developing potential therapeutics and vaccines to counter this emerging pandemic. Annals of Clinical Microbiology and Antimicrobials. 2020;**19**(1):40

[40] Mangla S, Zohra Makkia FT, Pathak AK, Robinson R, Sultana N, Koonisetty KS, et al. COVID-19 vaccine hesitancy and emerging variants: Evidence from six countries. Behavioral Sciences (Basel, Switzerland). 2021;**11**(11):148

[41] Shrestha S, Khatri J, Shakya S, Danekhu K, Khatiwada AP, Sah R, et al. Adverse events related to COVID-19 vaccines: The need to strengthen pharmacovigilance monitoring systems. Drugs & Therapy Perspectives : for Rational Drug Selection and Use. 2021:1-7

[42] Rabaan AA, Al-Ahmed SH, Sah R, Al-Tawfiq JA, Al-Qaaneh AM, Al-Jamea LH, et al. Recent advances in vaccine and immunotherapy for COVID-19. Human Vaccines & Immunotherapeutics. 2020;**16**(12):3011-3022

[43] Patel SK, Pathak M, Tiwari R, Yatoo MI, Malik YS, Sah R, et al. A vaccine is not too far for COVID-19. Journal of Infection in Developing Countries. 2020;**14**(5):450-453

[44] Schlagenhauf P, Patel D, Rodriguez-Morales AJ, Gautret P, Grobusch MP, Leder K. Variants, vaccines and vaccination passports: Challenges and chances for travel medicine in 2021. Travel Medicine and Infectious Disease. 2021;**40**:101996

[45] Urrunaga-Pastor D, Bendezu-Quispe G, Herrera-Añazco P, Uyen-Cateriano A, Toro-Huamanchumo CJ, Rodriguez-Morales AJ, et al. Cross-sectional analysis of COVID-19 vaccine intention, perceptions and hesitancy across Latin America and the Caribbean. Travel Medicine and Infectious Disease. 2021;**41**:102059

[46] Poudel S, Ishak A, Perez-Fernandez J, Garcia E, León-Figueroa DA, Romaní L, et al. Highly mutated omicron variant sparks significant concern among global experts – What is known so far? Travel Medicine and Infectious Disease. 2021:102234

[47] Sah R, Khatiwada AP, Shrestha S, Bhuvan KC, Tiwari R, Mohapatra RK, et al. COVID-19 vaccination campaign in Nepal, emerging UK variant and futuristic vaccination strategies to combat the ongoing pandemic. Travel Medicine and Infectious Disease. 2021;**41**:102037

[48] Rodriguez-Morales AJ, Franco OH. Public trust, misinformation and COVID-19 vaccination willingness in Latin America and the Caribbean: today's key challenges. The Lancet Regional Health - Americas. 2021;**3**:100073

[49] Alvarado-Socarras JL, Vesga-Varela AL, Quintero-Lesmes DC, Fama-Pereira MM, Serrano-Diaz NC, Vasco M, et al. Perception of COVID-19 vaccination amongst physicians in Colombia. Vaccine. 2021;**9**(3):287

[50] Checcucci E, Piramide F, Pecoraro A, Amparore D, Campi R, Fiori C, et al. The vaccine journey for COVID-19: A comprehensive systematic review of current clinical trials in humans. Panminerva Medica. 2022;**64**(1):72-79

[51] Ong E, Wong MU, Huffman A, He Y. COVID-19 coronavirus vaccine design using reverse vaccinology and machine learning. Frontiers in Immunology. 2020;**11**:1581

[52] Xing K, Tu XY, Liu M, Liang ZW, Chen JN, Li JJ, et al. Efficacy and safety of COVID-19 vaccines: A systematic review. Zhongguo dang dai er ke za zhi = Chinese Journal of Contemporary Pediatrics. 2021;**23**(3):221-228

[53] Dagan N, Barda N, Kepten E, Miron O, Perchik S, Katz MA, et al. BNT162b2 mRNA Covid-19 vaccine in a Nationwide mass vaccination setting. The New England Journal of Medicine. 2021;**384**(15):1412-1423

[54] Solante R, Alvarez-Moreno C, Burhan E, Chariyalertsak S, Chiu NC, ChuenkitmongkolS,etal.Furtherimplications on the global real-world vaccine effectiveness against SARS-CoV-2. Expert Review of Vaccines. 2022;**21**(9):1355-1357

[55] Patwary MM, Bardhan M, Al Imran S, Hasan M, Imam Tuhi F, Rahim SJ, et al. Psychological determinants of COVID-19 vaccine acceptance among urban slum dwellers

of Bangladesh. Frontiers in Public Health. 2022;**10**:958445

[56] Ngonghala CN, Taboe HB, Safdar S, Gumel AB. Unraveling the dynamics of the omicron and Delta variants of the 2019 coronavirus in the presence of vaccination, mask usage, and antiviral treatment. Applied Mathematical Modelling. 2023;**114**:447-465

[57] Chua JX, Durrant LG, Chok YL, Lai OM. Susceptibility to SARS-CoV-2 omicron following ChAdOx1 nCoV-19 and BNT162b2 versus CoronaVac vaccination. iScience. 2022:105379

[58] Hueda-Zavaleta M, de la Torre JC G, Cáceres-Del Aguila JA, Muro-Rojo C, De La Cruz-Escurra N, Arenas Siles D, et al. Evaluation of the humoral immune response of a heterologous vaccination between BBIBP-CorV and BNT162b2 with a temporal separation of 7 months, in Peruvian healthcare workers with and without a history of SARS-CoV-2 infection. Vaccines (Basel). 2022;**10**(4)

[59] Sapkota B, Saud B, Shrestha R, Al-Fahad D, Sah R, Shrestha S, et al. Heterologous prime-boost strategies for COVID-19 vaccines. Journal of Travel Medicine. 2022;**29**(3)

[60] Choudhary OP, Priyanka AJQ, Mohammed TA, Singh I, Rodriguez-Morales AJ. Heterologous prime-boost vaccination against COVID-19: Is it safe and reliable? Human Vaccines & Immunotherapeutics. 2021;**17**(12):5135-5138

[61] Edgar M, Selvaraj SA, Lee KE, Caraballo-Arias Y, Harrell M, Rodriguez-Morales AJ. Healthcare workers, epidemic biological risks - recommendations based on the experience with COVID-19 and ebolavirus. Le Infezioni in Medicina. 2022;**30**(2):168-179

[62] Rodriguez-Morales AJ, Paniz-Mondolfi AE, Faccini-Martínez ÁA, Henao-Martínez AF, Ruiz-Saenz J, Martinez-Gutierrez M, et al. The constant threat of zoonotic and vector-borne emerging tropical diseases: Living on the edge. Frontiers in Tropical Diseases. 2021;**2**:676905

[63] Bonilla-Aldana DK, Aguirre-Florez M, Villamizar-Pena R, Gutierrez-Ocampo E, Henao-Martinez JF, Cvetkovic-Vega A, et al. After SARS-CoV-2, will H5N6 and other influenza viruses follow the pandemic path? Le Infezioni in Medicina. 2020;**28**(4):475-485

[64] León-Figueroa DA, Bonilla-Aldana DK, Pachar M, Romaní L, Saldaña-Cumpa HM, Anchay-Zuloeta C, et al. The never-ending global emergence of viral zoonoses after COVID-19? The rising concern of monkeypox in Europe, North America and beyond. Travel Medicine and Infectious Disease. 2022;**49**:102362

[65] Sah R, Reda A, Abdelaal A, Mohanty A, Siddiq A, Alshahrani NZ, et al. A potential monkeypox pandemic: Are we making the same mistakes as COVID-19? New Microbes and New Infections. 2022;**49**:101030

[66] Suárez-Rodríguez GL, Salazar-Loor J, Rivas-Condo J, Rodríguez-Morales AJ, Navarro JC, Ramírez-Iglesias JR. Routine immunization programs for children during the COVID-19 pandemic in Ecuador, 2020-hidden effects, predictable consequences. Vaccines (Basel). 2022;**10**(6):857

[67] Garout MA, Saleh SAK, Adly HM, Abdulkhaliq AA, Khafagy AA, Abdeltawab MR, et al. Post-COVID-19 syndrome: Assessment of short- and long-term post-recovery symptoms in recovered cases in Saudi Arabia. Infection. 2022:1-9

Chapter 2

Perspective Chapter: Analysis of SARS-CoV-2 Indirect Spreading Routes and Possible Countermeasures

Cesare Saccani, Marco Pellegrini and Alessandro Guzzini

Abstract

The research community agrees that the main indirect way the severe acute respiratory syndrome coronavirus 2 (SARS-CoV-2) spreads among people who do not keep social distance is through the emission of infected respiratory droplets. Infected people exhale droplets of different sizes and emission velocities while breathing, talking, sneezing, or coughing. Complex two-phase flow modeling considering evaporation and condensation phenomena describes droplets' trajectories under the specific thermofluid dynamic boundary conditions, including air temperature, relative humidity, and velocity. However, public health organizations simply suggest a safe distance in the range of 1–2 m regardless of the effect of boundary conditions on droplets' motion. This chapter aims to highlight open research questions to be addressed and clarify how framework conditions can influence safe distance in an indoor environment and which technical countermeasures (such as face masks wearing or heating, ventilation, and air conditioning (HVAC) control) can be adopted to minimize the infection risk.

Keywords: SARS-CoV-2, droplets, airborne, aerosol, face masks, HVAC system, safe distance, contagion prevention

1. Introduction

Regardless of whether vaccination is efficient and effective [1, 2], a good knowledge of the mechanisms underlying infection among people would have helped against severe acute respiratory syndrome coronavirus 2 (SARS-CoV-2) spreading by minimizing lockdown measures. The scientific community has largely investigated how an infected person transmits pathogens to a susceptible person [3]. What is known is that an infected person emits a certain number of droplets. Some of these droplets, defined as infected, carry a certain number of virions or viral particles that can potentially infect target host cells if reached. The literature also shows that the emission of droplets can occur in different ways, for example, through speech, breathing, coughing, and sneezing. What is still not commonly agreed upon is related to the i) number, ii) size distribution, and iii) emission velocity of the potentially infected droplets for each of these emission modes. After the seminal papers of Wells [4] and Duguid [5], many investigators have grappled with the issue showing broad differences in the experimental results [6]. The reasons can be identified in i) a not full understanding of the physics underpinning the formation of respiratory droplets, ii) the absence of a common methodology, being the different experiments performed by using different techniques and under different ambient conditions, iii) the lack of a rigorous presentation of data, which is often not provided, and iv) the natural variability across individuals.

In addition, the conditions of the ambient air in which these droplets move have also to be considered. Knowing this information is essential to studying the mechanisms that govern the motion of potentially infected droplets. Safe distance, defined as the average distance to which, ideally, a negligible infection probability exists, can be identified once the emitted infected droplets' trajectory is known. However, rigorous terminology and definitions are needed to investigate droplets' motion based on the scientific method. To date, instead, a lack of unambiguous and agreed terminology exists. For example, terms commonly used for direct transmissions, such as "*droplets*," "*aerosol*," and "*airborne*," have been often used with various meanings by several authors. Tang et al. [7] highlighted how significant confusion over the definition and application of relevant terms among professionals (i.e., clinicians versus aerosol scientists) and the general public generates problems in mutual understanding. A second example is the lack of a distinction between solid and liquid carriers, i.e., droplets. Without it, the impact of the thermohygrometric conditions of the ambient air, i.e., relative humidity and temperature, is not adequately considered when studying particles' motion and viral load (defined as the number of copies of ribonucleic acid (RNA) detected in a certain volume). Solid particles that carry viral charges on their surface do not change size or shape along their trajectory except in particular environmental conditions, i.e., if they are condensation nuclei. On the other hand, droplets emitted with a certain viral load reduce their volume through evaporation along their trajectory, resulting in the variation of the balance of forces and viral load. Although experimental results demonstrated that a SARS-CoV-2 viral load lower than 100,000 virions per cubic centimeter (cc) corresponds to a negligible risk of infection [8, 9], to date, the infection risk as a function of the infected droplets' viral load along their trajectory has not yet been sufficiently investigated.

This chapter underlines what are the unsolved research questions (RQs) crucial for a full understanding of SARS-CoV-2 spreading routes and relative countermeasures. Nevertheless, this chapter proposes rigorous terminology and reports evidence to minimize the risk of SARS-CoV-2 infection based on the existing knowledge. The study demonstrates why an effective strategy cannot disregard, at least, i) the use of the facial mask, ii) the control of the thermohygrometric conditions of the ambient air, and iii) the maintenance of the safe distance. In particular, the simplified model shows that the facial mask acts as a first physical barrier against the larger droplets, which can reach very high viral loads in the case of incomplete evaporation. On the other hand, the control of the thermohygrometric conditions acts as a second immaterial barrier that guarantees the complete evaporation of the smaller droplets that come out of the mask before reaching any susceptible subject. Once droplets are completely evaporated, the virions are released into the surrounding environment, where the viral load is low enough to be unlikely to infect.

2. Size distribution of the infected droplets and calculation of the number of virions emitted

Many studies are available in the literature focusing on analyzing the dimensional distribution of the droplets emitted for different possible emission mechanisms such as breathing, speech, cough, and sneezing. However, since no universally accepted standard test identifies the instrumentation and the procedure to investigate the topic, the results are difficult to compare with each other. For example, if a single cough event is considered, [10] states that the droplets in the submicron range represent 97% of the exhaled droplets, while [11] reports only less than 4% and [5] measures not even a single droplet within submicron range. Therefore, the first unsolved research question RQ1 is the standardized characterization of the sizes and the distribution of the exhaled droplets for all the expulsion processes.

Since a standard characterization of the initial distribution of droplet sizes is missing, in the following evaluation, the data reported by [12] were used. [12] has been selected as a data source due to the high number of citations, the robust methodology adopted, and the quality of exposure. The following results are affected by the data source selected; nevertheless, the focus of this chapter is more on the suggested methodology to assess SARS-CoV-2 spreading mechanisms and the related comparison. In [12], only droplets with a diameter greater than 20 microns were considered, although a "*16-channel dust monitor*" was available. Furthermore, only speech and cough mechanisms were investigated. In the first case, the involved subjects were asked to count from 1 to 100. Therefore, assuming that about 100 seconds are necessary to complete the count, the emission rate is calculated by dividing the droplets counted by this time interval. Moreover, the individuals were asked to make 20 coughs each to simulate the cough mechanism.

Since the data refer to a group of people, the average number of droplets $N_{\text{droplet},\mu}$ emitted by a subject for each jth-dimensional interval [drops/individual] is calculated as

$$N_{\text{droplet},j,\mu} = \frac{\sum_{i=1}^{N} N_{\text{droplet},j,i}}{N_{\text{sample}}} \tag{1}$$

where $N_{\text{droplet},i}$ is the number of droplets emitted by the ith individual [droplets/person], while N_{sample} is the number of people who participated in the test. The number of droplets emitted by 99% of individuals, assuming a Gaussian distribution with a standard deviation σ_j, for the jth interval is equal to

$$N_{\text{droplet},j,99\%} = N_{\text{droplet},j,\mu} + 2.58 * \sigma_j \tag{2}$$

The total number of droplets emitted $N_{\text{droplet},\mu}$ and $N_{\text{droplet},99\%}$ are, respectively, computed as

$$N_{\text{droplet},\mu} = \sum_{j=1}^{M} N_{\text{droplet},j,\mu} \tag{3}$$

$$N_{\text{droplet},99\%} = \sum_{j=1}^{M} N_{\text{droplet},j,99\%}. \tag{4}$$

where M is the number of dimensional intervals on which the range has been divided.

The definition of the initial viral load of emitted droplets and the relationship with the viral load present in oronasopharyngeal (ONP) swabs represents the second RQ2. To calculate the number of virions emitted, it was assumed that all the infected droplets had the same initial viral load λ_0 [RNA copies/mL]. This simplifying hypothesis is necessary since the topic is still under investigation and without clear results [13]. There is evidence that viral load in emitted droplets should be lower than in ONP swabs: for example, [14] detected RNA copies of SARS-CoV-2 in exhaled breaths (EBs), which was three to four orders of magnitude lower than the RNA detected in the same participants' ONP swabs and with no correlation among EB and ONP. Nevertheless, since the results may vary based on the methodology applied, in the following assessment, it is conservatively assumed that the initial viral load λ_0 is equal to the one present in ONP swab.

Defined V_j as the average volume of a droplet emitted in the jth dimensional interval [mL], the released virions are calculated as in Eq. (5), while in Eq. (6), the worst case is defined

$$N_{\text{virions},\mu} = \sum_{j=1}^{M} N_{\text{droplet},j,\mu} \times \left(V_j || \times \lambda_0\right) \tag{5}$$

$$N_{\text{virions},99\%} = \sum_{j=1}^{M} N_{\text{droplet},j,99\%} \times \left(V_j || \times \lambda_{\text{viral}}\right). \tag{6}$$

To calculate the emission rate in the case of speech, the values are multiplied by 0.6 to have [virions/min]. In the cough case, the values are divided by 20 to have an emission rate in [virions/cough].

3. Calculation of the infected droplets' trajectory and viral load

To calculate droplets' trajectory and viral load variation, the model proposed by [15] was considered. However, a premise must be highlighted. Only part of the volume of the infected droplets is occupied by saliva, as virions occupy the remaining part. For example, considering the voidage ratio (i.e., the difference between the droplet's volume and the sum of the virions' volumes, divided by the volume of the infected droplets) in analogy with similar physical problems, only a part of the infected droplets' volume consists of a liquid that can evaporate. However, to date, the literature has no answer to RQ3: What effect the virions can induce on the droplet evaporation process? Therefore, it cannot be excluded that an infected droplet evaporates faster than a pure water droplet and that the evaporation time is proportional to the voidage ratio. On the other hand, it is not known, for example, if the virions hinder the mass transfer phenomenon by retaining water in the droplet. Similarly, virions' heat capacity is unknown, i.e., how long the virions take to reach thermal equilibrium with the water surrounding them. Therefore, due to the existing research gaps, the following assumption was made: the reduction of the infected droplet's evaporation time due to the lower volume of aqueous solution contained is counterbalanced by the potential obstacle the virions could cause during the evaporation mechanism. Therefore, the mass variation due to evaporation is calculated as

$$\frac{dm_G}{dt} = \frac{2\pi p D_G M_V D_\infty C}{R_0 T_\infty} ln\left(\frac{p - p_{va}}{p - p_{v,\infty}}\right). \tag{7}$$

where m_G is the mass of the droplet [kg], D_G is the diameter of the droplet [m], D_∞ is the vapor diffusion coefficient in the air surrounding the droplet [m^2/s], M_v is the molar mass of the vapor in [kg/kmol], R_0 is the universal gas constant in [J/kmolK], p_{va} and $p_{v,\infty}$ are, respectively, the partial pressure of the vapor on the surface of the droplet and far away in [Pa], and p and T_∞ are the air pressure [Pa] and temperature [K], respectively. C is a corrective coefficient that takes into account the presence of other constituents in human saliva different from pure water. The temperature variation T_G on droplet surface [K] due to the evaporation phenomenon is calculated as

$$m_G c_L \frac{dT_G}{dt} = 2\pi D_G^2 K_g \frac{T_\infty - T_G}{D_G} + r\frac{dm_G}{dt} - \pi\Gamma\left(T_G^4 - T_\infty^4\right). \tag{8}$$

where c_L is the specific heat in [kJ/kg·K], K_g is the thermal conductivity of the gas in [kJ/s·m·K], r is the latent heat of vaporization in [kJ/kg], Γ is the Stefan-Boltzmann constant in [kW/m^2·K^4]. In the second-member heat balance, therefore, there are three contributions, namely, heat conduction (first term), heat convection (second term), and heat radiation (third term). To calculate droplets' trajectory, the following equation was solved:

$$m_G \overrightarrow{a_G} = m_G \vec{g}\left(1 - \frac{\rho_a}{\rho_G}\right) - C_w A_G \rho_g \frac{{v_{\text{rel}}}^2}{2} \times \frac{\overrightarrow{v_{\text{rel}}}}{|v_{\text{rel}}|} \tag{9}$$

where a_G is the droplet's acceleration [m/s^2], g is the gravity acceleration [m/s^2], ρ_a and ρ_G are, respectively, the air and the droplet's densities [kg/m^3], C_w is the Stokes coefficient [−], A_G is the cross-sectional area of the droplet, and v_{rel} is the relative velocity between the drop and the surrounding air. Since the droplets' diameter along the horizontal distance is known, the droplet viral load [RNA copies/mL] is calculated as

$$\begin{cases} \lambda(x) = \dfrac{\lambda_0 D_{G,0}^3}{{D_G}^3(x)} \cdot \\ \lambda(x) = \lambda_{\max} \end{cases} \tag{10}$$

In Eq. (10), $\lambda_{\max}$ is calculated as the ratio between the number of virions and the volume of the minimum droplet in which they can be contained. Therefore, since virion volume is assumed to not change during droplets' evaporation, the voidage ratio decreases to a minimum, which corresponds to the maximum allowable concentration $\lambda_{\max}$. To date, no data about this maximum concentration exist. To cover the gap, the most conservative assumption is made. Specifically, the minimum voidage ratio of a bed of sphere, i.e., 39%, from [16] is considered. Therefore, the maximum viral load is equal to

$$\lambda_{\max} = \frac{\sum N_{\text{virions}}}{V_G} = \frac{(1-\varphi) \times \frac{V_G}{V_{\text{virions}}}}{V_G} = \frac{(1-\varphi)}{V_{\text{virions}}} = 1.165 \times 10^{15}\left[\frac{\text{RNAcopies}}{\text{mL}}\right]. \tag{11}$$

where N_{virions} is the number of virions contained in the droplet [#], V_G is the droplet's volume [mL], φ is the minimum void ratio (assumed equal to 39%), and V_{virion} is the mean virions' volume [mL]. For the analysis, an average virion diameter of 100 nm is assumed [17].

4. The proposed terminology for infectious droplets' transmission mode classification

The terminology suggested in [18] is adopted in this chapter, and it is the following:

- "Airborne transmission" is defined as the transport of solid particles in a fluid suspension in the examined environment, in whatever way they are carried, regardless of the carrying speed of the fluid current and, therefore, also including the transport of ultrafine particles (and, as such, virions as well) subject to Brownian motions;

- "Droplet transmission" is defined as the transport of droplets in the environment, regardless of how they are carried, including when they contain insoluble solid particles inside them (such as virions).

Figure 1 is an elaboration of the results calculated by [15]. The ordinate shows the vertical distance traveled by a droplet with an initial diameter of 20 microns (solid line) and by one of 40 microns (dashed line) falling from a height of 2 m. On the abscissa, the horizontal distance is shown. An air temperature equal to 20°C and an emission droplet velocity equal to 10 m/s are the boundary conditions. As shown, the time required for the complete evaporation (extreme points of the trajectories symbolized with a star), or the distance traveled, also depends on air relative humidity.

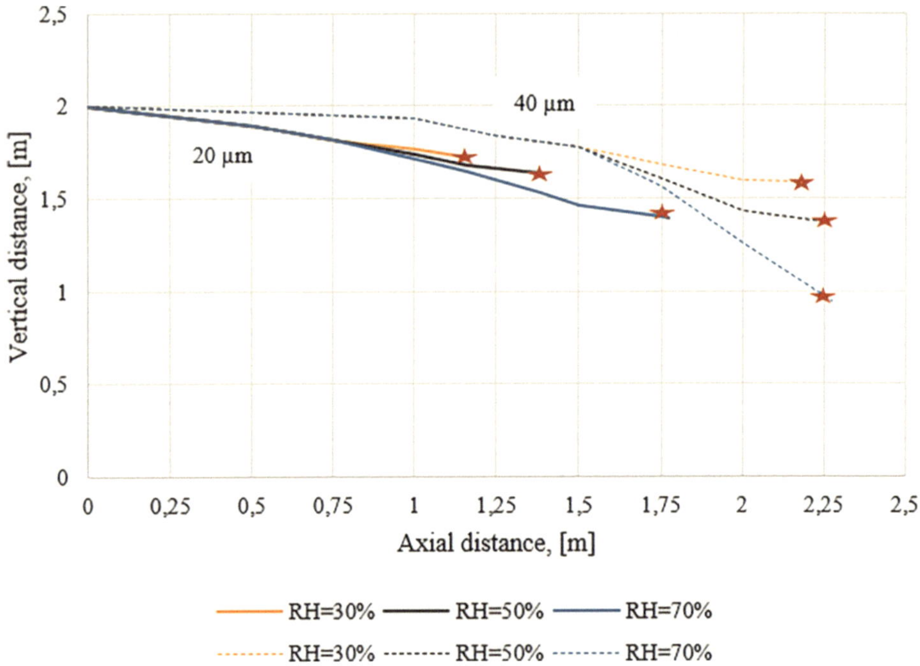

Figure 1.
Vertical and horizontal distance traveled by droplets with an initial diameter equal to 20 microns (continuous line) and 40 microns (dashed line) for three air relative humidity (RH) of 30%, 50%, and 70%. Air temperature and droplets' emission velocity equal to 20°C and 10 m/s (cough case) are considered boundary conditions. Figure elaborated from the results of [15].

Therefore, it is crucial to separate the two different transmission routes, since the evaporation of the infected droplet marks the boundary between two different modes of transport of the virions, i.e., through liquid or a solid carrier.

5. Methodology to compare droplet and airborne transmission modes

The data reported by [9], which identified and reported the link between ONP viral load and cell culture probability, were interpolated through the Matlab "curve fitting tool" by an interpolating equation of the fourth degree:

$$P(\lambda) = \alpha\lambda^4 + \beta\lambda^3 + \gamma\lambda^2 + \delta\lambda + \tau \tag{12}$$

where α, β, γ, δ, and τ are coefficients calculated equal to −0.3314, 9.34, −91.98, 385.2, and − 586.4, respectively. Based on these data, an R_2 equal to 0.9994 was calculated.

To compare airborne and droplet transmission modes, another relevant and open research question RQ4 is: What happens to viruses after complete droplet evaporation and if they retain their full potential for infection? The droplets produced from body secretions such as sneezing and coughing are not constituted of pure water and have a significant amount of residue or dissolved substances, including virions. While pure droplets evaporate completely, the real droplet evaporates to form a solid droplet residue or droplet nucleus. The final size of the droplet nucleus, once the droplet has evaporated to its crystallization diameter, will depend on the amount of the material dissolved [19]. Those residues potentially give a means for the virus to be further transported, provided that it survives the drying process. There is evidence supporting that viruses coated by a lipid membrane tend to retain their infectivity longer at low relative humidity [20]. However, the opposite is true in relevant counterexamples as discussed by [21]. There are many literature examples, in which virions' spreading after droplet evaporation is modeled by considering the virions i) entrapped in the droplet nuclei and ii) preserving their infectivity [22, 23]. Nevertheless, since there is no empirical evidence that i) virions are entrapped in the droplet nucleus, ii) multiple droplet nuclei can be generated by one droplet, and iii) dissolved substances (including virions) can be expelled by the droplet during evaporation, in this chapter, a different approach is suggested to compare droplet and airborne transmission modes. The idea is to compute the number of total droplets that an infected subject should emit to have the same number of airborne virions that touch the host surface in Brownian motion as those that impact the same surface being carried on a droplet of diameter D_G characterized by a medium concentration λ_0. Virions must traverse the distance to the target cell to infect it [24]. The same authors, to support the hypothesis of diffusion-limited infection, declared that it is not the amount of virus in a medium overlay in a culture well that determines the infectivity but the viral load.

Although several complex models exist to investigate the results of the impact of a droplet against a surface [25], it is assumed, for simplicity, that the impact area on which the virions are deposited is equal to the cross-sectional area of the droplet. Therefore, in the proposed model, the impact area is expressed as

$$S = \frac{\pi}{4} {D_G}^2. \tag{13}$$

The number of virions deposited by the droplet $N_{\text{virions,droplet}}$ [RNA copies] on the surface S is calculated as

$$N_{\text{virions,droplet}} = \frac{\pi}{6} D_{G,0}{}^{6} \times \lambda_0. \tag{14}$$

Since the average SARS-CoV-2 virion diameter is 100 nm, the virions motion follows the Brownian mechanism once released from the droplet in the surrounding air. For the comparison, it is assumed that virions are dispersed in the volume of inhaled air: the underlying hypothesis is that all the virions can infect but are released in the air as single particles after droplet drying. Virions that can come into contact with the surface S are contained in a control volume V_c [m^3], defined as

$$V_c = S \times dz \tag{15}$$

where dz is the average diameter of the virion in [m]. The airborne viral load $\lambda_{\text{airborne}}$ [RNA copies/mL] required to deposit the same number of virions as those contained by a droplet of diameter D_G can be found as

$$\lambda_{\text{airborne}} = \frac{N_{\text{virions,droplet}}}{V_c}. \tag{16}$$

It is assumed that the droplet's diameter distribution remains the same over time. Therefore, the time required to achieve the airborne viral load $\lambda_{\text{airborne}}$ is calculated as

$$t = \frac{\lambda_{\text{airborne}} \times V}{\sum_{j-1}^{M} N_{\text{droplet},j,\mu} \times \left(V_j || \times \lambda_0\right) \times 0.6}. \tag{17}$$

where 0.6 is the correction factor used to convert the values in [droplets/(person × minute)] in the case of speech. The volume V, conservatively, can be assumed to equal the volume that a person emits during a conversation, which is 11.7 L/min, or 11,700 mL/min [26].

6. Strategies against SARS-CoV-2 direct transmission within confined spaces

The strategy to minimize the risk of virus spreading must avoid the viral load reaching the susceptible subject. Alternatively, any viral load that comes into contact with the host surface should be responsible for a negligible risk of infection, i.e., equal to or less than 10^5 virions/mL [9]. As for industrial practice where filtration processes are carried out in two stages, in an enclosed space where at least one infected subject and other susceptible occupants are present, the infection risk is minimized by adopting two filters. The first filter is the mask or any other barrier that physically blocks with sufficient effectiveness the larger droplets that are the droplets that, statistically, contain the greatest number of virions. **Figures 2** and **3** schematically represent, respectively, two subjects with and without the facial mask. Once emitted, droplets' trajectory toward the susceptible subjects depends on ambient air fluid dynamic and thermohygrometric conditions. Assuming the experimental data of [12], an infected subject who does not wear a mask emits during a conversation, on

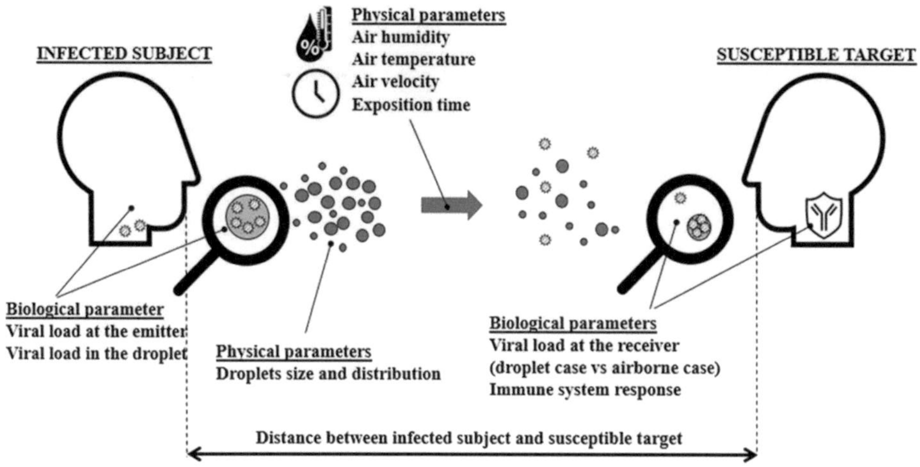

Figure 2.
Direct transmission occurring between infected and susceptible subjects that do not wear a mask or other physical barrier.

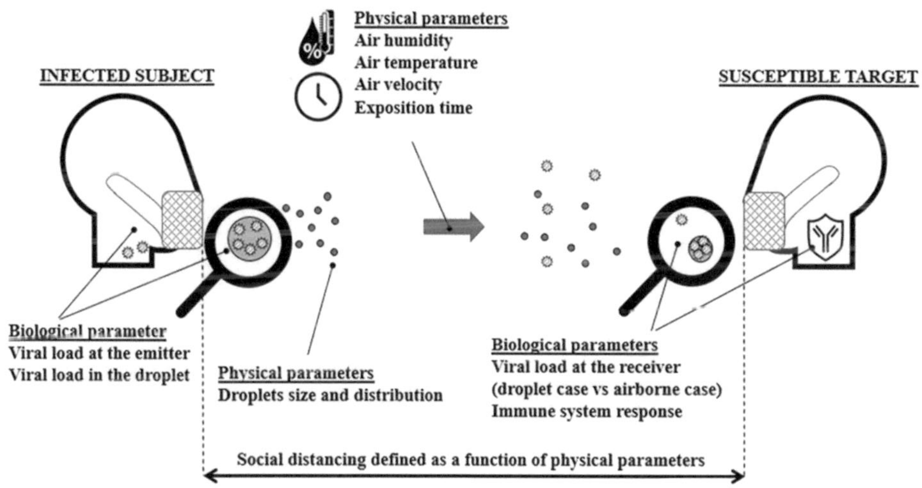

Figure 3.
Direct transmission occurring between infected and susceptible subjects that wear a mask or other physical barrier.

average, 460 droplets per minute whose size distribution is reported in **Figure 4**. In the worst case, the number of emitted droplets can be up to approximately 1850 per minute. On the other hand, conservatively, wearing a mask not all the droplets are captured, and vice versa, some of them escape due to the imperfect seal on the face [27]. Since no confirmation about the size of escaping particles is currently available, conservatively assuming a diameter less than or equal to 30 microns, for example, the rate of emitted droplets is about 10 times lower than the previous case. If higher tightness is achieved, a lower emission rate would be possible. For example, if the mask would block all the droplets with a diameter greater than 20 microns, the emission rate would be reduced by a factor of 30.

According to the shown data, coughing without a mask, almost 110 droplets per cough are emitted. Wearing a facial mask, the emission rate is reduced at least by a

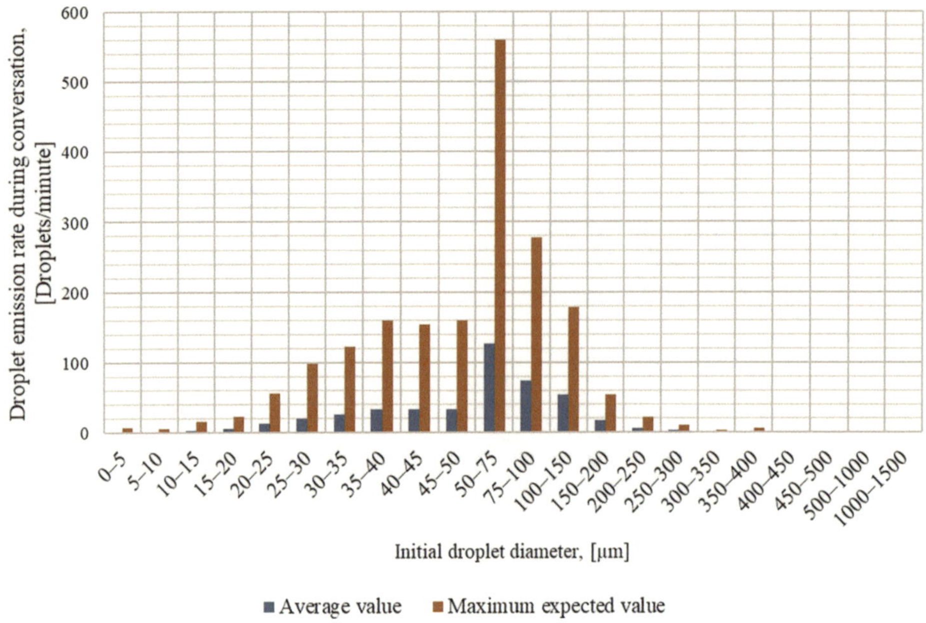

Figure 4.
Droplet rate emission during a conversation.

factor of 10. The role of the mask is even more evident considering the number of virions emitted in the environment. **Figure 5** shows that more than 87% of virions are emitted during speech within droplets having a diameter greater than 450 microns, i.e., 5% of the total emitted droplets. Therefore, assuming conservatively a threshold value of 30 microns (9% of the total emitted droplets), the droplets that can escape the facial mask during a speech carry, on average, about 0.0024% of the total virions. The same is for coughing. Better results would be achieved by tight facial masks. For example, let us assume a viral load at the emission equal to $10^{10.42}$ virions/mL. This value is the upper limit found in SARS-CoV-2 positive samples, and it refers to SARS-CoV-2 infection in the early stages of the COVID-19 pandemic [28]. If the same viral load characterizes all the droplets at the emission, the average virions emission rate is approximately 10 million virions per minute when no mask is worn. This value can achieve up to 45 million virions per minute for those infected subjects that emit more than the average, such as superemitters. Coughing without a mask, up to 58 million virions can be emitted per cough. Wearing a mask able to block droplets larger than 30 microns, the virions' emission rate can be reduced by a factor of 1000 or 50,000, respectively in the case of speech and cough.

Although the mask acts as the first element for reducing the risk of transmission of the infection, the infected droplets that escape are still a potential risk for susceptible individuals in the vicinity of an infected subject. Therefore, the second stage of filtration aims to minimize the infection risk occurring if the virion reaches the target negligible. The second barrier is immaterial and consists of the control of the air relative humidity and keeping a safe distance.

The safe distance is defined as the distance beyond which all the droplets have completely evaporated. The hypothesis is that all the carried virions are released into the surrounding ambient air and maintain their infectious potential. Therefore, droplet transmission is switched to airborne transmission. On the other hand, in the case of

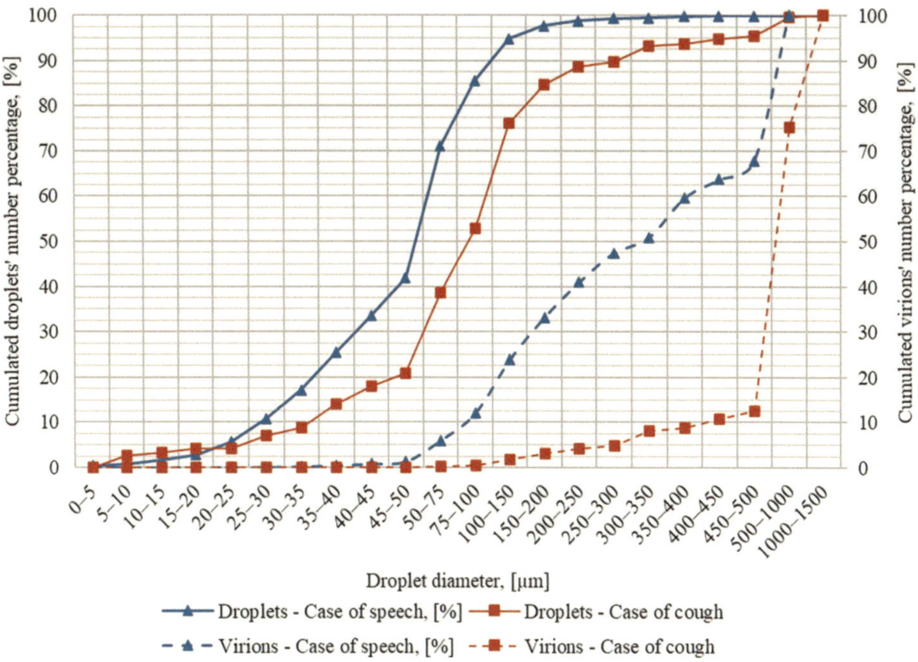

Figure 5.
Cumulative curves of the number of droplets (solid curve) and virions (dashed curve) during speech (blue) and cough (red).

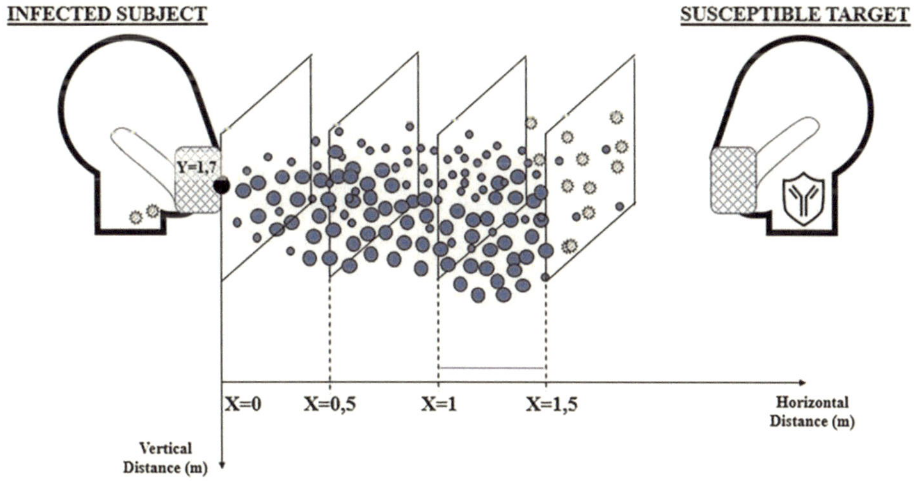

Figure 6.
Simplified scheme to investigate droplets' motion toward a susceptible target.

incomplete evaporation, the droplets reach the host surface at a viral load higher than the one they had at the emission. **Figure 6** shows infected and susceptible subjects, both equipped with masks. As the horizontal distance from the point of emission increases, the viral load of the infected droplets increases up to a maximum value calculated in Eq. (11). Regarding the scheme proposed in **Figures 6** and 7 shows the viral load of the droplets that come out of the mask with an initial diameter of 10

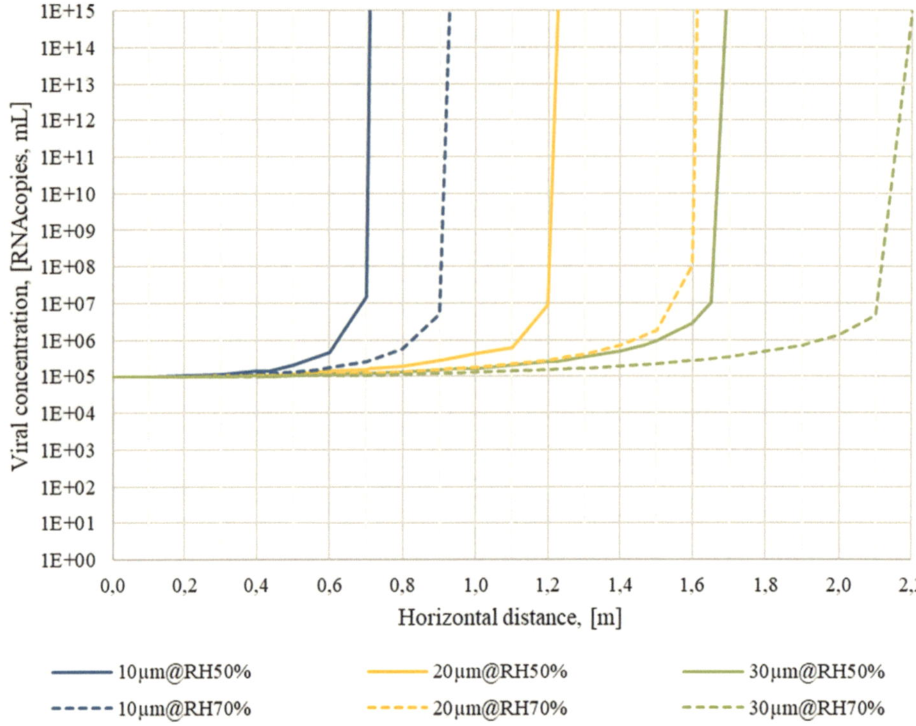

Figure 7.
The trend of the viral load through the horizontal distance from the infected subject. The continuous and dashed curves were calculated for 50% and 70% relative humidity, respectively.

microns, 20 microns, and 30 microns. The continuous curves refer to an air relative humidity equal to 50%, while the dashed ones refer to 70%. As the relative humidity increases, the front of the potential infection moves toward the susceptible subject. For example, the 30-micron droplets completely evaporate at 1.7 m for a relative humidity of 50%, while 2.2 m are necessary for a relative humidity of 70%. Therefore, at a distance of 1.8 m, an infected 30-micron droplet still conveys infecting particles with an air relative humidity of 70%.

Figure 8 shows in the ordinate axis the infection probability of the host surface when a 30-micron droplet deposits its viral load on it. The distance is shown on the abscissa axis. Two initial viral loads are examined: 10^5 virions/mL and 10^8 virions/mL, i.e., one thousand times greater. The second case simulates a variant of the original SARS-CoV-2 virus that causes a greater average viral load at emission [29]. Although an initial viral load equal to 10^5 virions/mL is responsible for a negligible viral replication probability, when air relative humidity is equal to 70%, the evaporation causes the increase of the viral load and so the infection probability. In the case of a higher viral load at the emission, the role of relative humidity concerning the risk of viral infection is even more evident. To control the relative humidity at 50% would guarantee the blockage of the infection front at a distance of almost 1.8 m from the infected subject. On the other hand, with increasing air relative humidity up to 70%, the 30-micron droplet completely evaporates at a distance of 2.2 m; furthermore, a viral load able to infect still exists between 1.8 and 2.2 m. Therefore, without the air relative humidity control, the infection front moves toward or away from the susceptible subject based on the existing environmental thermohygrometric conditions.

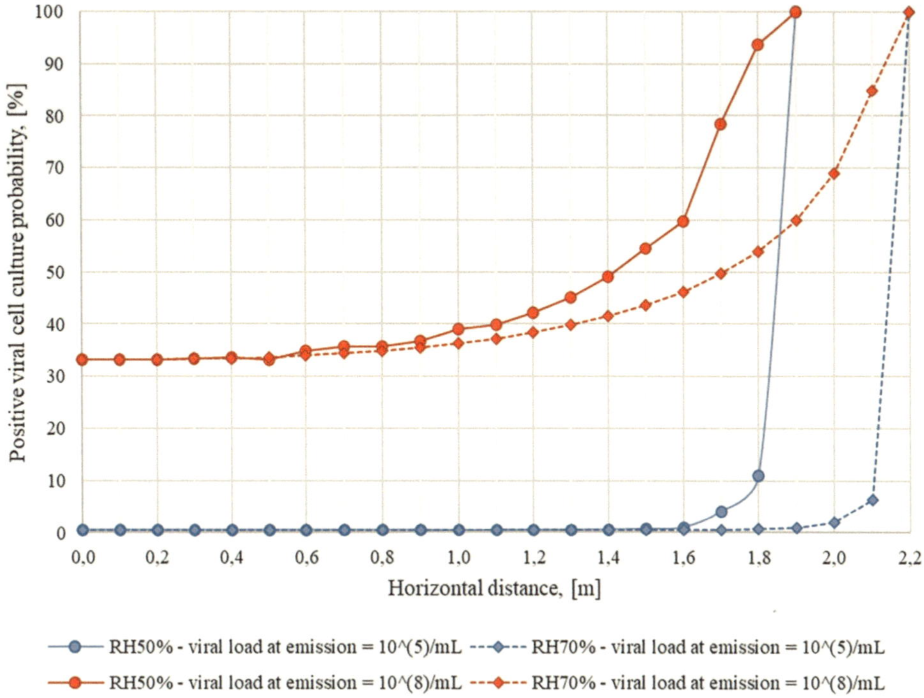

Figure 8.
Estimation of cell culture replication probability through horizontal distance. Initial viral load equal 10^8 virions/mL and 10^5 virions/mL are shown in red and blue, respectively. The continuous and dashed curves are calculated for 50% and 70% relative humidity, respectively.

Virions are released into the air when droplets completely evaporate. Since the virion's average size is 100 nm, Brownian motion occurs. Once released, the virions are wetted particles. However, the liquid film evaporates quickly since the ratio between the evaporating surface and the mass of water is high. In the specific case, since the mass of water does not fill the entire volume but only the external layer of the virions, airborne transmission occurs after the evaporation of the aqueous film. The authors conservatively assume that the minimum volume of air where the virions are released is equal to the volume of exhaled air. In the case of speech, it is 11.7 L/min [26]. Assuming two subjects, one of which is infected, who speak together, if all the droplets that escape the mask evaporate before reaching the host surfaces, the viral load in the volume is, on average, equal to 2.6×10^{-6} and 2.9×10^{-3} virions/mL, respectively, for an initial viral load of 10^5 and 10^8 virions/mL.

Based on these viral loads and the Brownian motion of the virions, airborne transmission causes a negligible infection risk. **Figure 9** shows that the virions that can reach the host surface are those inside the control volume highlighted in red, whose height is equal to the diameter of the virion (indicated as *dz*). Therefore, the probability of infection with the airborne transmission is much lower than for droplet one. In droplet transmission, infected droplets are blocked by the target surface through interception or impact mechanisms, thus determining a significant deposition of virions in terms of both number and load. For simplicity, it can be assumed that the target surface has a size equivalent to the cross section of the droplets, as shown schematically in **Figure 10**.

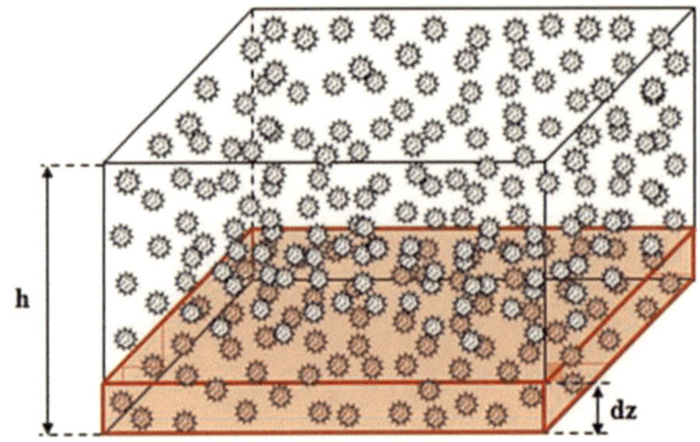

Figure 9.
The control volume where are located the virions that can touch the host surface is colored in red.

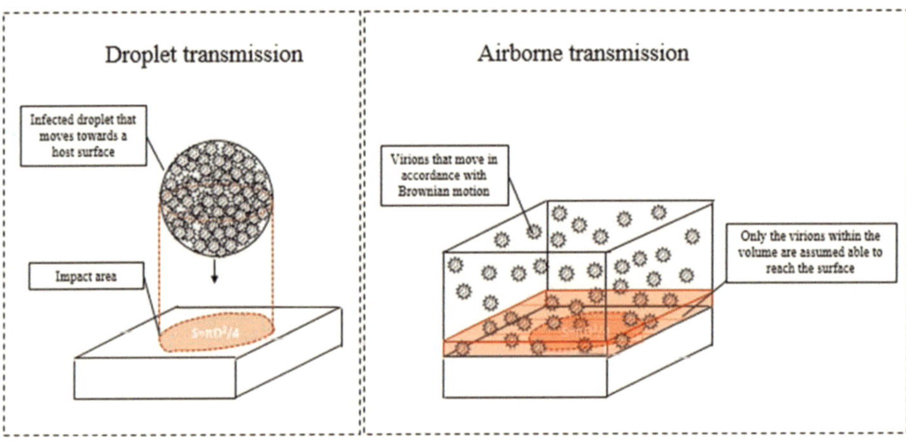

Figure 10.
Comparison between droplet transmission and airborne transmission.

To compare the airborne and droplet transmissions, the number of the infected droplets that have to evaporate to be equivalent to a single infected droplet that reaches the host surface before evaporating is calculated. **Figure 11** shows the results for a 10-micron droplet. The infected subject should emit 1.2×10^{14} droplets so that the number of virions that reach the host through airborne transmission is equivalent to the number released on the same surface by a 10-micron droplet. Assuming the worst case for the speech, i.e., an emission rate equal to 1850 drops per minute, it would take 6.5×10^{10} min for the infected subject to emit that number of drops, or a time interval several orders of magnitude longer than what, reasonably, two individuals employed to speech.

7. Conclusions

This chapter demonstrates that available knowledge is largely inadequate to make predictions on the reach of infectious droplets emitted during an emission

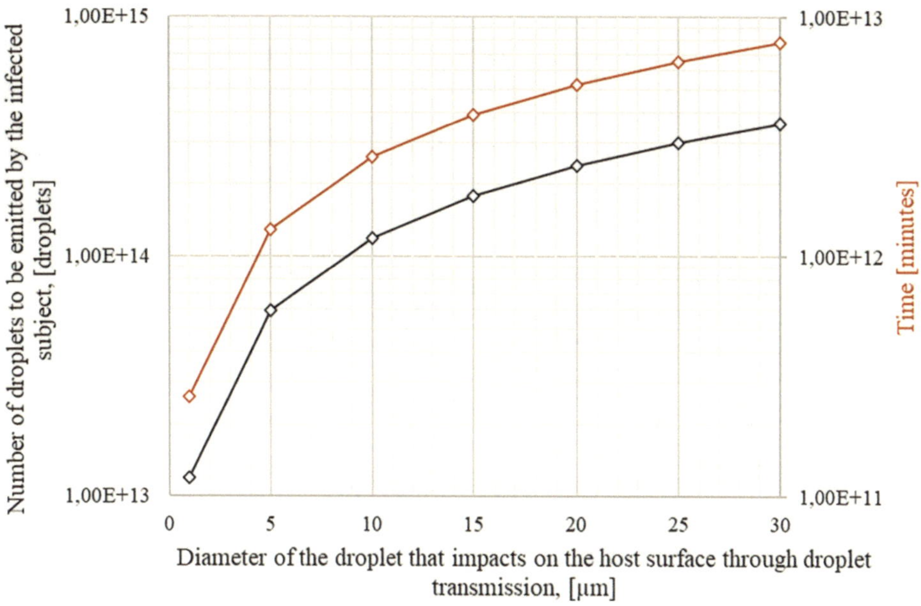

Figure 11.
Number of droplets that the infected subject must emit since the airborne transmission is equivalent to the droplet transmission of an infected droplet with a diameter between 1 and 30 microns.

phenomenon since several research questions still need to be properly addressed: i) standardized characterization of the sizes and distribution of the exhaled droplets for all the human expulsion processes; ii) definition of the initial viral load of emitted droplets and the relationship with the viral load present in oronasopharyngeal swabs; iii) the effect the virions can induce on the droplet evaporation process; and iv) what happens to viruses after complete droplet evaporation and if they retain their full potential for infection.

Nevertheless, in this chapter, some hypotheses have been described to model and compare different SARS-CoV-2 spreading routes. The results show that an effective preventive strategy against SARS-CoV-2 spread cannot neglect three elements: using the facial mask, controlling the relative humidity, and keeping social distance. Particularly, the control of air relative humidity in confined spaces is an essential element. The time an infected droplet takes to evaporate completely depends on the relative humidity of the ambient air. The droplet can move in suspension or settle on a surface, but it remains a potential danger until it completely evaporates. In this case, droplet transmission is substituted by airborne transmission, which should be associated with a modest risk of contagion. The use of the mask allows for blocking of the larger droplets; the control of the air relative humidity guarantees, as suggested in this chapter, that the escaping droplets evaporate until a defined time before reaching the susceptible target. On the other hand, the social distance concept loses its effectiveness. If there is high humidity in the environment, the droplets that escape the mask and that do not settle on the ground would remain in suspension without evaporating and for a relatively long time, significantly increasing the probability of infection [30]. In the worst case, i.e., in saturation conditions (relative humidity equal to 100%), evaporation time tends to infinity, making the concept of safe distance meaningless: at no point in the confined environment, it would be possible to guarantee the absence of virion-carrying droplets. Particular attention must be paid to avoid a susceptible individual coming into contact with droplets that have not completely evaporated. In such a case, cells' infection risk increases as the droplets' viral load is greater than the initial one. The contact with not completely evaporated droplets could explain, in the case of variants such as, for example, the delta variant, characterized by an average emission load higher by a factor of 10^3 than those of the original virus [29], the greater transmissibility. As the results show, the higher load at the emission determines an increase in the probability of infection of the susceptible targets' cells, especially in the case of high relative humidity conditions when the infection front moves forward. Although there are still many points to be clarified about virus transmission, only through the combined control of the air relative humidity, the social distance, and the wearing of the facial mask, it will be possible to ensure safe conditions in confined places and to minimize infection cases.

Conflict of interest

The authors declare no conflict of interest.

Author details

Cesare Saccani, Marco Pellegrini* and Alessandro Guzzini
Department of Industrial Engineering, University of Bologna, Bologna, Italy

*Address all correspondence to: marco.pellegrini3@unibo.it

References

[1] Olliaro P, Torreele E, Vaillant M. COVID-19 vaccine efficacy and effectiveness—The elephant (not) in the room. The Lancet Microbe. 2021;**2**:e279-e280. DOI: 10.1016/S2666-5247(21)00069-0

[2] Tartof SY et al. Effectiveness of mRNA BNT162b2 COVID-19 vaccine up to 6 months in a large integrated health system in the USA: A retrospective cohort study. Lancet. 2021;**398**:1407-1416. DOI: 10.1016/S0140-6736(21)02183-8

[3] Gralton J, Tovey E, McLaws ML, Rawlinson WD. The role of particle size in aerosolised pathogen transmission: A review. Journal of Infection. 2011;**62**:1-13. DOI: 10.1016/j.jinf.2010.11.010

[4] Wells WF. On air-borne infection: Study ii. Droplets and droplet nuclei. American Journal of Epidemiology. 1934;**20**:611-618. DOI: 10.1093/oxfordjournals.aje.a118097

[5] Duguid JP. The size and the duration of air-carriage of respiratory droplets and droplet-nuclei. The Journal of Hygiene. 1946;**44**:471-479. DOI: 10.1017/s0022172400019288

[6] Seminara G et al. Biological fluid dynamics of airborne COVID-19 infection. Rendiconti Lincei. Scienze Fisiche e Naturali. 2020;**31**:505-537. DOI: 10.1007/s12210-020-00938-2

[7] Tang JW et al. Dismantling myths on the airborne transmission of severe acute respiratory syndrome coronavirus-2 (SARS-CoV-2). The Journal of Hospital Infection. 2020;**110**:89-96. DOI: 10.1016/j.jhin.2020.12.022

[8] Wölfel R et al. Virological assessment of hospitalized patients with COVID-2019. Nature. 2020;**581**:465-469. DOI: 10.1038/s41586-020-2196-x

[9] van Kampen JJA et al. Duration and key determinants of infectious virus shedding in hospitalized patients with coronavirus disease-2019 (COVID-19). Nature Communications. 2021;**12**:267. DOI: 10.1038/s41467-020-20568-4

[10] Zayas G et al. Cough aerosol in healthy participants: Fundamental knowledge to optimize droplet-spread infectious respiratory disease management. BMC Pulmonary Medicine. 2012;**12**:1-12. DOI: 10.1186/1471-2466-12-11

[11] Yang S, Lee GW, Chen CM, Wu CC, Yu KP. The size and concentration of droplets generated by coughing in human subjects. Journal of Aerosol Medicine. 2007;**20**:484-494. DOI: 10.1089/jam.2007.0610

[12] Xie X, Li Y, Sun H, Liu L. Exhaled droplets due to talking and coughing. Journal of the Royal Society Interface. 2009;**6**:S703-S714. DOI: 10.1098/rsif.2009.0388.focus

[13] Johnson TJ et al. Viral load of SARS-CoV-2 in droplets and bioaerosols directly captured during breathing, speaking and coughing. Scientific Reports. 2022;**12**:3484. DOI: 10.1038/s41598-022-07301-5

[14] Malik M, Kunze AC, Bahmer T, Herget-Rosenthal S, Kunze T. SARS-CoV-2: Viral loads of exhaled breath and oronasopharyngeal specimens in hospitalized patients with COVID-19. International Journal of Infectious Diseases. 2021;**110**:105-110. DOI: 10.1016/j.ijid.2021.07.012

[15] Xie X, Li Y, Chwang ATY, Ho PL, Seto WH. How far droplets can move in indoor environments. Indoor Air. 2007; **17**:211-225. DOI: 10.1111/j.1600-0668. 2007.00469.x

[16] Benenati RF, Brosilow CB. Void fraction distribution in beds of spheres. AIChE Journal. 1962;**8**:359-361. DOI: 10.1002/aic.690080319

[17] Saccani C et al. Analisi della trasmissione di SARS-CoV-2: influenza delle condizioni termoigrometriche rispetto al rischio di diffusione del contagio. AMS Acta. 2020;**2020**:1-34. DOI: 10.6092/unibo/amsacta/6521

[18] Saccani C et al. Experimental testing of air filter efficiency against the SARS-CoV-2 virus: The role of droplet and airborne transmission. Building and Environment. 2022;**207**:108414. DOI: 10.1016/j.buildenv.2021.108414

[19] Morawska L. Droplet fate in indoor environments, or can we prevent the spread of infection? Indoor Air. 2006;**16**: 335-347. DOI: 10.1111/j.1600-0668.2006. 00432.x

[20] Sobsey MD, Meschke JS. Virus Survival in the Environment with Special Attention to Survival in Sewage Droplets and Other Environmental Media of Fecal or Respiratory Origin. Report for the World Health Organization: Geneva. Switzerland; 2003

[21] Yang W, Marr LC. Mechanisms by which ambient humidity may affect viruses in aerosols. Applied and Environmental Microbiology. 2012;**78**: 6781-6788. DOI: 10.1128/AEM.01658-12

[22] Stiti M, Castanet G, Corber A, Alden M, Berrocal E. Transition from saliva droplets to solid aerosols in the context of COVID-19 spreading. Environmental Research. 2022;**204**: 112072. DOI: 10.1016/j.envres.2021.112072

[23] Netz RR. Mechanisms of airborne infection via evaporating and Sedimenting droplets produced by speaking. The Journal of Physical Chemistry B. 2020;**124**:7093-7101. DOI: 10.1021/acs.jpcb.0c05229

[24] Klasse PJ. Molecular determinants of the ratio of inert to infectious virus particles. Progress in Molecular Biology and Translational Science. 2015;**129**:285-326. DOI: 10.1016/bs.pmbts.2014.10.012

[25] Moghtadernejad S, Lee C, Jadidi M. An introduction of droplet impact dynamics to engineering students. Fluids. 2020;**5**:107. DOI: 10.3390/ fluids5030107

[26] Gupta JK, Lin CH, Chen Q. Characterizing exhaled airflow from breathing and talking. Indoor Air. 2010; **20**:31-39. DOI: 10.1111/ j.1600-0668.2009.00623.x

[27] Cappa CD, Asadi S, Barreda S, Wexler AS, Bouvier NM, Ristenpart WD. Expiratory aerosol particle escape from surgical masks due to imperfect sealing. Scientific Reports. 2021;**11**:12110. DOI: 10.1038/s41598-021-91487-7

[28] Kleiboeker S et al. SARS-CoV-2 viral load assessment in respiratory samples. Journal of Clinical Virology. 2020;**129**: 104439. DOI: 10.1016/j.jcv.2020.104439

[29] Li B et al. Viral infection and transmission in a large, well-traced outbreak caused by the SARS-CoV-2 Delta variant. Nature Communications. 2022;**13**:460. DOI: 10.1038/s41467-022-28089-y

[30] Ou C et al. Insufficient ventilation led to a probable long-range airborne transmission of SARS-CoV-2 on two buses. Building and Environment. 2022; **207**:108414. DOI: 10.1016/j. buildenv.2021.108414

Chapter 3

Perspective Chapter: COVID-19 behind Ground Glasses

Bahadır Ertürk and Zamir Kemal Ertürk

Abstract

A hazy increase in opacity in the lung parenchyma without obscuring the underlying bronchovascular structures on chest CT is called a ground-glass pattern. Ground-glass opacities occur as a result of a wide variety of interstitial and alveolar diseases. It does not represent a specific finding. Coronaviruses are enveloped RNA viruses that can also infect many animal species. They also cause mild or severe respiratory infections in humans. The pandemic caused by SARS-CoV-2 has suddenly turned into the most important health problem of our day. Chest CT is frequently used due to the limited use of chest radiographs in COVID-19 disease. Thus, the ground glass pattern, which is the most common finding of this virus in CT, entered our lives intensively. In this article, we examined the concept of ground glass, its causes, and differential diagnosis.

Keywords: COVID-19, chest CT, ground-glass opacity

1. Introduction

In the last months of 2019, some viral pneumonia cases were detected in the city of Wuhan in China's Hubei Province. A new type of coronavirus has been identified in the etiology of these cases. The virus has spread rapidly. It has created an epidemic in China. Then it spread all over the world, causing a pandemic that continues today. In February 2020, the World Health Organization identified COVID-19, which means coronavirus 2019 disease [1]. The virus that caused this disease was named SARS-CoV-2. Coronaviruses are enveloped RNA viruses that can also infect many animal species. They also cause mild or severe respiratory infections in humans. Previously, Severe Acute Respiratory Syndrome Coronavirus (SARS-CoV) and Middle East Respiratory Syndrome Coronavirus (MERS-CoV) infected humans and caused epidemics in 2002 and 2012, respectively [2]. But the pandemic caused by the SARS-CoV-2 virus, which continues today, overwhelmingly outperformed these two viruses both in terms of the number of infected people and their spread around the world, according to the epidemics caused by SARS-CoV and MERS-CoV [3]. As of May 7, 2022, more than 516 million cases have been detected worldwide. More than 6.2 million patients died from this disease.

Some of the patients have the disease asymptomatically, while others have it symptomatically. Clinically objective abnormal findings are detected in some asymptomatic patients. In the study of Hu et al., thoracic tomography was performed on

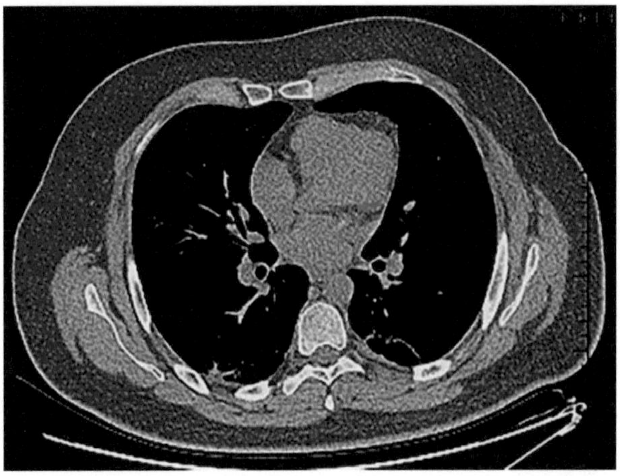

Figure 1.
A 31-year-old male with coronavirus disease 2019 pneumonia. Ground-glass opacities (GGO) and atelectasis.

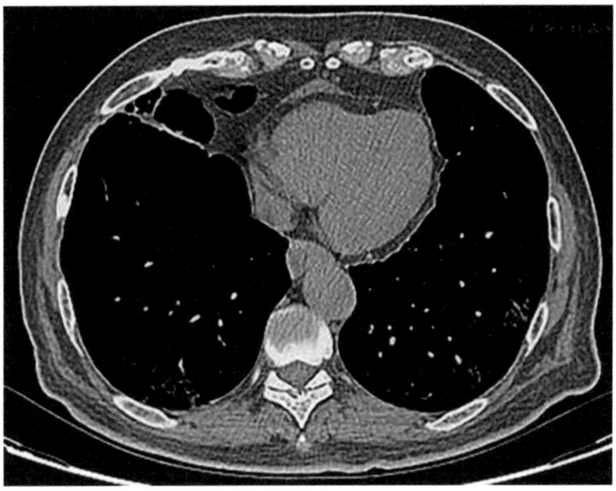

Figure 2.
A 65-year-old male with coronavirus disease 2019 pneumonia. Subpleural patchy infiltration.

patients with asymptomatic infection, and typical ground-glass opacities or patchy shadowing was detected in half of the patients, and atypical imaging abnormalities were detected in 20% (**Figures 1** and **2**), [4]. Some of the asymptomatic patients may become symptomatic over time.

Symptomatic disease can also be examined under three categories: mild illness, severe illness, and critical illness. There is a chance that mild disease accounts for the majority of cases. The incubation period for COVID-19 is within the first 14 days after exposure. In most cases, the disease occurs about 5 days after exposure [5]. Cough, myalgia, and headache are the most commonly reported symptoms in patients with symptomatic COVID-19. There are no specific symptoms to distinguish COVID-19 from other infectious diseases [6]. Symptoms such as fever and cough and parameters such as oxygen saturation and lung auscultation findings are the first and most easily accessible diagnostic information. Such information can be used to categorize COVID-19 disease and to select patients for further diagnostic testing. At the preanalytical stage, obtaining the appropriate respiratory tract sample at the right anatomical site at the right time is essential for the molecular diagnosis of COVID-19. At the analytical stage, real-time reverse transcription PCR (RT-PCR) tests are the preferred molecular test method for the etiological diagnosis of SARS-CoV-2 infection [7]. Pneumonia is a common serious symptom of infection, characterized mainly by fever, cough, dyspnea, and bilateral infiltrates on lung imaging. Methods such as chest radiography, chest computed tomography, and pulmonary ultrasonography are used for imaging the lungs.

2. Discussion

Although chest radiography is a low-cost and easily accessible method, it has low sensitivity in screening patients with COVID-19. It may be useful in the evaluation of complications such as pneumothorax and pleural effusion in the follow-up of hospitalized patients (**Figures 3** and **4**), [8]. Chest radiographs may be normal in early or mild disease.

Imaging plays an important role in the diagnosis and follow-up of thoracic diseases. Different imaging modalities have advantages and disadvantages. Today, there have been advanced developments in cross-sectional imaging methods. In many cases, cross-sectional methods for chest diseases have replaced radiography. However, chest radiographs continue to play a basic role. In the first step, the priority is always

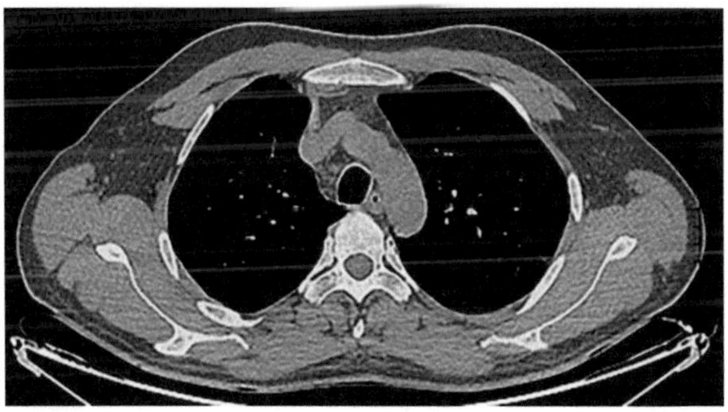

Figure 3.
A 44-year-old male with coronavirus disease 2019 pneumonia. Ground-glass opacities and crazy paving pattern.

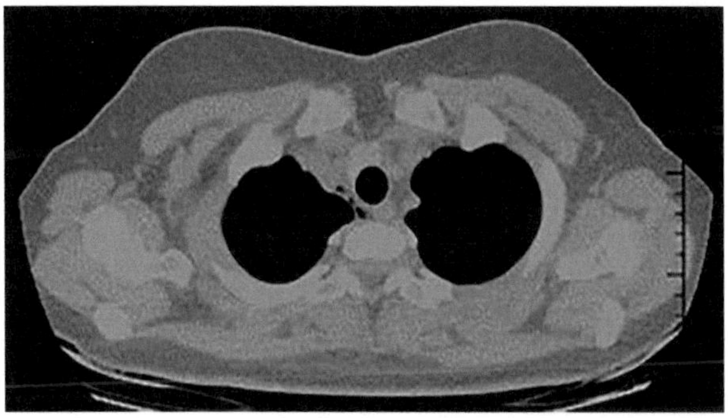

Figure 4.
A 47-year-old male with coronavirus disease 2019 pneumonia. Ground glass nodule (4 mm).

chest radiography. Imaging of the thorax involves difficulties due to differences in tissue density and thickness. Chest radiography is used with different indications in both acute and chronic lung diseases. One of the most important advantages of chest radiography is the low dose radiation exposure. In an outpatient patient, chest radiography usually involves imaging with posteroanterior and left lateral projections in the inspirium.

Although chest CT is highly sensitive, it has a low specificity. To facilitate interpretation and reduce the variability of radiological reports, there are some standardizations in the reports. Among the current classifications for COVID-19, it is possible to divide radiological findings into typical, indeterminate, atypical, and negative findings. The structured report also includes an estimate of the extent of lung involvement [8]. As with chest radiographs, thoracic CT may be normal soon after the onset of symptoms. According to the Fleischner consensus, CT in COVID-19 should be used as an aid in medical triage to determine the basic pulmonary condition in patients with moderate to severe disease, to detect underlying cardiopulmonary abnormalities, to determine the cause in case of clinical worsening, to find limited resources in patients at risk of disease progression [9]. A meta-analysis of Bao et al., which included 13 studies, examined the coronavirus findings of CT. Common findings were ground-glass opacities in 83%, mixed consolidation with ground-glass opacities in 58%, pleural thickening in 52%, interlobular septal thickening in 48%, and air bronchograms in 46% (**Figure 5**). Other less common findings were crazy paving pattern, bronchiectasis, pleural effusion, pericardial effusion, and lymphadenopathy (**Figures 6** and 7), [10].

Chest CT has managed to become one of the indispensable diagnostic methods of today. The main disadvantage is the relatively high radio exposure. The risk of carcinogenesis from a CT scan is much lower than the benefit of screening for the appropriate indication [11]. Therefore, physicians should not hesitate to have the necessary CT scans due to radiation concerns [12]. The thickness of routine CT scan sections ranges from 3 to 5 mm. Chest CT covers the entire thorax from the apex of the lungs to the posterior costophrenic angles. Screening is mostly done in the supine position. The vast majority of cases are shot without giving a contrast agent. However, contrast material is also used in some special indications (such as pulmonary embolism and aneurysm).

Pulmonary ultrasonography can be used to evaluate lung involvement in patients with suspected COVID-19 when other imaging sources are not available. Pulmonary

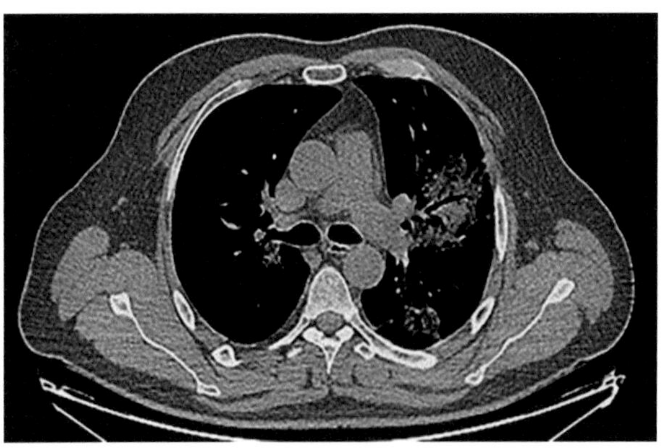

Figure 5.
A 43-year-old female with coronavirus disease 2019 pneumonia. Consolidation with air bronchograms.

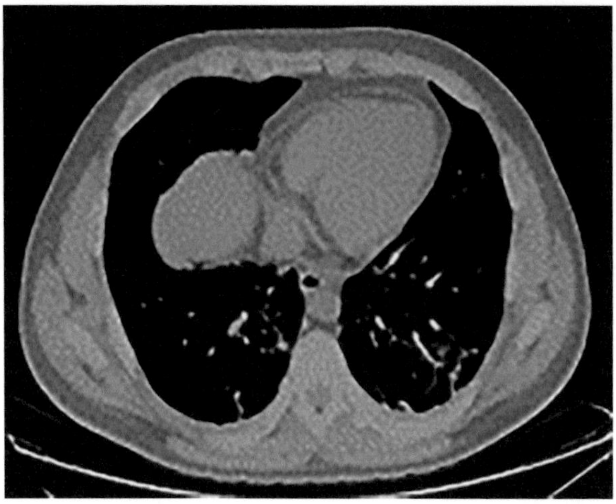

Figure 6.
A 56-year-old male with coronavirus disease 2019 pneumonia. Ground-glass opacification (GGO) and consolidation with air bronchograms.

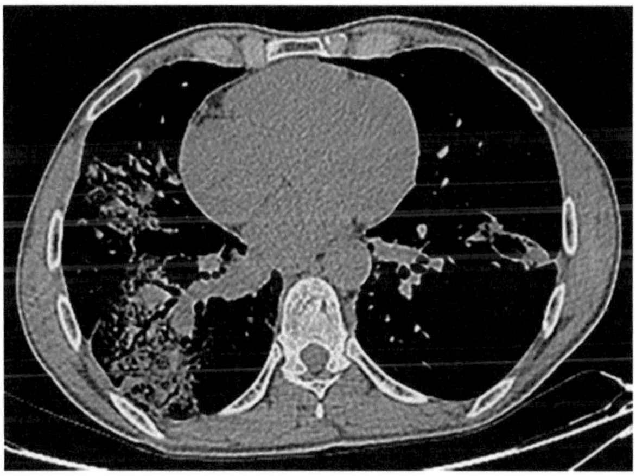

Figure 7.
A 40-year-old female with coronavirus disease 2019 pneumonia. Ground-glass opacification (GGO) with inter-intralobular septal thickening and crazy paving pattern.

ultrasonography can be a helpful method for monitoring in patients, especially in intensive care units where transfer to a tomography scanner is difficult [8].

Ultrasonography has benefits such as examining vascular, cardiac, and some mediastinal abnormalities, detecting the localization of pleural fluid and air collections and guiding appropriate interventions. Transesophageal ultrasonography allows examination of some mediastinal structures, heart and aorta. Endobronchial ultrasonography is used to evaluate mediastinal lymph nodes and guides biopsy for the staging of lung cancer. Transthoracic ultrasonography is used to examine the pleural and subpleural areas. It is used to detect and localize pleural effusion and to assist in thoracentesis.

A ground-glass pattern is considered to be present when there is a hazy increase in opacity in the lung parenchyma without obscuring the underlying bronchovascular

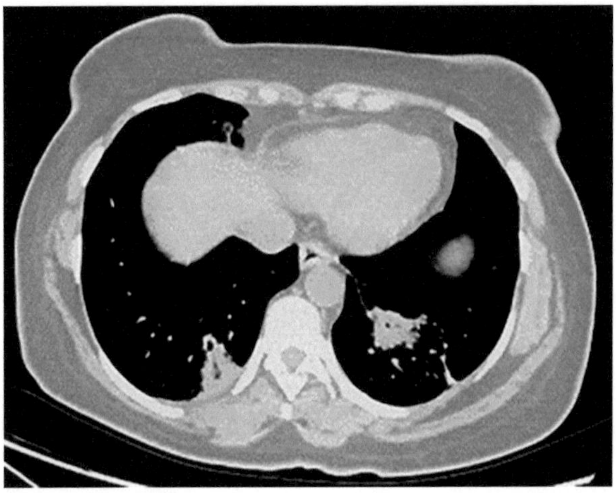

Figure 8.
A 37-year-old male with coronavirus disease 2019 pneumonia. Ground-glass opacification (GGO) with a peripheral distribution.

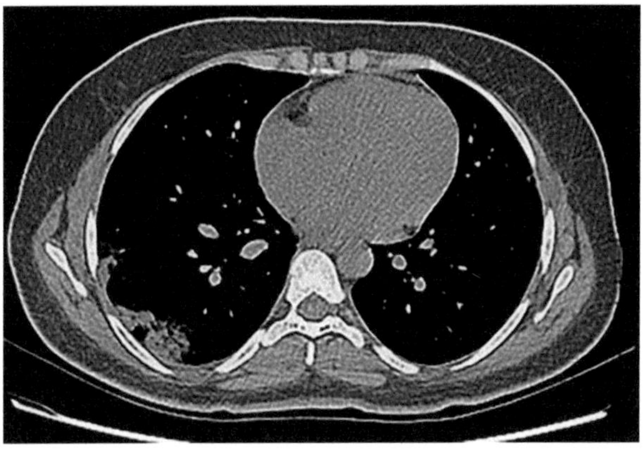

Figure 9.
A 62-year-old male with coronavirus disease 2019 pneumonia. Ground-glass opacification (GGO) with inter-intralobular septal thickening.

structures [13]. The increase in opacity in which bronchovascular structures are not observed is called consolidation (**Figure 8**) [14]. Pulmonary parenchymal opafication in CT scans is divided into ground glass and consolidation (**Figures 9** and **10**). Ground-glass opacities are a common and important finding on CT scanning but are often difficult to detect on chest radiography.

Ground-glass opacities are nonspecific and can occur in a variety of diseases (**Figure 11**). The differential diagnosis is related to the duration of the symptoms. Ground-glass opacities associated with acute symptoms usually indicate atypical pneumonia (such as Pneumocystis pneumonia or COVID-19 viral pneumonia), edema, bleeding, aspiration, or acute hypersensitivity pneumonia. Ground-glass opacities associated with chronic symptoms are usually associated with subacute hypersensitivity pneumonia, nonspecific interstitial pneumonia (NSIP), desquamative interstitial pneumonia (DIP), invasive mucinous adenocarcinoma, lipoid pneumonia, and pulmonary alveolar proteinosis.

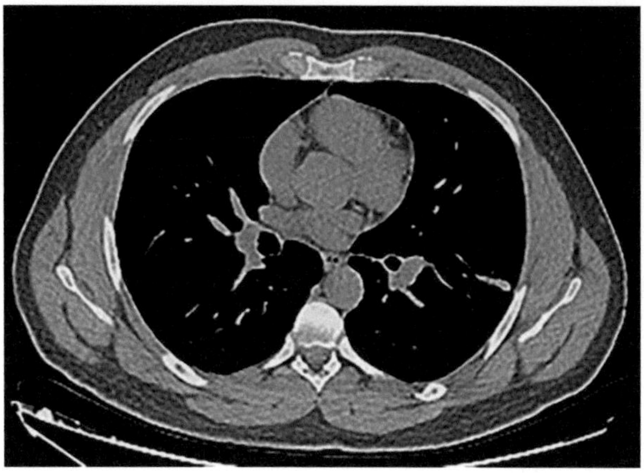

Figure 10.
A 56-year-old male with coronavirus disease 2019 pneumonia. Ground-glass opacities (GGO) with inter-intralobular septal thickening and cysts.

Although these opacities are not specific, differential diagnosis can be significantly reduced by evaluating the presence of associated signs such as concomitant nodules or reticulation (**Figure 12**). If the ground glass pattern does not include other interstitial or alveolar manifestations, it is called isolated. The ground-glass pattern, which includes most of both lungs, is also characterized as diffuse. Miller et al. emphasize that clinical knowledge is essential in the evaluation and differential diagnosis of patients with isolated and diffuse ground-glass patterns [15].

Ground-glass opacities may result from reduced air in alveolar air spaces, partial filling of alveolar air spaces, thickening of parenchymal interstitium and alveolar walls, relative increase in perfusion, or a combination of these factors [16]. Ground-glass opacities are classified into seven different groups according to their morphological patterns: diffuse, centrilobular, nodular, mosaic attenuation, crazy paving, halo sign, and reversed halo sign (**Figure 13**). The causes of isolated diffuse ground glass, which is also an important imaging finding of COVID-19, are shown in **Table 1**.

Chest CT findings are variable in COVID-19 pneumonia. The typical CT findings of COVID-19 are bilateral and peripheral ground-glass opacities (**Figures 14** and **15**). Features such as bilaterality, involvement of the lower lobes, and extension to the pleural surfaces can help distinguish COVID-19 pneumonia from other causes of lung diseases. It should be noted that the probability that CT findings represent COVID-19 is closely related to the prevalence of SARS-CoV-2 infection in society. The period at which the CT scan is performed has a direct relationship with the imaging findings. In COVID-19 pneumonia, ground-glass opacities, consolidations, posterior and lower lobes involvement, peripheral and bilateral involvement are widely monitored, while the unilateral and central involvement, nodules, Crazy Paving Pattern, and the reversed halo sign are less monitored (**Figures 16** and **17**). If the prevalence of disease in society is high, even atypical involvement is likely to represent COVID-19. Conversely, if the prevalence of the disease is low, the CT findings, which are quite typical for COVID-19, may have been caused by another disease [17].

Unlike COVID-19, bacterial pneumonias characteristically produce focal segmental or lobar pulmonary opacities. Complications such as cavitation, lung abscess, lymphadenopathy, parapneumonic effusions, empyema, and associated tomography findings are not monitored in COVID-19 unless patients are superinfected with

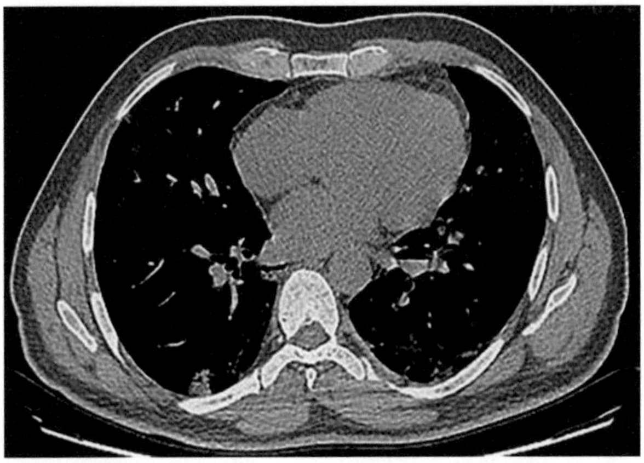

Figure 11.
A 27-year-old male with coronavirus disease 2019 pneumonia. Ground-glass opacification (GGO) with a peripheral distribution.

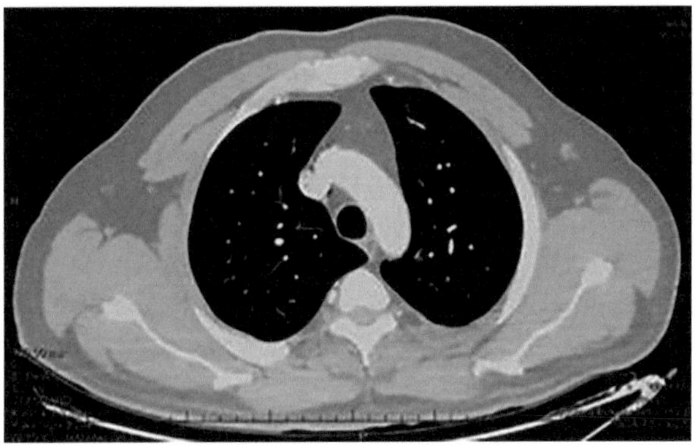

Figure 12.
A 41-year-old male with coronavirus disease 2019 pneumonia. Ground-glass opacities (GGO) and crazy paving pattern. Consolidation with air bronchograms and subsegmental atelectasis.

bacterial pneumonia. Therefore, these findings are distinctive in imaging [18]. Pneumocystis jirovecii is a common opportunistic infection that usually causes pneumonia in immunosuppressed patients. Pneumocystis jirovecii pneumonia has diffuse ground-glass opacities in CT. Unlike COVID-19, it occurs in immunosuppressed patients and more often in the upper lobes of the lungs.

Viruses are the most common cause of respiratory tract infections. The clinical signs and symptoms of viral pneumonia are diverse. The immunization status of the host is an important criterion for determining the prognosis of pneumonia. CT findings of viral pneumonias can be examined in four different categories: ground-glass opacities and consolidation, nodules, micronodules and tree-in-bud opacities, interlobular septal thickening, bronchial and/or bronchiolar wall thickening (**Figures 18** and **19**) [19]. One of these findings that may be confused with COVID-19 pneumonia is ground-glass opacities. Many viruses, such as cytomegalovirus (CMV), herpes simplex virus (HSV), respiratory syncytial virus, adenovirus, and influenza viruses, produce ground-glass opacities in CT.

Categories	Types of diseases and infections
Cause of pandemic	SARS-CoV-2 Pneumonia
Opportunistic infections	Pneumocystis Pneumonia (PCP)
	Cytomegalovirus Pneumonia (CMV)
	Herpes Simplex Virus Pneumonia (HSV)
	Respiratory Syncytial Virus Bronchiolitis
	Other
Chronic interstitial diseases	Hypersensitivity Pneumonitis (HP)
	Desquamative İnterstitial Pneumonia (DIP)
	Respiratory Bronchiolitis İnterstitial Lung Disease (RBILD)
	Nonspecific İnterstitial Pneumonia (NSIP)
	Acute İnterstitial Pneumonia (AIP)
	Lymphocytic İnterstitial Pneumonia (LIP)
	Sarcoidosis
Acute alveolar diseases	Pulmonary Edema
	Heart Disease
	Adult Respiratory Distress Syndrome (ARDS)
	Other
	Diffuse Alveolar Hemorrhage
Other causes	Drug Toxicity
	Pulmonary Alveolar Proteinosis (PAP)
	Bronchiolitis Obliterans with Organizing Pneumonia (BOOP, COP)
	Bronchoalveolar Carcinoma

Table 1.
Causes of isolated diffuse ground-glass opacity [15].

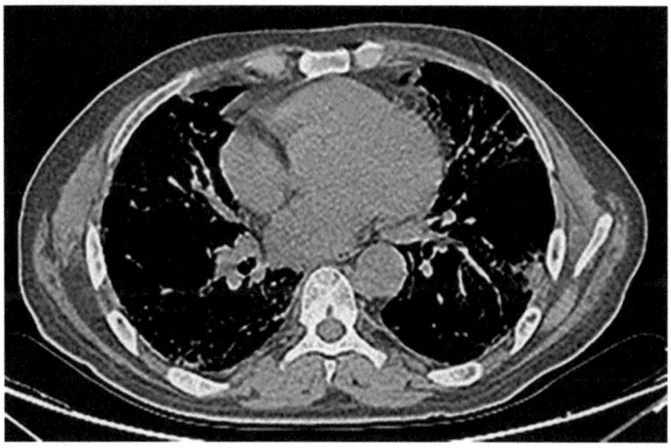

Figure 13.
A 63-year-old male with coronavirus disease 2019 pneumonia. Ground-glass opacification (GGO) with a peripheral distribution and crazy paving pattern.

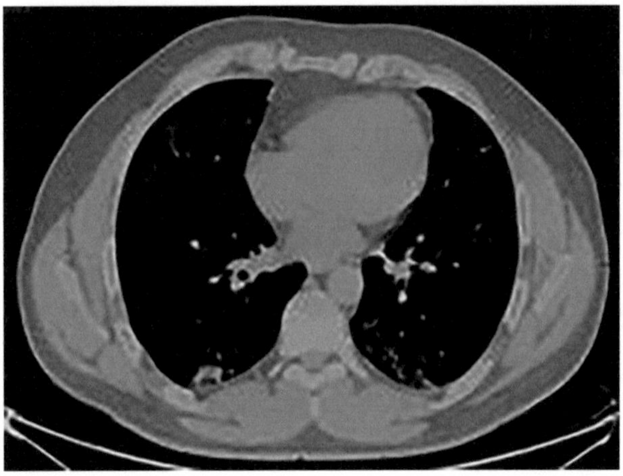

Figure 14.
A 45-year-old male with coronavirus disease 2019 pneumonia. Ground-glass opacification (GGO) with a peripheral distribution and pneumothorax.

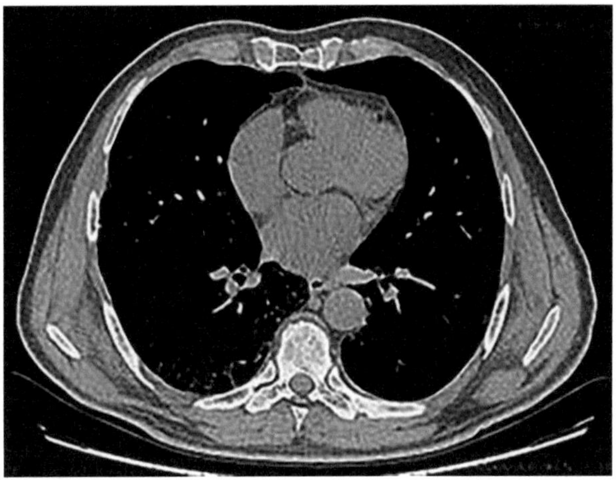

Figure 15.
A 21-year-old female with coronavirus disease 2019 pneumonia. Pneumomediastinum.

Hypersensitivity pneumonitis (HP), also called extrinsic allergic alveolitis, occurs as a result of inhalation of organic or inorganic particles by sensitive people [20]. In acute cases, the capillary permeability secondary to the allergy increases and leads to pulmonary edema. The disease is divided into acute, subacute, and chronic phases. In the acute phase, the ground-glass opacities are monitored as diffuse.

Desquamative interstitial pneumonia (DIP) is characterized by interstitial inflammation and fibrosis following the accumulation of alveolar macrophages [21]. CT scans show diffuse ground-glass opacities in many patients.

Respiratory-bronchiolitis-associated interstitial lung disease (RBILD) is a rare, mild inflammatory lung disease [22]. Central and peripheral bronchial wall thickening and centrilobular nodules are detected in CT, and ground-glass opacities associated with centrilobular emphysema are monitored in the upper lobes.

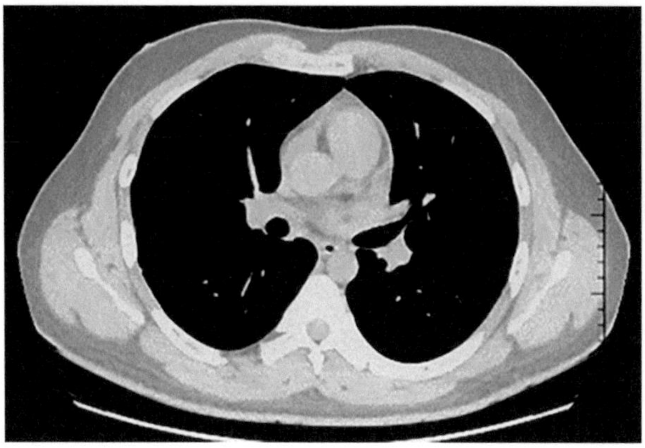

Figure 16.
A 28-year-old female with coronavirus disease 2019 pneumonia. Multilober ground-glass opacities (GGO) and subpleural consolidation.

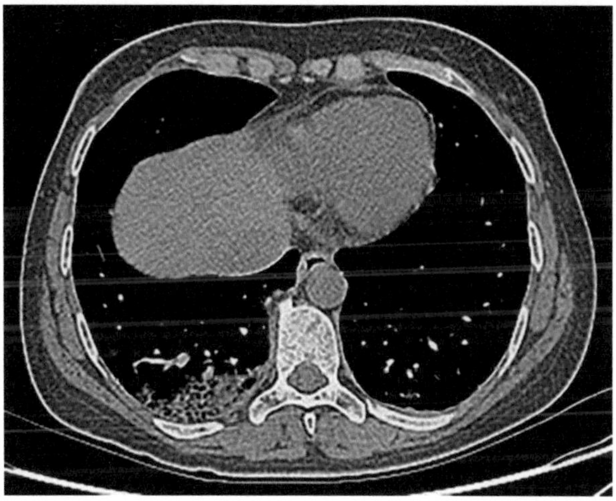

Figure 17.
A 40-year-old male with coronavirus disease 2019 pneumonia. Linear atelectasis.

Nonspecific interstitial pneumonia is a histological subtype of idiopathic interstitial pneumonia [23]. CT scans monitor ground-glass opacities, various amounts of interstitial changes, and honeycomb appearance in most patients.

Acute interstitial pneumonia (AIP) is an acute, fast-progressing idiopathic lung disease that often leads to fulminant respiratory failure and acute respiratory distress syndrome (ARDS) [24]. Ground-glass opacities and alveolar consolidations accompanied by traction bronchiectasis are monitored on CT.

Lymphocytic interstitial pneumonia (LIP) is a rare lung disease on the spectrum of benign pulmonary lymphoproliferative disorders. Ground-glass opacities, centrilobular and subpleural nodules, and randomly distributed thin-walled cysts are observed on CT [25].

Sarcoidosis is a multisystemic granulomatous disease that affects people of all ages, especially young adults [26]. Sarcoidosis has a wide range of CT findings. Ground-glass opacities are rarely detected.

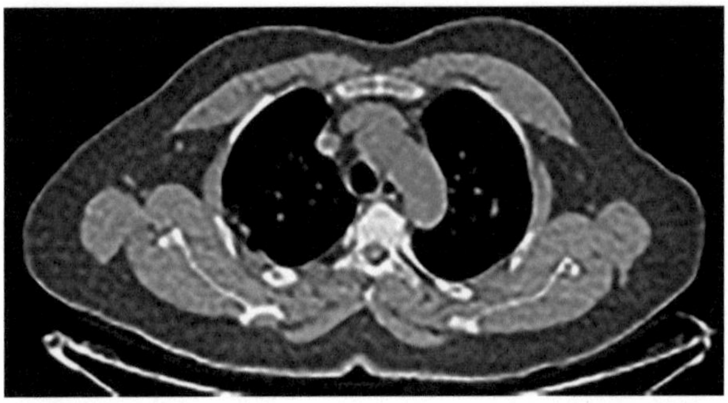

Figure 18.
A 32-year-old male with coronavirus disease 2019 pneumonia. Ground-glass opacification (GGO) with a peripheral distribution. Pleural effusion and fibroatelectatic bands.

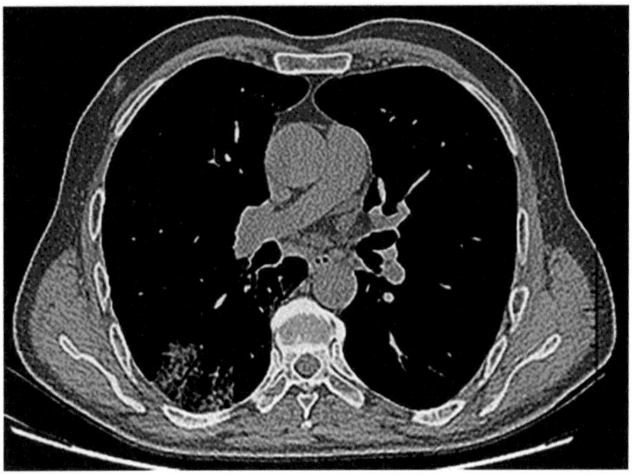

Figure 19.
A 61-year-old male with coronavirus disease 2019 pneumonia. Ground-glass opacification (GGO) with a peripheral distribution. Fibrosis and inter-intralobular septal thickening.

Pulmonary edema consists of imbalances in the starling forces that manage the transport of liquids between the vascular and interstitial gaps of the lung [15]. Pulmonary edema etiology is examined in two subcategories: hydrostatic pulmonary edema and edema due to increased permeability. Hydrostatic pulmonary edema is most commonly monitored in left heart failure. Pulmonary edema due to increased permeability is most often the result of Acute Respiratory Distress Syndrome (ARDS). The most common symptom of cardiogenic pulmonary edema on CT is isolated diffuse ground-glass opacities. ARDS is the most common cause of non-cardiogenic pulmonary edema. Bilateral ground-glass opacities and pulmonary consolidation are monitored on CT.

Diffuse alveolar hemorrhage is a potentially life-threatening clinical syndrome that leads to rare respiratory failure [27]. Diffuse ground-glass opacities and consolidation are often observed on CT.

Pulmonary drug toxicity is increasingly diagnosed as a cause of acute and chronic pulmonary disease. Drugs that can cause pulmonary edema due to increased permeability include cyclophosphamide, bleomycin, carmustine and methotrexate. The toxicity of these drugs causes ground-glass opacities on CT [28].

Pulmonary alveolar proteinosis (PAP) is a syndrome characterized by the accumulation of alveolar surfactants and dysfunction of alveolar macrophages [29]. Isolated diffuse ground-glass opacities and their associated interlobular septa thickenings are observed on CT.

Organized pneumonia is a consequence of the inability to fully resolve inflammation in the distal lung structures (alveoli, alveolar ducts, and respiratory bronchioles) [30]. Organized pneumonia with bronchiolitis obliterans is a histological pattern of lung damage. CT usually shows multifocal alveolar opacities scattered throughout the lungs. It is rarely accompanied by isolated diffuse ground-glass opacities.

The United States Preventive Services Task Force recommends screening for lung cancer with low-dose computed tomography (LDCT) in adults between the ages of 55 and 80 who have given up in the last 15 years or have a history of smoking 30 pack-years of smoking and still smoke [31]. Effective screening should be limited to individuals at high risk of death from lung cancer. It should be noted that false-positive results indicate a risk of harm due to overdiagnosis and unnecessary invasive tests. As a result of these scans, physicians will encounter more ground-glass opacities. In the study of Lee et al., it was revealed that a significant part of permanent ground-glass opacities may be adenocarcinoma, and the risk of invasion will increase as the diameter increases [32]. Predicting the biological behavior of a tumor based on the findings of computed tomography has significant effects on the choice of treatment. Patients with tumors with ground-glass opacity may be the group that benefits most from sublobar resection or, from another perspective, may not have to endure overtreatment with more extensive lung resection [33].

Bronchoalveolar carcinoma, a type of well-differentiated pulmonary adenocarcinoma, has a wide variety of radiographic appearances, including solitary pulmonary nodules, pneumonia-like focal alveolar opacities, ground-glass nodules, diffuse alveolar consolidation, and isolated diffuse ground-glass opacities [15].

The current staging system for lung cancer does not distinguish between tumors with and without ground-glass opacity. In the study of Watanabe et al., it was revealed that non-small-cell lung tumors with a solid component smaller than 3 cm accompanied by a ground glass component had a better prognosis compared with completely solid ones [34]. Therefore, clinical stage IA non-small-cell lung cancers should be evaluated separately as ground-glass opacity tumors and pure solid tumors. So if even the presence of a small ground-glass component in clinical stage I non-small-cell lung cancer is so protective, is this feature associated with a similar benefit in patients with larger tumors? [35]. Time and new studies will show that ground-glass opacities occur in many diseases. With the emergence of COVID-19, it has gained an important place in chest CT. In case of detection on CT, the morphology and distribution of these opacities should be revealed first. Then, a differential diagnosis should be made in the light of clinical history and examination findings. The use of such a systemic approach will play a key role in the success of diagnosis and treatment. It should be noted that the detection of this finding will also help in early diagnosis, differential diagnosis, and assessment of pulmonary activity.

In the twenty-first century, humans have three pandemics associated with coronaviruses: SARS, MERS, and COVID-19 [36]. Different strategies for effective vaccines and therapeutic combinations must be developed as soon as possible to deal with these viral pandemics. It will all become clear in time whether the SARS-CoV-2 virus will turn into an endemic virus. Lack of effective surveillance or adequate response could enable a new pandemic of SARS-CoV-2 [37]. There are many lessons to come out of this pandemic. But the most important one is to work together as a global community [38].

3. Conclusion

In summary, a hazy increase in opacity in the lung parenchyma without obscuring the underlying bronchovascular structures on chest CT is called a ground-glass pattern. Ground-glass opacities occur as a result of a wide variety of interstitial and alveolar diseases. The pandemic caused by SARS-CoV-2 has suddenly turned into the most important health problem of our day. Chest CT is frequently used due to the limited use of chest radiographs in COVID-19 disease. Thus, the ground glass pattern, which is the most common finding of this virus in CT, entered our lives intensively. Pneumonia is a common serious symptom of infection, characterized mainly by fever, cough, dyspnea, and bilateral infiltrates on lung imaging. Methods such as chest radiography, chest computed tomography, and pulmonary ultrasonography are used for imaging the lungs. Different imaging modalities have advantages and disadvantages. Today, there have been advanced developments in cross-sectional imaging methods. In many cases, cross-sectional methods for chest diseases have replaced radiography. However, chest radiographs continue to play a basic role. In the first step, the priority is always chest radiography. Although chest CT is highly sensitive, it has a low specificity. To facilitate interpretation and reduce the variability of radiological reports, there are some standardizations in the reports. Among the current classifications for COVID-19, it is possible to divide radiological findings into typical, indeterminate, atypical, and negative findings. Ground-glass opacities are classified into seven different groups according to their morphological patterns: diffuse, centrilobular, nodular, mosaic attenuation, crazy paving, halo sign, and reversed halo sign. New studies will both allow us to better recognize these viruses and improve the examination and treatment.

Author details

Bahadır Ertürk[1*] and Zamir Kemal Ertürk[2]

1 Ankara City Hospital, Ankara, Turkey

2 Etimesgut Martyr Sait Ertürk State Hospital, Ankara, Turkey

*Address all correspondence to: bahadirerturk@gmail.com

References

[1] Organization, W.H, WHO Director-General's remarks at the media briefing on 2019-nCoV on 11 February 2020. Available from: https://www.who.int/director-general/speeches/detail/who-director-general-s-remarks-at-the-media-briefing-on-2019-ncov-on-11-february-2020

[2] Cui J, Li F, Shi ZL. Origin and evolution of pathogenic coronaviruses. Nature Reviews. Microbiology. 2019;**17**(3):181-192

[3] Hu B et al. Characteristics of SARS-CoV-2 and COVID-19. Nature Reviews. Microbiology. 2021;**19**(3):141-154

[4] Hu Z et al. Clinical characteristics of 24 asymptomatic infections with COVID-19 screened among close contacts in Nanjing, China. Science China Life Sciences. 2020;**63**(5):706-711

[5] Li Q et al. Early transmission dynamics in Wuhan, China, of novel coronavirus-infected pneumonia. The New England Journal of Medicine. 2020;**382**(13):1199-1207

[6] Struyf T et al. Signs and symptoms to determine if a patient presenting in primary care or hospital outpatient settings has COVID-19 disease. Cochrane Database of Systematic Reviews. 2020;**7**(7):Cd013665

[7] Tang YW et al. Laboratory diagnosis of COVID-19: Current issues and challenges. Journal of Clinical Microbiology. 2020;**58**(6):e00512-e00520

[8] Farias LPG et al. Imaging findings in COVID-19 pneumonia. Clinics (São Paulo, Brazil). 2020;**75**:e2027

[9] Rubin GD et al. The role of chest imaging in patient management during the COVID-19 pandemic: A multinational consensus statement from the fleischner society. Radiology. 2020;**296**(1):172-180

[10] Bao C et al. Coronavirus disease 2019 (COVID-19) CT findings: A systematic review and meta-analysis. Journal of the American College of Radiology. 2020;**17**(6):701-709

[11] Brenner DJ, Hall EJ. Cancer risks from CT scans: Now we have data, what next? Radiology. 2012;**265**(2):330-331

[12] McCollough CH, Guimarães L, Fletcher JG. In defense of body CT. AJR. American Journal of Roentgenology. 2009;**193**(1):28-39

[13] Austin JH et al. Glossary of terms for CT of the lungs: Recommendations of the nomenclature committee of the fleischner society. Radiology. 1996;**200**(2):327-331

[14] Leung AN, Miller RR, Müller NL. Parenchymal opacification in chronic infiltrative lung diseases: CT-pathologic correlation. Radiology. 1993;**188**(1):209-214

[15] Miller WT Jr, Shah RM. Isolated diffuse ground-glass opacity in thoracic CT: Causes and clinical presentations. AJR. American Journal of Roentgenology. 2005;**184**(2):613-622

[16] El-Sherief AH et al. Clear vision through the haze: A practical approach to ground-glass opacity. Current Problems in Diagnostic Radiology. 2014;**43**(3):140-158

[17] Eng J, Bluemke DA. Imaging publications in the COVID-19 pandemic: Applying new research

results to clinical practice. Radiology. 2020;**297**(1):E228-e231

[18] Kanne JP et al. Essentials for radiologists on COVID-19: An update-radiology scientific expert panel. Radiology. 2020;**296**(2):E113-e114

[19] Parekh M et al. Review of the chest CT differential diagnosis of ground-glass opacities in the COVID Era. Radiology. 2020;**297**(3):E289-e302

[20] Spagnolo P et al. Hypersensitivity pneumonitis: A comprehensive review. Journal of Investigational Allergology & Clinical Immunology. 2015;**25**(4):237-250. quiz follow 250

[21] Chakraborty RK, Basit H, Sharma S. Desquamative interstitial Pneumonia, in StatPearls. In: StatPearls Publishing. Copyright © 2021. Treasure Island (FL): StatPearls Publishing LLC; 2021

[22] Sieminska A, Kuziemski K. Respiratory bronchiolitis-interstitial lung disease. Orphanet Journal of Rare Diseases. 2014;**9**:106

[23] Flaherty KR et al. Nonspecific interstitial pneumonia (NSIP). Seminars in Respiratory and Critical Care Medicine. 2001;**22**(4):423-434

[24] Mrad A, Huda N. Acute interstitial Pneumonia, in StatPearls. In: StatPearls Publishing. Copyright © 2021. Treasure Island (FL): StatPearls Publishing LLC; 2021

[25] Panchabhai TS, Farver C, Highland KB. Lymphocytic interstitial Pneumonia. Clinics in Chest Medicine. 2016;**37**(3):463-474

[26] Bargagli E, Prasse A. Sarcoidosis: A review for the internist. Internal and Emergency Medicine. 2018;**13**(3):325-331

[27] Alexandre AT, Vale A, Gomes T. Diffuse alveolar hemorrhage: How relevant is etiology? Sarcoidosis, Vasculitis, and Diffuse Lung Diseases. 2019;**36**(1):47-52

[28] Rossi SE et al. Pulmonary drug toxicity: Radiologic and pathologic manifestations. Radiographics. 2000;**20**(5):1245-1259

[29] Trapnell BC et al. Pulmonary alveolar proteinosis. Nature Reviews. Disease Primers. 2019;**5**(1):16

[30] Hansell DM. What are bronchiolitis obliterans organizing pneumonia (BOOP) and cryptogenic organizing pneumonia (COP)? Clinical Radiology. 1992;**45**(6):369-370

[31] Tanoue LT et al. Lung cancer screening. American Journal of Respiratory and Critical Care Medicine. 2015;**191**(1):19-33

[32] Lee GD et al. Lung adenocarcinoma invasiveness risk in pure ground-glass opacity lung nodules smaller than 2 cm. The Thoracic and Cardiovascular Surgeon. 2019;**67**(4):321-328

[33] Veeramachaneni NK. Commentary: Ground-glass opacity-an unexpected silver lining. The Journal of Thoracic and Cardiovascular Surgery. 2021;**161**(4): 1481-1482

[34] Watanabe Y et al. Clinical impact of a small component of ground-glass opacity in solid-dominant clinical stage IA non-small cell lung cancer. The Journal of Thoracic and Cardiovascular Surgery. 2020;**163**(3):791-801

[35] Brunelli A. Commentary: Ground glass opacity: Is it the Holy Grail? The Journal of Thoracic and Cardiovascular Surgery. 2021;**163**(3):802-803

[36] Khan M et al. COVID-19: A global challenge with old history, epidemiology and progress so far. Molecules. 2020;**26**(1):39

[37] Telenti A et al. After the pandemic: Perspectives on the future trajectory of COVID-19. Nature. 2021;**596**(7873):495-504

[38] Torbay R. Are we ready for the next pandemic? Health Affairs (Millwood). 2020;**39**(6):1104

Chapter 4

Perspective Chapter: SARS-CoV-2 Variants – Two Years Post-Onset of the Pandemic

Adekunle Sanyaolu, Aleksandra Marinkovic, Stephanie Prakash, Chuku Okorie, Abdul Jan, Priyank Desai, Abu Fahad Abbasi, Jasmine Mangat, Zaheeda Hosein, Kareem Hamdy, Nafees Haider, Nasar Khan, Rochelle Annan, Olanrewaju Badaru, Ricardo Izurieta and Stella Smith

Abstract

Since the pandemic began in China in December 2019, thousands of variants of SARS-CoV-2 have emerged globally since late 2020. The World Health Organization (WHO) defined the SARS-CoV-2 variant of concern (VOC) as a variant with increased transmissibility, virulence, and decreased response to available diagnostics, vaccines, and therapeutics. Areas of the emerging variant of concern arise from countries like the United Kingdom, South Africa, Brazil, and India. These mutations carry a lineage from N501Y, D614G, N439K, Y453F, and others, which are globally dominated by clades 20A, 20B, and 20C. SARS-CoV-2 VOC emerged after 11 months of evolution since the onset through massive human-to-human transmission with five major VOCs recognized by the WHO, namely Alpha, Beta, Gamma, Delta, and Omicron. Their emergence could be attributed to changing immunological dynamics in the human population, which has resulted in resistance or escape from neutralizing antibodies, or to mutations and/or recombinations that increase transmission or pathogenicity. This literature review intends to identify and report on SARS-CoV-2 variants that have evolved two years post-onset of the pandemic and their disease implications.

Keywords: COVID-19, SARS-CoV-2, variants of interest, variants of concern, genetic variations, genetic mutations, alpha, Beta, gamma, Delta, and omicron variants

1. Introduction

Severe acute respiratory syndrome coronavirus 2 (SARS-CoV-2) a member of the Coronaviridae family emerged in late 2019 in Wuhan, China, and has caused a global pandemic of acute respiratory disease in all ages of the population, ranging from mild symptoms to mortality [1]. It belongs to the family of coronaviruses (CoVs), sharing

79% of the genome sequence with SARS-CoV and 50% with Middle East respiratory syndrome coronavirus (MERS-CoV), while the rest of its structure is shared with other betacoronavirus [1]. In this enveloped positive sense, single-stranded ribonucleic acid (RNA) with crown-like S-shaped spiked proteins virus [2], there is an incubation period of 1–14 days with a median onset time of 8 days [1]. Transmission of SARS-CoV-2 is predominantly via droplets, aerosol, and airborne pathways [1]. It achieves invasion by using angiotensin-converting enzyme 2 (ACE2) receptors and human proteases as entry pathways, eventually fusing with the cell membranes in the lung [1]. Mild clinical presentations of this virus include fever, dry cough, and pneumonia [3]. Most patients with mild manifestations of this infection recover [3]. More severe cases cause other issues besides respiratory problems, such as injury to the myocardial cells and heart arrhythmias [3]. Other reported problems caused by this virus are in the central nervous system (CNS), gastrointestinal tract (GIT), musculoskeletal system, hypercoagulability leading to stroke, and organ failure [3]. In the most critical cases, end-organ failure and acute respiratory distress have led to death, especially in those with comorbidities such as hypertension and obesity [2, 3].

Coronaviruses continuously evolve due to mutations that occur during the replication of their genome [4]. Variants that emerged throughout the pandemic differ from each other due to one or more mutations, such as the number and location of substitutions in the spike (S) protein that makes each unique [4]. The United States SARS-CoV-2 Interagency Group (SIG) defines four classes of SARS-CoV-2 variants which are: variants being monitored (VBM), variants of interest (VOI), variants of concern (VOC), and variants of high consequence (VOHC) [4]. Thirteen variations in the S protein of coronavirus disease 2019 (COVID-19) have been detected by late November 2020 [3]. On November 30, 2021, SIG classified Omicron as a VOC, replacing the Delta variant [4]. Currently, there is no VOI and the VBM are Alpha, Beta, Gamma, Epsilon, Eta, Lota, Kappa, 1.616.3, Mu, and Zeta [4].

Of the two VOCs, Delta and Omicron, the Delta variant has been shown to cause a more severe illness in the unvaccinated as compared to the vaccinated [5]. November 2021, the Omicron variant was first discovered in Botswana [5]. Omicron was designated as a VOC by the World Health Organization (WHO), which stated that early research suggests that it carries a higher risk of reinfection than other variants [5]. Currently, in the United States, the Omicron variant is the most common [5]. In December of 2020, the Delta variant was first found in India but has since spread across 178 countries [5]. Changes to the S protein may render the Delta variant up to 50% more transmissible than other prior COVID-19 variants, according to research [5].

Significant advances have been made toward "real-time" generation and sharing of SARS-CoV-2 data throughout the pandemic [6]. As a result, a computational tool, Phylogenetic Assignment of Named Global Outbreak Lineages (Pangolin) was developed to assign the most likely lineage to a genome sequence for managing and interpreting the rapid generation and sharing of data worldwide, at either a national or regional level [6]. Hence this nomenclature was developed to name and track global transmission lineages of SARS-CoV-2 [6]. Nextstrain and GISAID focus on the prevalence and persistence of a variant by 'clades' [6]. Thus, the WHO has established a structure for nomenclature using GISAID, Nextstrain, and Pangolin (Pango) nomenclature, so that the scientific community may be able to name and track the variants of SARS-CoV-2 [7].

According to the WHO situation report as of March 22, 2022, there has been a 7% rise in COVID-19 positive cases for the week of March 14–20, 2022, versus the week before [8]. However, there has been a 23% decrease in mortality in comparison to the week before [8]. About 12 million new cases and slightly below 33 thousand deaths have been reported in this period among the six WHO regions [8]. Approximately 468,000,000 COVID-19 positive cases and slightly over 6,000,000 deaths have been disclosed universally as of March 22, 2022 [8].

COVID-19 has become a continuously evolving disease due to rapid changes in the viral variants and despite mitigation strategies such as facial masks, social distancing, hand hygiene, vaccine therapies, and other therapies [2]. One of the earliest VOCs was the Alpha variant (B.1.1.7), which had a high transmissibility rate [2]. Recently, Omicron (B.1.1.529) appears to be at least two times more transmissible than Delta, with Delta variations being 50–70% more transmissible than earlier variants such as Alpha [2]. VOCs remain prevalent, particularly among unimmunized persons [2]. VBM were more problematic earlier in the pandemic and were more notable for high transmission and increased virulence [2]. These include B.1.1.7 (Alpha), B.1.351 (Beta), and P.1 (Gamma), and of lesser concern, Epsilon (B.1.427 and B.1.429), Eta (B.1.525), Iota (B.1.526), Kappa (B.1.617.1), 1.617.3, Mu (B.1.621, B.1.621.1), and Zeta (P.2) [2].

The two other categories described by the WHO include VOI, which are variants that are widely circulating within a population or have the potential to have an impact on a population, and VOHC, which are mutations that elude vaccines and current therapies that are in place. Currently, there are no circulating VOI and VOHC [2]. Given the continuous evolution of SARS-CoV-2, the impact of variants on public health may be reclassified based on their attributes and prevalence. VOCs and VOIs may differ from those of other reporting agencies because of the impact the variants may cause by location. The purpose of this paper is to discuss the genetic lineages of SARS-CoV-2 that have emerged as variants and circulated globally during the 2 years since the onset of the COVID-19 pandemic.

2. Methodology

PubMed, Google Scholar, EBSCOhost, Mendeley, and MedLine Plus were used to conduct the electronic literature search. The search was confined to relevant publications and articles published between January 2020 and April 2022. If a manuscript was relevant to the issue of genetic mutations or variations of SARS-CoV-2, it was chosen. To narrow and guide the search process, the listed keywords were sought after. COVID-19, SARS-CoV-2, variants of interest (VOI), variants of concern (VOC), genetic variances, and genetic mutations are among them.

3. Variant being monitored

Viruses are known to change over time. SARS-CoV-2 has undergone multiple modifications since the start of the COVID-19 pandemic in Wuhan in late 2019 [9]. Comparing the SARS-CoV-2 pathogenic S protein sequence to the Wuhan-Hu-1 reference protein sequence showed about 96.5% of the original S protein sequence has undergone mutations [9]. These mutations lead to genetic differences, which results in the emergence of new variants of the virus [9]. Centers for Disease Control and Prevention (CDC), in collaboration with the SIG, added a fourth class of variant classification named VBM on September 21, 2021, as depicted in **Table 1** [22]. The other classes include VOI, VOC, and VOHC [22].

Lineage	Predominate Countries Affected	Date of Designation	Description
Alpha B.1.1.7 Q Lineages	United Kingdom (UK) 24.0%, United States of America (USA) 20.0%, Germany 9.0%, Sweden 6.0%, and Denmark 6.0%	September 3, 2020.	First detected in the UK and has spread to over 52 countries including the USA [10–12]
Beta B.1.351	South Africa 18.0%, Philippines 10.0%, USA 9.0%, Sweden 8.0%, and Germany 7.0%	September 9, 2020	South African lineage [10, 11, 13]
Gamma P.1	Brazil 56.0%, USA 29.0%, Chile 3.0%, Argentina 2.0%, and Spain 1.0%	October 1, 2020	Brazilian lineage with functionally significant spike mutations [10, 11, 13]
Epsilon B.1.429	USA 98.0%, Mexico 1.0%, Aruba 0.0%, and Argentina 0.0%	January 26, 2020	USA lineage, predominantly in California [10, 11, 14]
Eta B.1.525	Canada 20.0%, USA 15.0%, Germany 9.0%, France 8.0%, and Denmark 7.0%	March 25, 2020	International lineage [10, 11, 15]
Iota B.1.526	USA 97.0%, Ecuador 1.0%, Canada 1.0%, Puerto Rico 1.0%, and Spain 0.0%	January 28, 2020,	Predominately in New York, with S mutation E484K [10, 11, 16]
Kappa B.1.617.1	India 72.0%, UK 6.0%, Canada 6.0%, USA 5.0%, and Ireland 3.0%	March 3, 2020	Indian lineage [10, 11, 17]
N/A B.1.617.3	India 89.0%, UK 4.0%, USA 3.0%, Malawi 2.0%, and Russia 1.0%	January 1, 2021	Indian lineage [10, 11, 18]
Zeta P.2	Brazil 56.0%, USA 25.0%, Canada 5.0%, Argentina 2.0%, and Paraguay 2.0%	April 13, 2020	Brazilian lineage [10, 11, 19, 20]
Mu B.1.621	USA 42.0%, Colombia 27.0%, Chile 9.0%, Spain 5.0%, Mexico 3.0%	December 15, 2020	Predominantly in Columbia [10, 11, 21]

Note. *Researchers and public health authorities globally are using the Pango nomenclature to track the transmission and spread of SARS-CoV-2, including variations of concern and interest. This table contains information on various lineages and their distribution [10–21].*

Table 1.
Lineage list.

The VBM class includes variants under surveillance for mutations leading to increased receptor binding, reduced neutralization by host immune systems, decreased efficacy of treatments, and an increase in disease severity and transmissibility but have not yet been deemed a public health threat by SIG at this time [22]. The VBM class also includes previously designated VOIs and VOCs that are no longer detected or have a decreased prevalence in the population [22]. The variants belonging to the VBM class do not pose a significant risk to public health [22]. Regardless of the minimal risk presented by the VBM class, they are closely monitored for new data [22]. VBM class that warrants more concern can have their classification changed to VOI or VOC if required by SIG [2].

4. Variant of concern

4.1 Delta

Viruses constantly undergo mutations resulting in new variants [23]. **Table 2** shows the Delta variant of COVID-19, formally known as B.1.617.2 [4, 19]. Part of the AY lineage, this variant appeared in late 2020 from India and had spread to over 179 countries by late 2021 [4, 24]. By late 2021, the Delta variant was the most transmissible, spreading more easily than the first identified Alpha variant - roughly two times more contagious than the original virus [24]. Mutations of the S protein in the Delta variant have not been analyzed in detail, though the following substitutions identified are T19R, (V70F*), T95I, G142D, E156-, F157-, R158G, (A222V*), (W258L*), (K417N*), L452R, T478K, D614G, P681R, and D950N [4]. The Delta variant is thought to have a distinct receptor-binding interface than the other forms [24]. The replication capacity of the Delta variant has been noted to be more efficient, leading to increased rates of transmission, infectivity, and viral load in comparison to other strains [24].

Antiviral medication has been developed to minimize symptoms and lessen the duration of viral infection. There are no less than 13 vaccines against SARS-CoV-2 being used [25]. Each vaccine has been developed with the aim of the immune system recognizing the immunodominant S protein [26]. Although the development of vaccines has proven successful in decreasing fatalities, reports suggest that mutations continue to increase - proposing that the administration of these vaccines does not eradicate disease spread [24]. Therefore, the attributes for the Delta variant suggest that monoclonal antibody therapies with Emergency Use Authorization (EUA) are effective against nearly all Delta lineages [4]. The AY.1 and AY.2 lineages are resistant to several monoclonal antibody treatments [4]. In addition, research has shown a decrease in post-vaccination sera neutralization [4].

4.2 Omicron

The Omicron variant (B.1.1.529, BA lineages, and other recombinant lineages, respectively depicted in **Table 2**) of SARS-CoV-2 was initially reported to the WHO in late November 2021, by South Africa [4, 7, 27, 28]. By December 2021, the United States reported its first case of COVID-19 connected to the Omicron variant [4, 27, 28]. Numerous mutations not previously seen in the original SARS-CoV-2 strain have

Lineage	WHO Label	GISAID Clade	Nextstrain Clade
B.1.617.2	Delta	G/478 K.V1	21A, 21I, 21 J
B.1.1.529	Omicron	GR/484A	21 K → BA.1, BA.1.1 21 L → BA.2 Recombinant lineages → XE, XF, and XD

Note. *Data extracted and recreated from the WHO.*

Table 2.
Circulating variants of concern.

been recognized in Omicron [29]. Omicron possesses greater than 30 mutations on its surface within the S protein, one insertion, and three deletions which allows the virus to infect cells, rendering elusive characteristics [27, 29].

A substantial number of amino acid substitutions are in the receptor-binding domain (RBD) with several alternative changes in other genomic regions [27]. Mutations to the S protein of the Omicron variant increase the affinity of binding to receptors, allowing the virus to circumvent antibodies against previous variants and remain infectious [30]. Factors influencing the transmissibility and infectivity of the Omicron variant are dependent on genetic variability and the location of the mutation [31].

Monoclonal antibody treatments aid the immune system in recognizing and responding more effectively to the virus [32]. The attributes for the Omicron variant suggest that some monoclonal antibody treatments with EUA may reduce neutralization [4]. In addition, post-vaccination sera may also reduce neutralization [4]. A comprehensive list of the lineages can be cross-referenced from **Table 1** [4, 7].

5. Discussion

Viruses regularly undergo mutations, sometimes creating a lineage of virus progeny known as variants. SARS-CoV-2 has mutated several times since its discovery. Using the original Wuhan-Hu-1 protein as a reference, researchers discovered that the genes encoding the pathogenic S protein had mutated to the point that just 3.5% of the original coding sequence remains [9]. The SIG was founded by the United States Department of Health and Human Services (HHS). SIG and the CDC collaborated on a report that accounted for these variants and their classification [33]. In terms of population impact, the VBM are quite a minimal risk. Alpha, Beta, Gamma, Epsilon, Eta, Iota, Kappa, Mu, and Zeta are the varieties under the VBM class as of December 2021, with B.1.617.3's structure being unique when comparing other progenies: B.1617.1 and B.1.617.2 [2]. As per the CDC, the VBM class poses no significant and imminent risk to public health in the United States; in addition, there are no VOI or VOHC for SARS-CoV-2 [4].

Countries such as the United Kingdom, South Africa, Brazil, and India have growing variants of concern [23]. These mutations have a pedigree that includes N501Y (i.e., B.1.1.7 and several lineages), D614G (i.e., B.1 lineage and the initial dominant variant of 2020), N439K (i.e., arising from the B.1 lineage of the mutated D614G), Y453F (i.e., Cluster 5 and mink variant), and additional mutations that are dominated by clades [23]. Clades are classified according to the year they first appeared and are given a new alphabetical letter depending on their discovery: 19A (first emerging in 2019), 19B (appearing after 19A), 20A (new appearance at the start of 2020), 20B, and 20C, so on and so forth [23]. Delta (i.e., of clades 21A, 21I, and 21 J) and Omicron (i.e., of clades 21 K and 21 L) were designated as VOCs by the CDC and SIG in late 2021 [7]. The Delta variant was discovered to be the most infectious version, with an estimated transmission rate double that of the original virus. Its evolved receptor-binding interface may be the reason for its success when compared to the other variants [24]. Where Delta may have been the fastest transmissible variant, Omicron was the most clandestine [27, 29, 34]. First seen in late November of 2021, researchers found over 30 mutations within the S protein. These mutations increased the affinity of receptor binding, allowing the virus to circumvent antibodies against previous variants and remain infectious [30]. It was also reported that monoclonal antibody treatments were found to be effective against Omicron [34].

The S protein is found on the external surface of the virus and is categorized into two subunits, S1 and S2 [24]. The S protein is the main virulence factor that moderates host infection by binding to the ACE2 receptors prominent on type II alveolar epithelial cells found in the respiratory epithelium [24]. Once the S protein binds to the host cell, it undergoes a conformational change in its structure from the inactive "down" state into an active "up" state, which signals a cascade of cleavages to the S1/S2 subunits by the host enzymes and other proteases [24]. This change further alters the S protein into an amino N-terminal S1 subunit containing an RBD and a carboxyl (C)-terminal S2 subunit for virus and host cell membrane fusion [24]. Much of the SARS-CoV-2 genome is made of ORF1ab (one large open reading frame), and when the virus penetrates the host cell, it gets translated into polypeptides pp1a or pp1ab [24]. These polypeptides primarily make non-structural proteins nsp1-nsp16 that mediate ssRNA replication [24]. Approximately one-third of the SARS-CoV-2 genome is responsible for synthesizing structural proteins such as the S (spike) protein, E (envelope) protein, M (membrane) protein, and N (nucleocapsid) protein, as well as accessory proteins ORF3a, ORF6, ORF7a, ORF7b, ORF8, and ORF10 [24].

During viral replication, mutations in the ssRNA genome can be classified as synonymous with no changes to the amino acid being synthesized or non-synonymous with modifications to the amino acid [24]. The S protein has two regions that are susceptible to mutation, the N-terminal domain, and the receptor-binding domain, which directly interacts with host ACE2 and is a region that contains a heightened number of amino acid substitutions [24].

5.1 +S: K417N (Delta)

The mutation K417N has lysine (K) being substituted with asparagine (N) [35]. This mutation is found close to the RBD and has displayed the capability of impairing the RBD inactive "down" state [24]. Recent data also indicates that multiple combination mutations are possible and can generate an even more significant decline in neutralization attempts, such as mutation K417N in conjunction with mutations E484K and N501Y [24].

5.2 +S: E484K (Delta)

The mutation E484K has arisen from multiple lineages, such as Beta and Gamma [24]. This variant indicates an amino acid substitution in position 484 with glutamic acid (E) substituting for lysine (K) [35]. In addition, this mutation is close to the tip of the spike [24]. This substitution alters the shape of the S protein and grants resistance to several antibodies and the ability to evade the immune response [24].

5.3 +S: R346K (Omicron)

A recent study conducted by Lu et al., which used transmembrane protease serine 2 (TMPRSS2) to isolate variant Omicron strains HKU691, and HKU344-R346K from patients indicated that the Omicron variant has an extra spike R346K mutation that is seen in 8.5% of strains reported in the GISAID database [36]. The study also indicated that both strains were less susceptible to neutralization, and many patients did not demonstrate neutralizing antibodies to Omicron variant isolates [36]. The R346K mutation is also found in the receptor-binding domain and the mu variant [36].

Coronaviruses often recombine; therefore, a single phylogenetic tree will not necessarily depict SARS-CoV-2's evolutionary history accurately [10]. While this complicates the phylogenetic analysis, recombination is made possible with the approach of lineage nomenclature and assignment [10]. Conversely, the co-infection of both Delta and Omicron, although rare, happens [34, 36]. If a different recombination event initiates continuous transmission, it will result in the formation of a new viral lineage with a distinct common ancestor. Because this new lineage lacks a specific or clear ancestor, it will be given the next available alphabetical prefix [10]. For example, XE, a cross between two Omicron strains that are now well-known: BA.1 (the original Omicron strain) and BA.2 (the more contagious strain that is now prominent in the United States and other countries) [4, 7, 10].

6. Conclusion

SARS-CoV-2 first appeared in late 2019 in Wuhan, China, as a positive-sense, single-stranded RNA virus with crown-like S-shaped spiking proteins; and has since spread throughout the world, resulting in a global pandemic of acute respiratory illness in people of all ages, with symptoms ranging from mild to fatal. It can undergo mutations, creating a lineage of virus progeny. It has become a continuously evolving disease due to rapid changes in the viral variants. They differ from each other due to one or more mutations, such as the number and location of substitutions in the S protein that makes each unique. This article discusses the genetic lineages of SARS-CoV-2 that have emerged as variants and circulated globally during the two years since the onset of the COVID-19 pandemic. There are four classifications by SIG of which the most alarming is classified as VOC. Important VOCs are Alpha, Beta, Gamma, Delta, and Omicron. Some of the lineages of these mutations are N501Y, D614G, N439K, Y453F, and others, which are globally dominated by clades 20A, 20B, and 20C. Of these, Alpha was the earliest and most infective initially. Variants have mostly emerged from countries like the United Kingdom, South Africa, Brazil, and India. The mutations are thought to appear due to massive human-to-human transmission, which is why prevalence is particularly higher among unimmunized persons. Other classifications are defined as VBM, VOI, VOC, and VOHC but most of these are at lower risk for infectivity, although they are still being monitored for new data. To date, no SARS-CoV-2 variants are designated as VOI or VOHC. Of note, further research is required to fully understand these variants and increase the accuracy of treatments. The public should consider vaccination along with preventative measures, such as wearing a mask, washing hands frequently, and practicing social distancing for the best chance of avoiding contact and increase in the variants.

Conflict of interest

The authors declare no conflict of interest.

Author details

Adekunle Sanyaolu[1*], Aleksandra Marinkovic[2], Stephanie Prakash[2], Chuku Okorie[3], Abdul Jan[4], Priyank Desai[5], Abu Fahad Abbasi[6], Jasmine Mangat[7], Zaheeda Hosein[7], Kareem Hamdy[2], Nafees Haider[8], Nasar Khan[4], Rochelle Annan[9], Olanrewaju Badaru[10], Ricardo Izurieta[11] and Stella Smith[12]

1 Federal Ministry of Health, Abuja, Nigeria

2 Saint James School of Medicine, Anguilla, BWI

3 Union County College, Plainfield Campus, New Jersey, USA

4 Windsor University School of Medicine, Cayon, Saint Kitts, and Nevis

5 American University of Saint Vincent School of Medicine, Saint Vincent and the Grenadines

6 Loyola University Medical Center, Maywood, IL, USA

7 Caribbean Medical University School of Medicine, Curacao

8 All Saints University School of Medicine, Dominica

9 University of Health Sciences Antigua School of Medicine, Antigua and Barbuda

10 Nigeria Centre for Disease Control, Abuja, Nigeria

11 Global Communicable Diseases, College of Public Health, University of South Florida, Tampa, FL, USA

12 Nigerian Institute of Medical Research, Lagos, Nigeria

*Address all correspondence to: sanyakunle@gmail.com

References

[1] Hu B, Guo H, Zhou P, Shi ZL. Characteristics of SARS-CoV-2 and COVID-19. Nature Reviews. Microbiology. 2021;**19**:141-154. DOI: 10.1038/s41579-020-00459-7

[2] Auwaerter PG. Coronavirus COVID-19 (SARS-CoV-2). Johns Hopkins ABX Guide. Baltimore, MD; 2022. https://www.hopkinsguides.com/hopkins/view/Johns_Hopkins_ABX_Guide/540747/all/Coronavirus_COVID_19__SARS_CoV_2

[3] Wang MY, Zhao R, Gao LJ, Gao XF, Wang DP, et al. SARS-CoV-2: Structure, biology, and structure-based therapeutics development. Frontiers in Cellular and Infection Microbiology. 2020;**10**:2235-2988. DOI: 10.3389/fcimb.2020.587269

[4] CDC. SARS-CoV-2 Variant Classifications and Definitions. Centers for Disease Control. Atlanta, GA; 2022. https://www.cdc.gov/coronavirus/2019-ncov/variants/variant-classifications.html

[5] Nazario B. Variants of Coronavirus. WebMD. Atlanta, GA; 2022. https://www.webmd.com/lung/coronavirus-strains#1-1

[6] O'Toole A, Scher E, Underwood A, Jackson B, Hill V, et al. Assignment of epidemiological lineages in an emerging pandemic using the pangolin tool. Virus. Evolution. 2021;7(2):veab 064. DOI: 10.1093/ve/veab064

[7] WHO. Tracking SARS-CoV-2 Variants. Washington, DC: World Health Organization; 2022. https://www.who.int/en/activities/tracking-SARS-CoV-2-variants/

[8] WHO. Weekly Epidemiological Update on COVID-19 - 22 March 2022. Washington, DC: World Health Organization; 2022. https://www.who.int/emergencies/diseases/novel-coronavirus-2019/situation-reports

[9] Guruprasad K. Mutations in human SARS-CoV-2 spike proteins, potential drug binding and epitope sites for COVID-19 therapeutics development. Current Research in Structural Biology. 2022;**4**:41-50. DOI: 10.1016/j.crstbi.2022.01.002

[10] Rambaut A, Holmes EC, O'Toole Á, Hill V, McCrone JT, et al. A dynamic nomenclature proposal for SARS-CoV-2 lineages to assist genomic epidemiology. Nature Microbiology. 2020;**5**:1403-1407. DOI: 10.1038/s41564-020-0770-5

[11] Pango. Pango lineages: Latest epidemiological lineage of SARS-CoV-2. Pango. Network. 2022. [Accessed on April 10, 2022]. https://cov-lineages.org/index.html#cite

[12] Roquebert B, Trombert-Paolantoni S, Haim-Boukobza S, Lecorche E, Verdurme L, et al. The SARS-CoV-2 B.1.351 lineage (VOC β) is outgrowing the B.1.1.7 lineage (VOC α) in some French regions in April 2021. Euro Surveillance. 2021;**26**(23):2100447. DOI: 10.2807/1560-7917.ES.2021.26.23.2100447

[13] Franceschi VB, Caldana GD, Perin C, Horn A, Peter C, et al. Predominance of the SARS-CoV-2 lineage P.1 and its sublineage P.1.2 in patients from the metropolitan region of Porto Alegre, southern Brazil in march 2021. Pathogens. 2021;**10**(8):988. DOI: 10.3390/pathogens10080988

[14] Carroll T, Fox D, van Doremalen N, Ball E, Moris MK, et al. The B.1.427/1.429 (epsilon) SARS-CoV-2 variants are

more virulent than ancestral B.1 (614G) in Syrian hamsters. PLoS Pathogens. 2022;**18**(2):e1009914. DOI: 10.1371/journal.ppat.1009914

[15] Janik E, Niemcewicz M, Podogrocki M, Majsterek I, Bijak M. The emerging concern and interest SARS-CoV-2 variants. Pathogens. 2021;**10**(6):633. DOI: 10.3390/pathogens10060633

[16] Padilla-Rojas C, Jimenez-Vasquez V, Hurtado V, Mestanza O, Molina IS, et al. Genomic analysis reveals a rapid spread and predominance of lambda (C.37) SARS-CoV-2 lineage in Peru despite circulation of variants of concern. Journal of Medical Virology. 2021;**93**:6845-6849. DOI: 10.1002/jmv.27261

[17] Cascella M, Rajnik M, Aleem A, Dulebohn SC, Di Napoli R. Features, Evaluation, and Treatment of Coronavirus (COVID-19). Treasure Island, FL: StatPearls; 2022. https://www.ncbi.nlm.nih.gov/books/NBK554776/

[18] Kunal S, Aditi GK, Ish P. COVID-19 variants in India: Potential role in second wave and impact on vaccination. Heart & Lung. 2021;**50**(6):784-787. DOI: 10.1016/j.hrtlng.2021.05.008

[19] Levi JE, Oliveira CM, Croce BD, Telles P, Lopes ACW, et al. Dynamics of SARS-CoV-2 variants of concern in Brazil early 2021. Frontiers in Public Health. 2021;**9**:1-6. DOI: 10.3389/fpubh.2021.784300

[20] Islam S, Islam T, Islam R. New coronavirus variants are creating more challenges to global healthcare system: A brief report on the current knowledge. Clin Pathol. 2022;**15**:2632010X221075584. DOI: 10.1177/2632010X221075584

[21] Aleem A, Akbar Samad AB, Slenker AK. Emerging Variants of SARS-CoV-2 and Novel Therapeutics against Coronavirus (COVID-19). Treasure Island, FL: StatPearls; 2022. https://pubmed.ncbi.nlm.nih.gov/34033342/

[22] CDC. Lab Advisory: CDC Updates SARS-CoV-2 Variant Classifications. Centers for Disease Control and Prevention. Atlanta, GA; 2021. https://www.cdc.gov/csels/dls/locs/2021/09-22-2021-lab-advisory-CDC-Updates-SARS-CoV-2-Variant-Classifications_1.html

[23] Sanyaolu A, Okorie C, Marinkovic A, Haider N, Abbasi AF, et al. The emerging SARS-CoV-2 variants of concern. Therapeutic Advance in Infectious Disease. 2021;**8**:20499361211024372. DOI: 10.1177/2049936121102437

[24] Perez-Gomez. The development of SARS-CoV-2 variants: The gene makes the disease. Journal of Developmental Biology. 2021;**9**(4):58. DOI: 10.3390/jdb9040058

[25] Li DD, Li QH. SARS-CoV-2: Vaccines in the pandemic era. Military Medical Research. 2021;**8**(1):1-15

[26] Chi X, Yan R, Zhang J, Zhang G, Zhang Y, et al. A neutralizing human antibody binds to the N-terminal domain of the spike protein of SARS-CoV-2. Science. 2020;**369**(6504):650-655. DOI: 10.1126/science.abc6952

[27] CDC. Science Brief: Omicron (B.1.1.529) Variant. Centers for Disease Control and Prevention. Atlanta, GA; 2021. https://www.cdc.gov/coronavirus/2019-ncov/science/science-briefs/scientific-brief-omicron-variant.html

[28] CDC. SARS-CoV-2 B.1.1.529 (omicron) variant - United States. MMWR Centers for Disease Control and Prevention. 2021;**70**(50):1731-1734

[29] Kwon D. Omicron's molecular structure could help explain its global takeover. Nature. 2022;**602**:373-374

[30] McCallum M, Czudnochowski N, Rosen LE, Zepeda SK, Bowen JE, et al. Structural basis of SARS-CoV-2 omicron immune evasion and receptor engagement. Science. 2022;**375**(6583):864-868. DOI: 10.1126/science. abn8652

[31] Hirabara SM, Serdan TDA, Gorjao R, Masi LN, Pithon-Curi TC, et al. SARS-CoV-2 variants: Differences and potential of immune evasion. Frontiers in Cellular and Infection Microbiology. 2022;**11**:1-17. DOI: 10.3389/fcimb.2021.781429

[32] CDC. Treatments your Healthcare Provider Might Recommend if you Are Sick. Centers for Disease Control and Prevention. Atlanta, GA; 2022. https://www.cdc.gov/coronavirus/2019-ncov/your-health/treatments-for-severe-illness.html

[33] Post D, DeGrace M, Bratt D. SARS-CoV-2 Assessment of Viral Evolution (SAVE) Program. NIH: National Institute of Allergy and Infectious Diseases; 2022

[34] Mohapatra RK, Tiwari R, Sarangi AK, Sharma SK, Khandia R, et al. Twin combination of omicron and Delta variants triggering a tsunami wave of ever high surges in COVID-19 cases: A challenging global threat with a special focus on the Indian subcontinent. Journal of Medical Virology. 2022;**94**(5):1761-1765. DOI: 10.1002/jmv.27585

[35] Khateeb J, Li Y, Zhang H. Emerging SARS-CoV-2 variants of concern and potential intervention approaches. Critical Care. 2021;**25**:244. DOI: 10.1186/s13054-021-03662-x

[36] Lu L, Mok BWY, Chen LL, Chan JMC, Tsang OTY, et al. Neutralization of severe acute respiratory syndrome coronavirus 2 omicron variant by sera from BNT162b2 or CoronaVac vaccine recipients. Clinical Infectious Diseases. 2021:ciab1041. DOI: 10.1093/cid/ciab1041. https://academic.oup.com/cid/advance-article/doi/10.1093/cid/ciab1041/6463504

Chapter 5

SARS-CoV-2 Mutation Mechanism, Features, and Future Perspective

Tahereh Alinejad, Danial Zareh, Zuo Hao, Tengfei Zhou and Cheng-shui Chen

Abstract

Over two years, the SARS-CoV-2 virus has evolved by producing several variants by RNA polymerase mutation. This mutation created many virus variants that five of them are designated by WHO. These are Alpha, Beta, Gamma, Delta, and Omicron, among them Alpha, Delta, and Omicron spread faster. Coronaviruses (CoVs) are enveloped in positive-sense RNA viruses and contain huge RNA virus genomes. RNA polymerase controls the replication in which the genomic material is copied, and it often makes errors that lead to create a new mutation. Most mutations create a virus that cannot replicate and spread among people. However, some mutations lead to a virus that can replicate and create a variant. This chapter will discuss the mechanism of the mutations during the last two years and the future of these mutations in SARS-CoV-2.

Keywords: SARS-Cov-2 mutation-biochemical mechanisms, RNA polymerase

1. Introduction

To begin, most known human-associated coronaviruses have caused colds, therefore, to date, this family of viruses has not been extensively researched and is still very unknown to humanity, and only a number of severe human diseases have been attributed to this family.

However, in 2003, a virus from this family, which was responsible for severe acute respiratory syndrome (SARS) appeared and spread rapidly among humans and was the starting point for research into coronaviruses [1]. In addition to the 2003 SARS outbreak, coronaviruses (CoVs) have had two other large-scale outbreaks in the last two decades: middle eastern respiratory syndrome (MERS) and now COVID-19. Current coronavirus (COVID-19) originates from a cluster of pneumonia related to the seafood market in Wuhan City, Hubei Province, China [2]. With the occurrence of the MERS and the SARS outbreaks within the past couple of decades combined with the ongoing pandemic, coronaviruses are now considered "emerging pathogens" [1, 3–5]. In (**Figure 1**), you can have a better understanding of the types of diseases and viruses that cause the disease, as well as their relationship and year of spread.

In addition, CoVs disease (COVID-19) caused by severe acute respiratory syndrome coronavirus 2 (SARS-CoV-2) is an infectious disease [6]. SARS-CoV-2

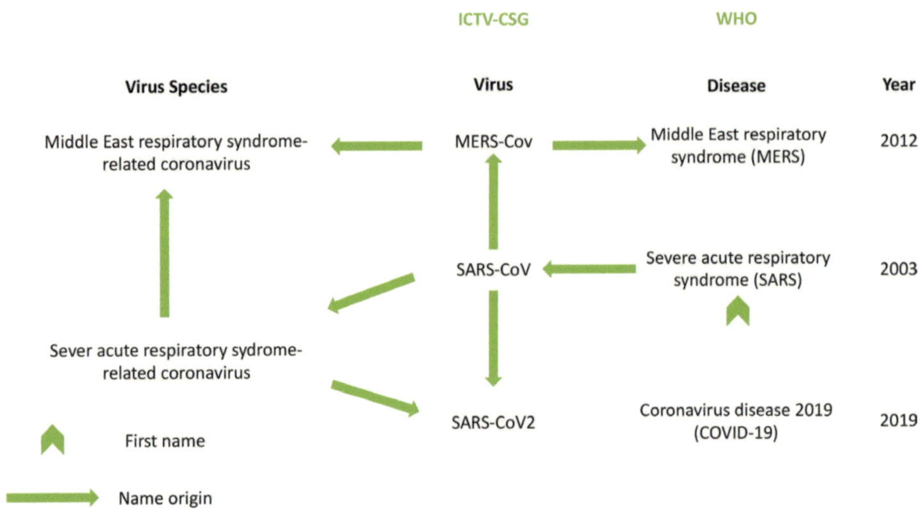

Figure 1.
History of coronavirus naming during the three zoonotic outbreaks in relation to virus taxonomy and diseases caused by these viruses. According to the current international classification of diseases, MERS and SARS are classified as 1D64 and 1D65, respectively.

belongs to the betacoronavirus genus [1]. As mentioned above, the third highly pathogenic coronavirus to enter the human population is SARS-CoV-2, which is more contagious and has a broad tissue tropism that is likely to increase the prevalence [7].

In December 2019, the SARS-CoV-2 first spread to Wuhan, China, and the rapid spread of the virus sounded the alarm around the world and all countries were on alert. The World Health Organization (WHO) declared the outbreak an epidemic, and several countries quickly confirmed several cases. By May 4, 2020, more than 3.3 million cases had been diagnosed with the disease, a staggering number. It was a concern for governments and humanity [8].

The first observations showed that the virus is transmitted from a carrier to a healthy person through close contact, such as shaking hands and kissing, and by small droplets produced during sneezing, coughing, and talking [9].

Most researchers and scientists are now focused on identifying different types of coronaviruses and in particular the regular identification of new types of mammalian coronaviruses. For example, in 2018, the HKU2-associated coronavirus of bat origin was identified as responsible for the deadly acute diarrhea syndrome in pigs **Figure 1** [5].

1.1 SARS-CoV-2 genome and structure

Coronaviruses (CoVs) of the family Coronaviridae are enveloped, positive-sense single-stranded RNA genomes ranging from 26 to 32 kilobases in length, which replicate in the cytoplasm [1, 3–5]. All of the highly pathogenic CoVs, including SARS-CoV-2, belong to the betacoronavirus genus, group 2. The SARS-CoV-2 genome sequence shares ~80% sequence identity with SARS-CoV and ~50% with MERS-CoV [3, 4]. Its genome comprises 14 open reading frames (ORFs), two-thirds of which encode 16 nonstructural proteins (nsp 1–16) that make up the replicase complex, whereas the remaining one-third encodes the structural proteins envelope (E), spike (S), nucleocapsid (N), and membrane (M). [1, 4, 5].

1.2 Entry mechanism of SARS-CoV-2

All external agents that want to enter the host cell have their entry mechanism, and the covids have their mechanism. All covids first bind to the host cell receptor by a surface glycoprotein called spike, which is encoded by themselves, and whose main job is to mediate entry into the host cell. Covids transfer their nucleocapsid to the host cell cytoplasm when their coating fuses with the host cell layer. This occurs in acidic endosomal portions or, in some cases, in the plasma membrane. The route of infection is driven by the spike glycoprotein (S), which is also a major determinant of cellular tropism. This protein is a class I combination protein and plays a key role in binding the virus to the corresponding receptor at the surface of the host cell, also the role of interference between the host membrane and the virus in the cycle is driven by critical structural changes in the spike protein. For beta-coronaviruses, there is a receptor-binding region (RBD) in the spike protein that is involved in binding to the host cell receptor. This occurs when the spike is cleaved by the proximal host protease, then the spike combination peptide is released to facilitate virus entry. ACE2 for SARS-CoV and dipeptidyl peptidase-4 (DPP4) for MERS-CoV have identified receptors. Past investigations have announced that RBDs from the heredity B of beta covids can be arranged into practically distinct clades. Those from clade 1, which incorporates SARS-CoV-2 can enter cells expressing ACE2. This has been tentatively approved by a few investigations exhibiting the crystal construction of the RBD of the spike protein with that of ACE2. ACE2 is enhanced in the ciliated bronchial epithelial cells, which have all the major targets of being significant focuses of SARS-CoV-1 and -2, though DPP4 is advanced in the unciliated epithelial cells, which act as target cells for MERS disease. The two receptors are expressed in the sort II pneumocytes, which are contaminated by both infections. Aside from the ACE2 receptor, neuropilin-1 has been as of late distinguished as an entry factor that functions in concert with ACE2 to facilitate SARS-CoV-2 entry. In any case, expression of ACE2 in the mix with a host transmembrane serine protease has been displayed to confer susceptibility to SARS-CoV-2 [1].

Like other covids, the SARS-CoV-2 section happens by means of a multi-step interaction of cell surface connection, receptor commitment, proteolytic cleavage, and membrane combination that includes a few particular domains on the spike protein [1], which is shown clearly in (**Figure 2**).

As mentioned, the function of the RBD receptor plays the most important role in the virus entering the host cell. Researchers have also recently realized that protease plays a key role in facilitating virus entry, processing covid results, and as a potential barrier to species. Research shows that the entry of the virus SARS-CoV-2 is increased following the external expansion of trypsin. The most colorful role among host proteases is the serine transmembrane protease Tmprss2, although it should be noted that different types of this family, as well as certain cathepsins, are involved. Although the spike protein has been shown to be cleaved by host proteases, there is further evidence that this protease acts on the receptor and activates it [1].

SARS-CoV-2 is different from SARS-CoV-1 and other SARS-related types due to the presence of a furin cleavage (FCS) site containing the PRRAR multi-basic amino acid in the S1/S2 convergence of the viral spike protein (S). Although FCS is present in other relatives of CoVs, such as HKU1-CoV, MERS-CoV, and OC43-CoV. However, SARS-CoV-2 has a growth-enhancing function and it is assumed that other vital factors accompany it and the rate of infection and contagion in these factors is higher [10].

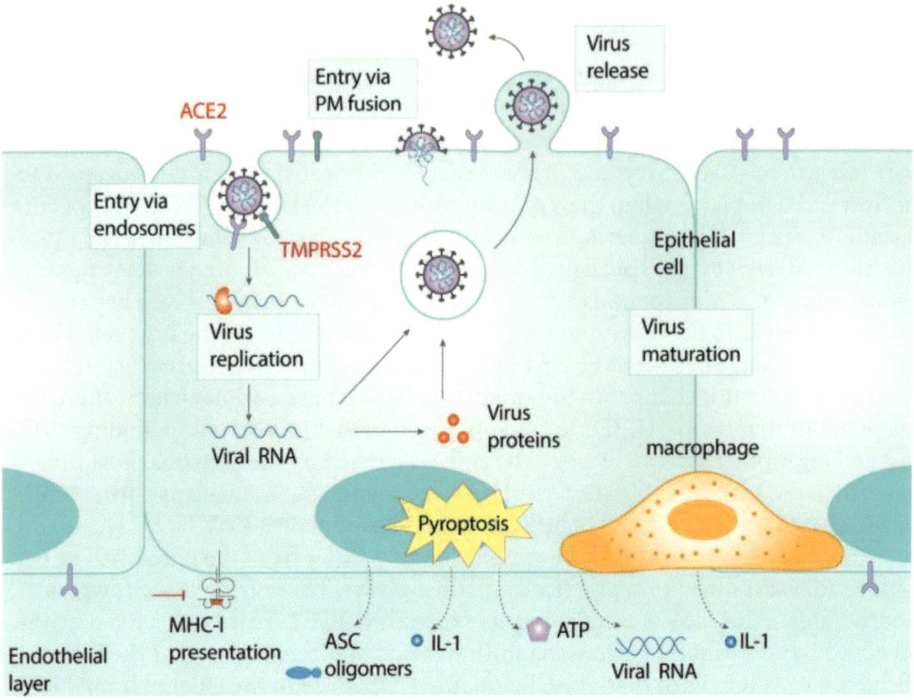

Figure 2.
Schematic of the intracellular lifecycle of SARS-CoV-2 and related immunopathology.

FCS is a known factor in influenza infections and appears to increase destruction and infection. Of course, it should be noted that it has not yet been determined whether this pathogenic function is also present in the SARS-CoV-2 virus [10].

Although various proteases, such as TMPRSS2 and cathepsin-B or -L (CTS-B or -L), cause cleavage at the S1/S2 site of the SARS-CoV-2 virus, the presence of FCS can have benefits for the SARS-CoV-2 virus, although research is needed to prove this. A new report by Johnson et al. shows that a SARS-CoV-2 virus that mutates and lacks FCS in its spike protein reduces the proliferation of Calu3 cells in a human respiratory cell line, thus weakening the disease in the hamster pathogenesis model. Preliminary observations suggest that FCS in the SARS-CoV-2 virus may play an important role in degradation [10].

Observations show that the ACE2 receptor and the TMPRSS2 serine protease are the main factors determining the entry of SARS-CoV-2 into cell tropism. It should be noted that the cells that express these two proteins are always defending against the SARS-CoV-2 virus [1].

Taking into account all the mentioned cases and points, we find that the SARS-CoV-2 virus has higher infectivity and higher transmissibility than previous types of coronavirus, and escapes from the host's immune system and delayed its function, for example, by disabling the system of long-term antibody formation against the virus. They control and direct subatomic pathways in host cells that reduce cell growth and damage in lung epithelial cells. These new discoveries are very large and effective in helping to interpret the basic pathomechanisms in Covid-19 and in particular cause immune disorders **Figure 2** [10].

The cells encoding TMPRSS2 and the angiotensin-converting enzyme 2 (ACE2) are infected by the SARS-CoV-2 virus (severe acute respiratory syndrome coronavirus 2), which causes it to pass into the host cell through endocyte machinery or fuse into the plasma membrane. The genetic material (genome) of the virus is released into the cytosol of the host cell and transcription, replication, assembly, and translation. Viral progenies are produced and released into the extracellular space through undiscovered mechanisms. Arrival and amplification of the viral lead to cell pyroptosis and arrival of harm-related atomic examples, including ASC oligomers, ATP, and nucleic acids. This is joined by the discharge of supportive pro-inflammatory cytokines and chemokines culminating in a cytokine storm. Then again, MHC-I limited antigen releasing is down-regulated in all probability by binding of the viral Orf8 protein, bringing about lessened T-cell activation.

1.3 The origin and evolution of SARS-CoV-2

Researchers have identified and sequenced the complete sequence of the SARA-CoV-2 genome and other beta-coronavirus genomes. The results show that SARS-CoV-2 is 96% similar to covid strain bat Cov RaTG13. And this research clearly shows that SARA-CoV-2 may have originated in bats, and may also have evolved from bat Cov RaTG13 [11].

The genomic RNA of SARS-CoV-2 encodes four driving structural proteins which are known as spike (and which likewise contains the receptor-binding domain [RBD] through which the infection ties to its natural receptor at have cell surface), the envelope (E) protein, the membrane (M) protein, and the nucleocapsid (N) protein. The genome of SARS-CoV-2 likewise contains extra genes, like that encoding for the RNA-dependent RNA polymerase (RdRP). This enzyme is fundamental for replicating viral RNA and for transcription of all RNA virals, both bearing negative and positive-sense RNA. In positive-sense single strand RNA virals, for example, SARS-CoV-2, the enzyme straightforwardly transcribes the positive-sense RNA, which acts precisely like a messenger RNA, yet additionally twofold convert positive-sense RNA into negative-sense RNA and then again in positive-sense RNA, to be gathered in the last viral particle [12].

Researchers demonstrate that an isolate numbered EPI_ISL_403928 shows different hereditary distances of the entire length genome and different phylogenetic trees, the coding sequences of nucleoprotein (N), spike protein (S), and polyprotein (P) from other SARS-CoV-2, with 2, 4, and 22 varieties in N, S, and P at the level of amino acid residues respectively. The outcomes show that at least two SARS-CoV-2 strains are involved in the outbreak [11].

Among the 103 strains, a sum of 149 mutations is distinguished and populace hereditary investigations demonstrate that these strains are predominantly isolated into two kinds. Results recommend that 101 of the 103 SARS-CoV-2 strains show considerable linkage between the two single nucleotide polypeptides (SNPs). The main kinds of SARS-CoV-2 (L sort and S type) are distinguished by two SNPs which situate at the destinations of 8,782 and 28,144. L sort contains 70% of the 103 strains and S type contains 30%, showing that L sort is more prevalent than the S type. Notwithstanding, the S type is the ancestral version of SARS-CoV-2. Until today, 13 mutations in the spike protein have been recognized [11].

1.4 Emergence of SARS-CoV-2 variants and how they mutate

Changes and causes of created virus types are caused by nucleotide changes that usually occur in the virus genome sequence during replication. It should be noted that these changes are faster in RNA viruses than in DNA viruses. However, the rate of nucleotide changes in CoVs is usually slower than in other RNA viruses, due to the presence of an enzyme that plays a role in correcting defects created during replication. This enzyme is called non-structural protein 14 (nsp14) which has the function exoribonuclease (ExoN) which causes it to play a role in "editing." It is also detrimental to the replication of SARS-CoV-2 and MERS-CoV if this function is inactivated. Nucleotide changes in the genome sequence increase with respect to viral replication, transmission, and escape from the immune system due to natural selection in a population. For example, when a virus is detected by the immune system and its chances of survival are reduced, it is naturally eliminated, so the virus in which the nucleotide change occurred and caused it to escape the immune system and be safe has a better chance of survival. In general, genomic changes that affect viral health can randomly increase or decrease the frequency. Various treatments, such as monoclonal antibodies (mAb), convalescent plasma and vaccines, and even environmental factors, are important factors that have a significant impact on the genomic changes of viruses and cause the continuation of these changes and the emergence of new strains. In the event that variations evidently change the phenotype (transmission and virulence) of a viral, they are alluded to as a strain [13].

Of course, it should be noted that not only the changes that occur during replication and the specified host stresses, not only the formation of different species but also RNA editing or RNA modification can cause the formation of new types of SARA-CoV-2 Be. For example, the replacement of cytosine nucleotides by uracil and adenosine by inosine has been observed in SARS-CoV-2 genome sequence research. These events occur by RNA-editing enzymes, which include apolipoprotein B mRNA editing catalytic polypeptide-like enzyme (APOBEC) and adenosine deaminase RNA specific 1 enzyme (ADAR1) respectively. Host cells have enhanced these editing enzymes as innate viral sensory defense mechanisms; however, viruses can use these mechanisms to evolve. In Covid-19 patients, alterations in the structure of viruses have been observed within the host and are likely to occur by the same RNA-editing enzymes, but how exactly is SARS-CoV-2 altered and manipulated using these enzymes to nucleotide changes is not yet known [13].

Another factor in the development of the new SARS-CoV-2 species is recombination, which occurs in infected cells where the inherited substance of the two types is packaged in a single virion and causes different changes in the sequence of the virus genome. Recently, evidence has shown that a person can be infected with two different types of SARA-CoV-2 at the same time. In this case, the new species resulting from recombination can each have different pathogenic properties and have serious consequences for SARS-CoV-2 interactions, especially when this new species can move away from normal and stimulated antibody resistance. Overall, CoVs have a high recombination rate, and so far, conflicting data on SARS-CoV-2 recombination have been reported and its exact nature is still unclear [13].

An increase in the rate of viral evolution and a decrease in the rate of repulsion of the replicable virus has been observed in immunocompromised individuals with SARS-CoV-2 disease. Several studies during the treatment of this disease with plasma recovery method and mAb treatment have shown that the emergence of various viruses is associated with reduced sensitivity to neutralizing antibodies. However, in patients infected with the human immunodeficiency virus (HIV), an increase in changes in the genomic sequence of the virus has been observed. Single nucleotide polymorphism (SNP) examination distinguished a few varieties, frequently bringing about amino acid changes in the S protein related to immune evasion tracked down in variations of concern. Beta, for example, was first seen in South Africa and was thought to have evolved through the evolution of a virus within at least one host with delayed viral replication, such as in a person with HIV or immunodeficiency. Intra-host evolution is by all accounts more articulated in immunocompromised populaces, which could act as a drawn-out wellspring of new SARS-CoV-2 variations, but it stays unclear whether basic co-morbidities assume the main part in the development of viral variations [13]. All in all, various factors change the genome and create a new type of virus and disease, as mentioned above, not only the structure and editing enzymes and proteins involved in replication but also the host's immune system and the host body's enzymes and antibodies, which are injected through vaccines, can also be effective in mutation.

1.5 Currently circulating SARS-CoV-2 variants

SARS-CoV-2 variations are classified by the CDC (Center for Disease Control and Prevention) and the WHO into two sorts: variants of concern (VOC) and variants of interest (VOI). A few VOC have emerged from the first wild-type strain detached in Wuhan since the outbreak initially started in December 2019. As indicated by the Center for Disease Control (CDC), a VOC is one that has expanded contagiousness, expanded destructiveness, resistance to the vaccine, or acquired immunity from the previous infection, and can escape symptomatic recognition. The VOCs are classified by the WHO as Beta (B.1.351), Alpha (B.1.1.7), Delta (B.1.617.2), and Gamma (P.1) [13, 14].

2. SARS-CoV-2 variants

2.1 D614G variant

At the beginning of February, a new strain of the disease began to spread in Europe, and the first species to rapidly dominate the world was the D614G strain, which underwent a change in the S protein and caused the disease to become more infectious, but still, It was treatable by neutralizing with recovery serum [13]. This species rapidly replaced the original and weaker species, a mutation that increased replication capacity and sensitivity in both human and animal models. SG614 is more steady than SD641 and less S1 shedding is noticed, so the SARS-CoV-2 with SG614 could transmit more efficiently. One review shows that in different cell lines, the SARS-CoV-2 containing the D614G change is eight times more effective at transducing cells than wild-type spike protein, providing evidence that the D614G mutation in SARS-CoV-2 spike protein could increase the transduction of multiple human cell types. TheD614G in the furin binding is a conspicuous common mutation depicted in nearly all of the new variations. The D614G mutation could decrease neutralization sensitivity to the sera of convalescent COVID-19 patients [11, 13, 14].

2.2 Alpha variant (B.1.1.7 lineage)

In late December 2020, a new strain of the disease was identified that quickly became dominant in the UK, called alpha (B.1.1.7). This species of SARS-CoV-2 is highly contagious. The alpha species (B.1.1.7) is caused by a receptor-restricting space (RBD) in the spike protein. As mentioned earlier, it is important to identify the original genomic sequence of the SARS-CoV-2 virus to control the epidemic and identify how new species formed, and find a way to treat and prevent further changes or predict the next mutation. The researchers identified seventeen mutations in the viral genome sequence in which eight mutations occurred in the spike (S) protein, such as Δ144 cancellation, Δ69–70 deletion, A570D, N501Y, D1118H, S982A, T716I, and P681H. Another important mutation that increases the incidence of the disease and binds the spike protein to the ACE 2 receptor is the N501Y mutation, which accelerates and improves the viral binding and thus cells entry. This species was seen in Britain and the United States in September and December 2020, respectively. The death rate was seen to be high in B.1.1.7 variant tainted patients and the changed peril proportion was examined as 1.67, 95% CI 1.34–2.09. The B.1.1.7 predominant variation SARS-CoV-2 strain is flowing in different nations worldwide. Research has shown that people who have been vaccinated have each been somewhat resistant to the species. The following results show some data. Those who received the BNT162b2 vaccine had a significant reduction in the neutralization titer against the alpha species (B.1.1.7). Individuals vaccinated with the Janssen vaccine (Ad26.COV2-S) had a moderate effect *in vitro* against alpha species (B.1.1.7) but were less effective than against the reference strain. In the case of individuals who had been vaccinated with Novavax (NVX-CoV2373), the data showed that they were 96% effective against the first strain and 86% effective against the alpha species (B.1.1.7). In Phase III clinical trial in the United Kingdom containing 15,000 members (18 to 84 years old), AZD1222 was 70% effective in alpha (B.1.1.7) infected individuals and 77% effective in non-alpha species was observed. Studies have identified a variety of amino acid changes in the spike protein of the alpha species (B.1.1.7). The reason for these changes is N501Y, P681H, 69/70, ORF8, and E484K mutations. In addition to the above, another F888L mutation in protein (S) has been identified in the Nigerian species alongside E484K. This mutation increases the virus's permeability to the host cell by hydrolysis by TMPRSS2 to alter the biological efficacy of SARS-CoV-2. Every one of the above examinations was completed with their restrictions regarding methodology, sample size, and immune reaction [13, 14].

2.3 Beta (B.1.351 Lineage)

In October 2020, a new species called beta (B.1.351) was identified for the first time and quickly became the dominant strain, causing the second wave of epidemic in South Africa [13]. This species is caused by E484K mutations and has more side effects than other species. New mutant species are more resistant to species originating in Britain and South Africa but are less effective against vaccines. The K417N and E484K mutations give rise to the V2.501 variant seen earlier in South Africa, which is more contagious and has a strong correlation with the parent strain. E484K mutation also assumes a significant part in immune component, host receptor affinity, and infectivity. Starting discoveries have demonstrated that the Oxford-AstraZeneca immunization has shown an extensive decrease in inadequacy against these variations and was checked on by the WHO. Novavax vaccine can protect to a moderate level, while the Pfizer-BioNTech and Johnson and Johnson vaccines immunizations likewise have diminished the viability against the β-variant (B.1.351) [14].

2.4 Lineage B.1.258

In late 2020, the species B.1.258 was first identified in the Czech Republic and Slovakia, it had a greater ability to escape the immune response, as well as a more acute infection in the host. The N439K mutation in the terminal region of the spike glycoprotein has given rise to this species, although 69–70 deletions in the receptor-binding domain (RBD) have been observed to be modified. Also, due to the change of antigenic peptides in the amino-terminal region, neutralizes this species when exposed to vaccine and serum [14].

2.5 Gamma variants (P.1 or 20 J/501Y.V3)

In January 2021, four Brazilians traveling to Japan brought a new strain of the disease with them to the Brazilian city of Manaus, where it was first found, and named it the gamma species (P.1). The disease has exacerbated the number of cases in Brazil [13].

This new species of gamma (P.1) is caused by 11 mutations in the spike protein. Researchers have been conducting extensive research on SARA-CoV-2 cases since December 2021, and about 42% of cases have infections of the gamma species (P.1). Mutations that cause this species have increased the infectivity rate of the disease to +160% and caused them to better escape from the immune system due to antibody-mediated. Statistics also show that this variant is more lethal and can kill up to 2.2 times more people. Gamma and quasi-gamma variants (P.1 and P.1-like) are more common and contagious among younger people. P.1 or 20 J/501Y.V3 were classified as gamma mutations (K417T, N501Y, and E484K) in the RBD domain. In November 2020 and January 2021, it has been seen that the Gamma variant is 1.4–2.2 times more infectious than the baseline [14].

2.6 Delta (Lineage B.1.617 and B.1.617.2)

Delta (B.1.617.2) was first identified in December 2020, which quickly became the dominant species, causing a second wave of pandemics in India, which was catastrophic and even resumed. The strictures became in the United States [13].

This type of delta (B.1.617 and B.1.617.2) is caused by three mutations of the alternative type, these mutations include P681R, L452R, and E484Q. Of these three mutations, two were seen in the RBD domain and the other near the furin that binds to the host. This species is up to 64% more transmissible than the previous, has also increased the number of hospitalizations by 85%, and even affected natural immunity. However, the risk of re-infection in patients is lower than before. Among the 15 mutations found in Delta species are spike protein mutations E484Q, D111D, P681R, and G142D, which have been shown are caused to escape antibody neutralization [14].

2.7 Lineage B.1.168

In West Bengal, a new variant has been found that was created by the deletions of the two amino acids His146 and Tyr145 and the mutations D618G and E484K, called B.1.168. These changes can escape convalescent plasma and numerous monoclonal antibodies [14].

2.8 Variant Omicron (B.1.1.529)

As of late designated VOC by the WHO, was first identified in November 2021 by world-class genomic surveillance laboratories in South Africa and has been tracked down in numerous nations all over the planet. The rise of these variants is disturbing since they might affect viral transmissibility, virulence, and rate of reinfection by escaping natural and vaccine-induced immunity [13]. The Omicron SARS-CoV-2 variant shows in excess of 30 mutations prompting amino-acid changes in the spike sequence, 15 of them situated in the receptor-binding domain (RBD), which is key for viral-cell association interceded by ACE2 receptor. Deductions to decide transmission rate have endeavored from the Omicron spike quality arrangement. This information revealed a bunch of mutations at the S1–S2 furin cleavage site, which might upgrade viral infectivity. Additionally, docking studies showed that a blend of mutations in the RBD would yield a high binding proclivity with human ACE2 of this variation [15].

2.9 Other VOIs

Numerous other VOI has been accounted for which are just anticipated to influence transmission, virulence, and acquired or vaccine immunity. The VOI and variants being checked to incorporate; **Epsilon (B.1.427/B.1.429)** was first found in California, and research has shown that it is the result of several mutations in the spike protein and ORF1ab. These include the I4205V, D1183Y, and L452R, S13I, and L452R mutations in which the first two mutations occur in ORF1ab and the next three mutations occur in the spike protein, also known as CAL.20C, CA VUI, 21C or 20C/S: 452R. In November 2020, the CAL.20C variant was differentiated in California and eventually named Epsilon [14].

Zeta (P.2) was identified in Brazil, and has key spike mutations (T20N; L18F; F157L; P26S; D614G; E484K; V1176F; and S929I) [12–24]. **Eta (B.1.525)** is recognized in Nigeria and the UK and Iota (B.1.526.1/B.1.526) is distinguished in New York, both have key spike mutations (B.1.525: Δ69/70, A67V, Δ144, D614G, E484K, F888L, Q677H; B.1.526: T95I, (L5F*), D253G, (E484K*), (S477N*), (A701V*), D614G [12–24]. **Theta (P.3)**, additionally called GR/1092K.V1 distinguished in the Philippines were accounted for on February 18, 2021, with two mutations N501Y and E484K. Theta variants were likewise distinguished in Japan, the United Kingdom, and Malaysia in July 2021. Theta variants vanished by July 2021 [13, 14]. **Kappa (B.1.617)** harbor key transformations (G142D, (T95I), E154K, E484Q, L452R, D614G, Q1071H, and P681R) and same as Delta Plus (B.1.617.2.1) distinguished in India [12–24]. **Lambda** (C.37) is distinguished in Peru and Mu (B.1.621) is recognized in Colombia [13].

Eleven COVID-19 vaccines (mRNA-1273 (Moderna), BNT162b2 (Pfizer/BioNTech), ChAdOx1 (AstraZeneca/Oxford), Ad26.COV2.S (Janssen), NVX-CoV2373 (Novavax), BBV152 (Bharat Biotech), CoronaVac (Sinovac), BBIBP-CorV (Sinopharm), SCB-2019, CVnCoV, and HB02)) [25, 26]. Full vaccination of COVID-19 antibodies is highly compelling against Alpha variant, and moderate viable against Beta, Gamma, and Delta variants. A booster vaccination is more powerful against Delta and Omicron variants. mRNA vaccines appear to have higher vaccine effectiveness (VE) against Alpha, Beta, Gamma, and Delta variants over others [26]. So far, we have described all the variants that mutated and spread, mentioning the cause of the mutation and the first place they discovered it. This is definitely not the end of the story, and like all other microorganisms and diseases, they always mutate and adapt to new enemies which are dangerous to their survival.

3. Implications of variants on transmission and virulence

Again, a brief overview of the important issues mentioned above: Spike protein binds to the ACE2 receptor and accelerates the entry of the virus into the host cell.

Replacement and change in amino acids in spike protein, especially in RBD, directly affect the mechanism of virus entry into the host cell and cause many concerns. The N501Y mutation is very common among a variety of alpha, beta, and gamma species, and is also known to enhance cellular infection in animal models. One of the most important amino acids associated with ACE2 receptor binding is asparagine, which is located at position 501 (N501). Replacing this amino acid with the amino acid tyrosine (Y) increases the affinity for binding to the host receptor. This makes the coronavirus more contagious, found in both alpha and beta species. Research in the UK has shown that the alpha type does not essentially increase the risk of hospitalization. Despite this research, further studies have shown that this species increases the mortality rate by up to 61% and the severity of the disease is higher in this species. In addition to the above, the alpha type has the P681H mutation, which is located in the area near the site of the furin incision, and this mutation plays an important role in increasing infection and transmission. Another factor that increases viral infection *in vitro* is the deletion ΔH69/V70, which binds to specific receptors and manages to detect glycoprotein S [13].

In the beta type, the amino acid substitution in the spike protein is higher than in the alpha type. The RBD-ACE2 interaction complex has been examined fundamentally utilizing in silico strategies to evaluate the effect of the K417T, N501Y, and E484K replacements. The N501 residue is significant for ACE2 collaboration, while E484 and K417 are not anticipated to assume a significant part. The last two residues may as a matter of fact diminish binding fondness, which shows that the expansion in contagiousness found in the Beta variation is because of N501Y or different modifications in the viral. Among people infected with the SARS-CoV-2 virus in South Africa in October 2020, only 11% were infected with the Beta, but in December of that year, the number of people infected with Beta increased to 87%. Also in Cape Town, the second wave of the Covid-19 epidemic with Beta variant took half the time compared to the cases of the wild-type variant in 100,000 cases. Also, the mortality rate in the second wave was significantly higher, although one of the reasons could be amazing health care services at that time. Pearson et al. affirmed these outcomes utilizing an adjusted model which showed that this variation has expanded contagiousness and destructiveness [13].

In late 2020 in Brazil, a new strain of the SARS-CoV-2 virus called gamma caused a new wave of epidemics that disrupted health services. The gamma type has 17 amino acid substitutions, which in three cases are similar to the substitutions in the beta-type spike protein. Reports have shown that this species is 1.4–2.2 times more transmissible to the host than the wild type. Doctors' reports indicate that this species could be more serious, as the infected cases were mostly young people with high levels of infection who became infected with the virus. Comparison of the first and second wave data between adults aged 20–39 years showed that this type has increased the mortality rate by 2.7 times and even increased the rate among all people in any age group by 1.15 times. In addition to the gamma type, another type called delta is responsible for the emergence of the second strong wave in India, this dominant type has spread to other countries with eight changes in the spike protein. It also triggered a third wave in South Africa, rapidly weakening and replacing Beta in about three months. One of the reasons was its higher transferability (46%) than Beta. It even eradicated the alpha type in Britain and delayed community activities in June 2021 as the incidence increased, especially at gatherings of young people and unvaccinated people. In this type of mutation, two amino acid substitution mutations have been discovered, one L452R, which occurs in the RBD region, and the other, P681R, which occurs at the site of the furin cleavage of the spike protein. It should be noted that in addition to the Delta type, the P681R mutation has also been seen in the Alpha type, which increases the binding to the host cell receptor, which directly causes infection and the prevalence rate. Although the P681R mutation has recently been identified as a fixed mutation that alone is not able to change the rate of transmission and infection, several mutations cause this action. Reports indicate that the Delta type is more contagious than both the wild type and other variants. Even doctors' observations and reports indicate that the Delta type has doubled the risk of hospitalization compared to the Alpha type and that patients with the Delta type have a more acute illness and the mortality rate in the hospital emergency room is significantly higher. In addition to all of the above, researchers are analyzing epidemiological data to estimate the transmissibility and rate of Omicron infection. Preliminary reports predict that this type could trigger a new wave of Covid-19 epidemics, especially in South Africa. November 2021, in South Africa, the Omicron type is found in 76% of people infected with the SARS-CoV-2 virus, just where the Delta type was most prevalent recently. Of course, the important point in this type is data from emergency clinics in South Africa that the Omicron type causes less infection and disease than the Delta type [13]. In total, we have so far gained a vast chunk of the sea of information and mechanisms that cause mutations in the structure of viruses. And we have explained to you the most important and main ones that have been proven so far, although as you know, science is always evolving and full of behaviors that have not yet been discovered.

3.1 Future prediction

Our understanding according to other studies that have been done and are mentioned earlier that RNA viruses, such as HIV, can use more than one host receptor to intervene in cell intrusion. Like other CoVs, for example, SARS-CoV and MERS-CoV, it is thought that SARS-CoV-2 may likewise foster the capacity to infect host cells by means of the S protein binding to receptors other than its primary receptor of passage as the viral keeps on developing wellness improving varieties. *In vitro* examinations have proposed that the transmembrane glycoprotein CD147 could act as an elective receptor for SARS-CoV-2. These glycoprotein capacities as a receptor for cyclophilin A, which assumes a part in the provocative reaction by going about as a chemotactic factor for leukocytes and moreover enacts antiviral reactions. Despite the fact that proof is as yet expected for the job of integrins, which are CD147 interacting proteins, they have additionally been conjectured to be SARS-CoV-2 host passage receptors. Neuropilin-1 (NRP-1) and NRP-2 contain a space succession, which as per sub-atomic demonstrating and *in vitro* examinations, could act as a binding site for the SARS-CoV-2 furin cleavage site in this manner going about as a potential co-receptor for viral entry.

4. Lung cancer

The second most common and malignant cancer among men and women worldwide is lung cancer, the leading and most dangerous cause of lung cancer is smoking. There are two types of lung cancer: small cell lung cancer and non-small cell lung cancer, which make up 15% and 85% of all lung cancer patients, respectively. Histological studies and hereditary characteristics of lung cancer are needed to make the right treatment and prevention methods. The SARS-CoV-2 virus, which causes the Covid-19 epidemic, has severely affected people with lung cancer and how they are treated. Pressures over care frameworks have prompted demonstrative deferrals, the need to sort out for the administration of foundational therapies, yet in addition to oral therapies, lastly postpones in the administration of medical procedures and radiation therapy. It does not give the idea that lung malignant is a considerable risk factor for vulnerability to Covid-19 or deteriorating of contamination, at least not similarly to other comorbidities, such as cardiovascular illness, diabetes, and constant obstructive pneumonic sickness. Interestingly, apparently, when tainted, patients with lung cancer have a higher gamble of deteriorating [22]. Coronavirus is more serious in patients with lung cancer. Patient-specific features, instead of malignant growth explicit highlights or treatments, are the best determinants of seriousness [21].

Severe Covid-19 can be considered a hyperinflammatory issue described by gigantic resistant cell enactment. Accordingly, this might make sense of more awful results in more established individuals and cancer patients. While it very well may be conjectured that the brought down resistance prompted by malignant growth itself or its treatment could be a defensive component against the significant safe response seen in Covid-19, there is natural reasoning for rejecting this proposal. An increase in inflammation is normal during aging and has been characterized as "inflamm-aging." Constant irritation, including from malignant growth and progress in years, as well as immune checkpoint inhibitors (ICIs) can cause a flood in proinflammatory immune responses, prompting upgraded creation of cytokines from T cells and phagocytes, specifically in lung cancer, there is chronic pulmonary inflammation, both from the tumor microenvironment (TME) and the successive hidden lung pathology. This immune deregulation observed in older, lung cancer, or ICI-treated patients might drive the serious pathogenesis of Covid-19 in these exceptional populaces. Additionally, T cells produce proinflammatory cytokines with multiple functions, for example, selecting monocytes and neutrophils to the site of disease and activating other downstream cytokine and chemokine overflows [18].

As of late researchers considered an over-portrayal of cancer patients in the Covid-19 companion. In that, lung cancer was the most frequent sort (5 of 18 patients). In view of their outcomes, the authors have proposed three significant procedures for patients with malignant growth in this Covid-19 emergency: 1- To delay all adjuvant foundational treatment or elective medical procedures for stable cancer in endemic regions. 2- To increment personal protection provisions for patients with malignant growth and in-danger disease survivors. 3- To strengthen surveillance in disease patients tainted with SARS-CoV-2. Albeit these suggestions came from a little example size with a lot of heterogeneity, there is a rising agreement to change our standard administration during this pandemic. Patients with lung cancer are prone to serious entanglements, for example, admission to the emergency unit for invasive ventilation, or demise, from Covid-19. Smoking has additionally been distinguished as an autonomous risk factor in serious Covid-19 cases [19]. Along this line, it has been noticed a relationship between the severity of Covid-19 and subjects with a high-level period of malignant growth illness and a poor ECOG execution status. Furthermore, aging, heftiness, and metabolic condition are inclining factors for disease and address comorbidities that might impact defenselessness to SARS-CoV-2 infectious and the severity of its confusions. A review examination revealed an expected gamble of disease to SARS-CoV-2 and serious or deadly complexities of around 2.31 times higher in lung cancer patients than overall public or contrasted with patients with different malignancies [16].

A study and report published in the Medical Oncology Department of Wuhan University Zhongnan Hospital on 1524 cancer patients admitted to the same hospital on March 25, 2020, reports the consequences of Covid-19. This report shows that people with cancer are more at risk for infection with the SARS-CoV-2 virus than healthy people. This risk is increased in all people with cancer, even those undergoing anti-cancer treatment. The most likely to develop Covid-19 were patients with non-small cell lung cancer (NSCLC) and above the age of 60 [20].

A major challenge in the Covid-19 pandemic comprises making a fast and right differential finding among SARS-CoV-2 prompted pneumonitis and medication incited lung poisonousness. For sure, this might give side effects frequently not explicit, comprising fundamentally of cough (or get worse), dyspnea, chest agony, and fever, which are basically the same as those saw in the SARS-CoV-2 disease. Along this line, likewise, radiological imaging of medication-related poisonousness might cover that run-of-the-mill of Covid-19-initiated pneumonia, accordingly impeding the separation of these clinical elements. Chest computed tomography (CT) is the imaging methodology of decision, for the assessment of pneumonitis in patients with lung cancer who went through target treatment or immunotherapy, and it is likewise the most touchy strategy for the conclusion of Covid-19 pneumonitis, even in the underlying phases of the disease. Concerning ICI-related lung harmfulness, a wide range of imaging signs has been accounted for, for example, ground glass (GG) regions or potentially combinations that happens in roughly 70–80% of cases, as a rule with no particular dispersion, septal thickening, and foothold bronchiectasis in around 15–20% of patients, or elements of acute interstitial pneumonitis (AIP), including consolidations and volume loss that depend on the severity of toxicity; additionally, sores are for the most part multifocal and include the lower lobes [16].

Another challenge of Covid-19 in patients treated with chemoradiotherapy for a locally progressed cancer is likewise the presence of differential findings with different reasons for radiological irregularities, such as radiation-prompted pneumonic fibrosis, which is a typical complication of thoracic radiotherapy for lung cancer. Radiation-prompted aspiratory fibrosis prompts irreversible obliteration of lung engineering and interruption of gas exchange. Immunotherapy could all the while support cytotoxic T lymphocyte insusceptible response against infection contaminated and neoplastic cells. This immune stimulation might cause exacerbate the disease, however, a new report has shown the contrary that proceeding with proceeded with utilization of PD-1 barricade during the Covid-19 pandemic is protected. It is vital to recognize Covid-19 pneumonia from other lung pathologies for the right treatment and right on time as conceivable [22].

Lobectomies, autopsies, and biopsies have yielded information about the histologic impression of the pathophysiology of Covid-19. An especially fascinating report concerns two patients with lung cancer treated with lobectomy, retrospectively diagnosed to have Covid-19, offering a brief look into the early pathologic show of this illness. As in the first SARS illness, Covid-19 can prompt exudative as well as proliferative lung injury in an intense setting. Today, we realize that the super histological discoveries in Covid-19 lung sores are commonplace indications of alveolar harm, including the triad of injury to type II pneumocyte hyperplasia, alveolar epithelial cells, and hyaline membrane development. The hallmark hyaline membrane arrangement found in SARS and seen in resulting pathologic examines of Covid-19 were lacking with regards to, revealing insight into the order of intense lung injury. For this situation, this constellation was reasonable on the grounds that these patients were operated on at a presymptomatic stage. An outstanding perception was a plentiful invasion of mononuclear inflammatory cells and alveolar macrophages. Strangely, the authors bring up that while clinically asymptomatic, these patients gave leukocytosis lymphopenia, showing the immune reaction was in progress at this early illness stage. Similarly, radiographic changes can go before side effects and should be deciphered circumspectly during an epidemic [18].

Lung cancer patients have a higher death rate than the overall public. Joined azithromycin and hydroxychloroquine treatment appear to be a decent treatment choice [17].

Today, different suggestions have arisen about fitting disease treatments, including for NSCLC, to the truth of the Covid-19. The foundation of these is to diminish unnecessary exposure, accordingly decreasing the risk of transmission. For lung cancer patients, this likewise implies cautiously gauging the risk to benefit proportion of every treatment. While ICI-prompted pneumonitis might look like Covid-19, the two on a pathophysiological and clinical level, there is no proof recommending patients getting these medicines are at increased risk of severe Covid-19 confusions, contrasted and those on other oncological treatments. Also, no information exists about the possible collaboration between SARS-CoV-2 and tyrosine kinase inhibitors. Once more, regardless of whether drug-prompted pneumonitis is thought, Covid-19 ought to be rejected. For all NSCLC patients, the component to remember; notwithstanding, is to be receptive. While anticipating viral swab affirmation, one ought to hinder cytotoxic treatment ought to natural, radiological, or clinical tests be reminiscent of Covid-19 [18].

A group from Milan created, as per clinical information and restorative modalities, a very intriguing help algorithm. This algorithm laid out from sex, PS, age, sex BMI, comorbidities, treatment or not corticosteroids, and tumor characteristics and treatments, arranges patients into three risk classes:

1. A low-risk category that permits keeping up with cancer on the board as arranged before the pandemic, delaying or decreasing the quantity of visits to the medical clinic, utilizing teleconsultation instruments, or utilizing foundational oral therapies.

2. A halfway risk class where the organizing of the illness is efficiently viewed as postponed.

3. A high-risk class that requires intense therapy, yet additionally closer checking of clinical and biological signs.

In that series, the treatment modalities (history of surgery, history of irradiation, systemic treatment) do not seem to affect the seriousness of Covid-19 contamination. The authors found no biological variable especially fundamentally connected with severity. Current treatment choices include medical procedure chemotherapy, radiotherapy, designated treatment, and immunotherapy [23].

5. Conclusion

As you know, the coronavirus epidemic has been affecting all countries financially and socially for almost two years, and like all other viral diseases, it will certainly not be eradicated soon, but it will threaten humanity in a new way each time. In the last

20 years, three CoVsubspecies transmitted to humans, and established researchers must continue to further develop identification and observation methods to prevent such adverse effects in the future.

Worldwide routine observation of SARS-CoV-2 variations and their consequences for destructiveness and right now utilized therapeutics will permit researchers to evaluate on the off chance that immunizations and different treatments are expected to be refreshed occasionally. New variations might infiltrate group invulnerability and taint unvaccinated people or work with immunization escape, which can incline these people toward extreme illness or passing. Nonetheless, most investigations have proposed that antibodies are as yet viable against the now coursing variations and can safeguard against extreme to direct illness results. Proof supporting the utilization of even a single vaccination dosage in keeping serious sickness from the Delta variation in the UK has featured the requirement for quicker immunization arrangement and rollout in more unfortunate areas like Africa. It is trusted that the in-house assembling of Covid-19 immunizations will help South Africa as well as the remainder of the African mainland to accomplish this objective. Also, more examinations are expected to assess the purpose for leading-edge diseases and the chance of winding down resistance to SARS-CoV-2 as well as the job that booster immunization dosages could play in counteraction. To lessen the risk of new and possibly more malicious variants from arising, health specialists ought in on vaccinating people as quickly as could be expected and ought to keep on underscoring the significance of mask-wearing and social distancing. A multipronged treatment approach ought to keep on being carried out in nations, for example, South Africa has a high predominance of co-morbidities, for example, HIV, which might add to the rise of variations. This would not just save lives, yet additionally, give restricted space for the viral to develop. While it may not be imaginable to foresee what the following VOC will be, we can gain from previous encounters and difficulties to more likely adapt to the situation at hand. SARS-CoV-2 is not supposed to vanish soon, however, will probably turn into a (the) essential medical care issue from now on, and as such will stay a challenge.

Besides, the amount of information on the connections between lung cancer and Covid-19 contamination has become richer, mainly because of studies on several patients in multicenter. It is, in this way, vital to make a protected medical care framework during the Covid-19 pandemic and it is fundamental to support clinical service conveyance to patients with lung cancer. One of the hypotheses about the SARS-CoV-2 virus is that it can change the mechanism of its entry into the host cell, that is, the binding to the host receptor no longer occurs through the spike protein and occurs by another method, and, in that method, new mutations occur that make it harder for researchers to find a treatment for this disease, like many other diseases, will be inexhaustible and will constantly evolving.

Author details

Tahereh Alinejad[1*], Danial Zareh[2], Zuo Hao[1], Tengfei Zhou[1] and Cheng-shui Chen[1*]

1 The Key Laboratory of Interventional Pulmonology of Zhejiang Province, Department of Pulmonary and Critical Care Medicine, The First Affiliated Hospital of Wenzhou Medical University, Zhejiang, People's Republic of China

2 Faculty of Biological Sciences, Department of Cell and Molecular Biology (Genetic), Sistan and Baluchestan – Zahedan University, Zahedan, Iran

*Address all correspondence to: talinejad698@gmail.com and wzchencs@163.com

References

[1] Sanyal S. How SARS-CoV-2 (COVID-19) spreads within infected hosts—What we know so far. Emerging Tropical Life Science. 2020;**4**(4):371-378

[2] Zhou P, Yang XL, Wang XG, Hu B, Zhang L, Zhang W, et al. A pneumonia outbreak associated with a new coronavirus of probable bat origin. Nature. 2020;**579**(7798):270-273

[3] Coronaviridae Study Group of the International Committee on Taxonomy of Viruses. The species Severe acute respiratory syndrome-related coronavirus: Classifying 2019-nCoV and naming it SARS-CoV-2. Nature Microbiology. 2020;**5**(4):536-544

[4] Lu R, Zhao X, Li J, Niu P, Yang B, Wu H, et al. Genomic characterisation and epidemiology of 2019 novel coronavirus: Implications for virus origins and receptor binding. Lancet. 2020;**395**(10224):565-574

[5] Zhou P, Fan H, Lan T, Yang XL, Shi WF, Zhang W, et al. Fatal swine acute diarrhoea syndrome caused by an HKU2-related coronavirus of bat origin. Nature. 2018;**556**(7700):255-258

[6] Lai CC, Shih TP, Ko WC, Tang HJ, Hsueh PR. Severe acute respiratory syndrome coronavirus 2 (SARS-CoV-2) and coronavirus disease-2019 (COVID-19): The epidemic and the challenges. International Journal of Antimicrobial Agents. 2020;**55**(3):105924

[7] Harrison AG, Lin T, Wang P. Mechanisms of SARS-CoV-2 Transmission and Pathogenesis. Trends in Immunology. 2020;**41**(12):1100-1115

[8] World Health Organisation. Coronavirus disease (COVID-19) outbreak situation. 2020. Available from: https://www.who.int/emergencies/diseases/novel-coronavirus-2019

[9] Sethi BA, Sethi A, Ali S, Aamir HS. Impact of Coronavirus disease (COVID-19) pandemic on health professionals. Pakistan Journal of Medical Science. 2020;**36**:S6-S11

[10] Kumar A, Prasoon P, Kumari C, Pareek V, Faiq MA, Narayan RK, et al. SARS-CoV-2-specific virulence factors in COVID-19. Journal of Medical Virology. 2021;**93**(3):1343-1350

[11] Wang MY, Zhao R, Gao LJ, Gao XF, Wang DP, Cao JM. SARS-CoV-2: Structure, biology, and structure-based therapeutics development. Frontiers in Cellular and Infection Microbiology. 2020;**10**:587269

[12] Lippi G, Mattiuzzi C, Henry B. Updated picture of SARS-CoV-2 variants and mutations. Diagnosis. 2022;**9**(1):11-17

[13] Mistry P, Barmania F, Mellet J, Peta K, Strydom A, Viljoen IM, et al. SARS-CoV-2 variants, vaccines, and host immunity. Frontiers in Immunology. 2022;**12**:809244

[14] Singh DD, Parveen A, Yadav DK. SARS-CoV-2: Emergence of new variants and effectiveness of vaccines. Frontiers in Cellular and Infection Microbiology. 2021;**11**:777212

[15] Ferré VM, Peiffer-Smadja N, Visseaux B, Descamps D, Ghosn J, Charpentier C. Omicron SARS-CoV-2 variant: What we know and what we don't. Anaesthesia Critical Care Pain Medicine. 2022;**41**(1):100998

[16] Calabrò L, Rossi G, Covre A, Morra A, Maio M. COVID and lung

cancer. Current Oncology Reports. 2021;**23**(11):134

[17] Rogado J, Pangua C, Serrano-Montero G, Obispo B, Marino AM, Pérez-Pérez M, et al. Covid-19 and lung cancer: A greater fatality rate? Lung Cancer. 2020;**146**:19-22

[18] Addeo A, Obeid M, Friedlaender A. COVID-19 and lung cancer: Risks, mechanisms and treatment interactions. Journal for Immunotherapy of Cancer. 2020;**8**(1):e000892

[19] Liang W, Guan W, Chen R, Wang W, Li J, Xu K, et al. Cancer patients in SARS-CoV-2 infection: A nationwide analysis in China. The Lancet Oncology. 2020;**21**(3):335-337

[20] Yu J, Ouyang W, Chua MLK, Xie C. SARS-CoV-2 transmission in patients with cancer at a tertiary care hospital in Wuhan, China. JAMA Oncology. 2020;**6**(7):1108-1110

[21] Luo J, Rizvi H, Preeshagul IR, Egger JV, Hoyos D, Bandlamudi C, et al. COVID-19 in patients with lung cancer. Annals of Oncology. 2020;**31**(10):1386-1396

[22] Haineala B, Zgura A, Badiu DC, Iliescu L, Anghel RM, Bacinschi XE. Lung cancer, Covid-19 infections and chemotherapy. In Vivo. 2021;**35**(3):1877-1880

[23] Ciceri F, Castagna A, Rovere-Querini P, De Cobelli F, Ruggeri A, Galli L, et al. Early predictors of clinical outcomes of COVID-19 outbreak in Milan, Italy. Clinical Immunology. 2020;**217**:108509

[24] Aleem A, Akbar Samad AB, Slenker AK. Emerging Variants of SARS-CoV-2 And Novel Therapeutics Against Coronavirus (COVID-19). Treasure Island (FL): StatPearls Publishing; 2022

[25] Ghasemiyeh P, Mohammadi-Samani S, Firouzabadi N, Dehshahri A, Vazin A. A focused review on technologies, mechanisms, safety, and efficacy of available COVID-19 vaccines. International Immunopharmacology. 2021;**100**:108162

[26] Zeng B, Gao L, Zhou Q, Yu K, Sun F. Effectiveness of COVID-19 vaccines against SARS-CoV-2 variants of concern: A systematic review and meta-analysis. BMC Medicine. 2022;**20**(1):200

Chapter 6

Panama: Scope and Psychosocial Challenges Two Years after the COVID-19 Pandemic

Ericka Matus and Lorena Matus

Abstract

It is a review of the challenges that Panama faced during the two years of the COVID-19 pandemic, in terms of mental health. From social psychology, some of the research that provided a vision of the effects in the short, medium, and long term is shown. Finally, social psychology is proposed as a reference framework for the study of the phenomena associated with the pandemic.

Keywords: social psychology, pandemic, COVID-19

1. Introduction

On January 16, 2020, an epidemiological alert for coronavirus was issued urging members of the World Health Organization (WHO) to guarantee updated information on the new coronavirus due to the increase in positive acute respiratory syndrome cases. The etiology was unknown. At that time, twenty-seven patients were detected in Wuhan (China on December 31, 2019), one patient in Thailand (January 13, 2020), and another in Japan (January 14, 2020) [1].

By January 20, 198 positive cases and three deaths from coronavirus had already been added in China, two cases in Thailand, one case in Japan, and one case in the Republic of Korea, so the WHO suggests isolation and follow up on these. In this scenario, the experience gained during the SARS and MERS epidemics was particularly useful in limiting international health care and alert protocols [1].

On January 27, WHO reported 2801 cases of coronavirus worldwide, of which eighty died. The health alert was intensified, considering that China reported 2761 cases. An additional forty cases were confirmed in eleven countries (Australia, Canada, France, Japan, Nepal, Malaysia, Republic of Korea, Singapore, Thailand, United States of America, and Vietnam) [2].

Under the established scenario, on January 30, WHO considered a Public Health Emergency of International Importance (PHEIC) due to coronavirus, then called COVID-19, and was categorized as a pandemic on March 11, 2020. More than 9700 positive cases were in China and 106 in nineteen other countries [3].

On January 20, Panama's Ministry of Health (MINSA) monitored the international situation due to the COVID-19 alert. Biosafety measures were implemented in hospitals, including a national health care campaign based on physical distancing and frequent hand washing prevention. As of that date, MINSA disclosed the concrete actions and guidelines to face the Pandemic.

On March 9, the first confirmed case of COVID-19 in Panama was announced. With it, the "Plan Protect yourself Panama" was implemented to deal with the situation, based on the preparations made during the previous months and the experiences from different countries.

As of March 24, the figures for the Pandemic established 422,829 positive cases of COVID-19, in 197 countries, with 18,907 deaths. Panama reported 443 positive cases and eight deaths, which yielded a quarantine from March 25 [4]. As of March 26, the country reported 674 cases, nine deaths, and a transmissibility rate, R_0, between 1.5 and 2.5 [5–7].

The health measures included a sanitary fence that implied staying at home, and teleworking formats were activated for those activities. This measure provided the population with the protection of their health and family; however, it was not easy for the people or the authorities because isolation favors sensory deprivation, fear, and defenselessness.

2. COVID-19 as a social phenomenon

According to Van Zoonen & Van der Meer [8], there are three response strategies to a crisis: denial, reduction, and reconstruction. The best of these is the third because it offers symbolic support that reduces uncertainty, fear, and anger, minimizes rumors, and generates an imprint of credibility of the source and content of the speech.

Faced with the chaotic situation, due to being confined at home, a small part of the world's population focused on the alternative personal and family "reconstruction" strategy; that is, a distant turn was required from the direction that had been maintained at least in the last century of civilization. They are small groups of influence with credibility, far from the political, economic, and religious sectors; they are responsible and committed professionals, civil organizations, and academics who have maintained a proactive behavior that Moscovici [9] called active minorities.

The majority, who also perceived a chaotic situation in the face of the crisis, still use "denial" or "decrease" strategies, according to Van Zoonen & Van der Meer [8]. Society's behavior during the Pandemic in the world is essential to go back to the thinkers of the beginning and middle of the previous century, even earlier, since the Greeks also elucidated social exercise.

One proposal is to section off areas to clarify people's behavior. So that one section would correspond to the social framework seen from the individuality, that is, through motivation, stress, attitude, confidence, uncertainty, adaptation, and another from the group itself, such as with social influence, communication, the credibility of the source, the rumor, and the expression of the masses, among others.

There is a fear of freedom regarding the social subject's role in his individuality (Fromm) [10]. The challenges are so overwhelming that thinking about it causes significant uncertainty in the human being that turns into anguish. Hence, he does not wish to exercise it. In addition, and according to Freud [11], in the future of an illusion, culture restricts us from exploring other contexts. Those capable of doing so must consider that present comes from the past and impacts future decisions. These individuals will boldly seek to look beyond the obvious and face their success or failure. Yet, the discomfort will always be present. With the confinement situation as a measure of protection for physical health and defense against COVID-19, the uncertainty, anguish, and fear inherent to the human condition were exacerbated in all social groups.

Humans could glimpse their "self," explore emotions, confront identity. Yet, humans chose to move before thinking about what could have been an opportunity for evolution have been an opportunity for evolution. Humanity preferred defenselessness by contingency, because of the uncontrollable, and with it a low expectation of efficiency and response.

On the other hand, in the social sphere, human groups relate in a stereotyped way, look for similarities, and squeeze together to feel safe. Their reference groups are more present than ever, trying to maintain the status quo, despite the apparent signs of change. With this confinement scenario, the family group had to remain united with this confinement scenario, the family group had to remain united without leaving home, for at least twelve weeks, under a dry law regime and with restricted hours to buy groceries restricted hours to buy groceries.

The mandatory confinement triggered a massive change in the use and functionality of the areas, not counting the need for teleworking and distance education for at least three family members on average at the same time. Coexistence in common spaces deteriorated interpersonal relationships due to the time and type and the room it was established. In his field theory, Kurt Lewin sustains that each member requires a vital space: a physical area where a psychological environment was built, essential to perceive harmony, which has been challenging to achieve.

Under this circumstance, not only the family group that cohabited a space was disrupted, other reference groups such as friends (colleagues, coworkers, neighbors), also suffered distortion with respect to social perception, due to the low physical contact; to communication, since these media respond to the economy and not to mental health; leadership among its members, which involved skills in managing technology to continue being the protagonist or "influencer" virtually; to the exacerbated social influence due to uncertainty and the false belief that what is seen through social networks is genuine and who speaks is an expert, however, they contradict each other; to the mechanisms of obedience to the authority and credibility of the source, which in most cases prevented people from having a logical reasoning thought; to the locus of control, which has historically been external, generating greater defenselessness in the face of cognitive dissonance; and above all to rumor, which due to its characteristics tends to spread exponentially (being a trend) generating fear and more significant uncertainty, which has led the population into a spiral of social alterations.

Regarding the exercise of leadership, social construction presupposes autonomy and independence and the ability to influence the behavior of others [12], hence the need for a separation of the exercise of power.

Even before the arrival of COVID-19, submitting to the conformity process already allowed functional coexistence. Likewise, the phenomenon of social persuasion has guaranteed that behavior in groups is acceptable and appropriate. The social pressure to follow the rules confers a kind of shelter that protects the mass, the majority, but limits individuality. In Foucault's words [13] when this is not enough, power relations, control technologies, and the microphysics of power present in society use punishment as a social function to tame, configure and guide behavior.

This consensual social functioning makes individuals believe that they make their own decisions. Western thought inculcates the belief that he is the expert in his choices, opinions, and judgments about the world [14]. During the pandemic confinement, the group attraction that motivates cohesion was altered by the obstacle of physical proximity, especially in populations without internet access which generated alterations and psychosocial risks.

The population with Internet access suffered another type of damage: overexposure to information, difficulty in evaluating it, determining its truth or falsity, and social comparison with other locations, regions, hemispheres, and latitudes. Similarly, the possibility of scarcity led "civilized populations" to panic buying and compulsion to jealously guard personal hygiene and cleaning products more than food and pharmaceuticals.

These are not the only psychological alterations presented in the document. The efforts to understand the psychosocial processes and the variables that could establish a proposal to understand this atypical pandemic situation led a group of psychologists to make some measurements.

3. Psychological publications

From Psychology, a series of activities were developed, such as measurement scales and research on stress, anguish, confidence, and attitudes regarding the virus and the Pandemic. From a psychological perspective, a series of activities were developed, such as measurement scales and research on stress, anguish, confidence, and attitudes regarding the virus and the Pandemic. Likewise, prolonged isolation was studied, triggering panic attacks, distress, sleep disorders, domestic violence, eating disorders, and irritability.

Matus and Matus [15] developed a scale for measuring attitudes toward confinement by COVID-19. They consulted the extensive literature and began the process with the search for the social representation of the concept in the Panamanian population. Next, the categorization and analysis were conducted to elaborate on the tentative items or consider wording, semantics, clarity, specificity, precision, spelling, and idiomatic interpretation [16].

The tentative instrument was sent to a group of experts for review, who made observations and suggestions. Upon revision, the scale was applied to a group of twenty participants. Using the reagents' discrimination index, the number of items was reduced to thirty-six items on a Likert-type scale. A non-probabilistic snowball-type sample was redesigned and prepared through the Google© form to be distributed electronically.

Between April 17 and 30, 2020, 233 completed questionnaires from adults between 18 and 75. About 67.7% were women, and 33.3% were men. Up to 66.4% share a home with between 1 and 3 people. The psychometric characteristics were obtained with the SPSS 24© program through factorial analysis for validity and Cronbach's Alpha for reliability. Three factors were obtained: Cognitive, which integrates twelve items; Affective with fifteen; and Behavioral with nine (**Table 1**).

With the weighting and interpretation, the possibility of psychosocial risk was established (**Figure 1**).

Values up to twenty-four imply a high probability of contagion due to the lack of accurate information (elevated risk). The results of questions 1–12 were added. A score from 25 to 36 indicates that they have 50% of the knowledge (medium risk). From thirty-seven onwards, participants have sufficient knowledge to prevent contagion (minimal risk) (**Figure 2**).

Values from one to thirty indicate that affective management is healthy, so minimal risk is low. The results of questions 13–27 were added. A score from 31 to 45 indicates intermediate management of emotions. They are not sufficiently prepared in the affective area (medium risk). From 46 to 60, people do not have the necessary emotional tools to support or resist the Pandemic (elevated risk) (**Figure 3**).

The results from questions 28–36 were added. The evaluation between 1 and 18 represents a high probability of disruptive, untimely, or inadequate behavior

Structure of attitudes towards lockdown Covid-19			
No.	Items	r_{it}	Factorial weight
Factor 1. Cognitive (Alfa = 0.925)			
Explained Variance = 23.00%			
01	I inform myself about the Covid-19	0.81	0.84
02	I wash my hands	0.81	0.83
03	I know how Covid-19 is transmitted	0.82	0.81
04	I know what to do in case of get Covid-19	0.76	0.76
05	I talk to my family about Covid-19	0.70	0.74
06	I recognize Covid-19 symptoms	0.76	0.74
07	I comply with the quarantine	0.70	0.71
08	I watch news	0.63	0.68
09	I know the decrees of the Ministry of Health	0.69	0.68
10	I eat what is necessary	0.57	0.63
11	I work from home	0.52	0.63
12	I forward true information	0.60	0.62
Factor 2. Afectivo (Alfa = 0.927)			
Explained Variance = 21.34%			
13	I feel confused	0.76	0.81
14	I feel vulnerable	0.76	0.81
15	I feel defenseless	0.75	0.80
16	I feel overwhelmed	0.68	0.74
17	I feel in danger	0.72	0.73
18	I feel afraid	0.70	0.73
19	I feel upset	0.63	0.71
20	I feel isolated	0.64	0.69
21	I feel angry	0.61	0.69
22	I feel uncertain	0.65	0.69
23	I feel tired	0.63	0.68
24	I feel worried	0.65	0.67
25	I feel imprisoned	0.56	0.62
26	I feel at risk	0.57	0.60
27	I distrust of the authorities	0.44	0.48
Factor 3. Behavioral (Alfa = 0.849)			
Explained Variance = 5.51%			
28	I sing	0.61	0.78
29	I dance	0.56	0.72
30	I write	0.66	0.70
31	I do manual activities	0.57	0.63
32	I read	0.66	0.59
33	I exercise	0.53	0.56
34	I talk with friends	0.59	0.40
35	I watch TV	0.41	0.16
36	I study what I want	0.52	0.30

Table 1.
Cognitive factor.

1-12
Whitout Knowledge
13-24
Few Knowledge
25-36
Some Knowledge
37-48
Knowledge
49-60
Hi Knowledge

Figure 1.
Cognitive factor.

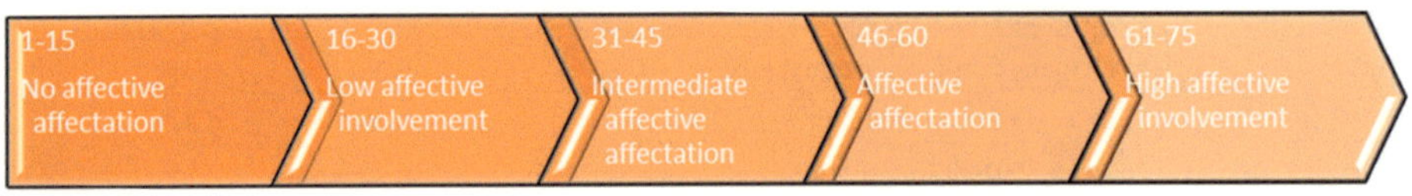

Figure 2.
Affective factor.

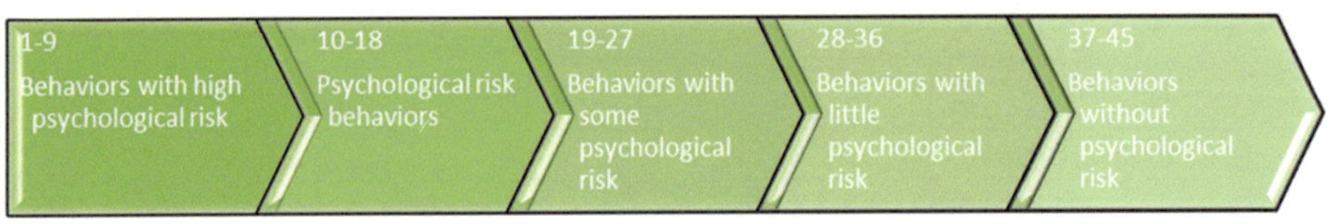
1-9
Behaviors with high psychological risk
10-18
Psychological risk behaviors
19-27
Behaviors with some psychological risk
28-36
Behaviors with little psychological risk
37-45
Behaviors without psychological risk

Figure 3.
Behavioral factor.

concerning the recommendations of the health institutions (elevated risk). Between 19 and 27 points, some inappropriate behaviors are expected (excessive purchases, too many hours in front of screens, etc.) medium risk. The score from 28 to 45 expresses adequate behavior management; its behavioral response is healthy (minimal risk). Furthermore, was publication Attitudes toward COVID-19 lockdown as a risk predictor in Panama [17].

On the other hand, and as part of the international project COVIDiSTRESS global survey [18], the digital instrument was distributed, and 765 questions were obtained from the Republic of Panama between March 30 and May 30, 2020. With the data obtained, Cronbach's Alpha was calculated. Likewise, the construct validity was calculated with the extraction method used as principal component analysis and the

Name	Items	Reliability	Validity	Factors
Perceived Stress (PSS10-UCLA).	13	α = 0.703	50.87%	○ Stress
				○ Loniless
Distress	24	α = 0.880	51.00%	○ Uncertainty
				○ Social Relations
				○ Adaptability
				○ Family Relationships
				○ Personal Economy
Confidence	8	α = 0.882	69.69%	○ Authorities/Institutions.
				○ People.

Varimax rotation method with Kaiser normalization for the factor analysis exposing the total percentage of explained variance. The following table shows the applied scales, the number of items, the reliability, the construct validity, and the factors that each of them obtained from the Panamanian population (**Table 2**):

Name	Items	Reliability	Validity	Factors
BFI-S15	15	$\alpha = 0.558$	60.65%	o Openness
				o Extraversion
				o Awareness
				o kindness
				o Neuroticism
Social Provisions Scale short (SPS-10).	10	$\alpha = 0.916$	67.21%	o Intrinsic
				o Extrinsic
Concern over coronavirus	5	$\alpha = 0.894$	54.30%	o Family and friends
				o Others
Coping	16	$\alpha = 0.783$	45.99%	o Participating
				o Getting informed
				o Entertaining myself
Information sources and media behavior	6	$\alpha = 0.778$	49.72%	o Information Search
Compliance with local prevention guidelines	6	$\alpha = 0.489$	54.82%	o Prevención
				o Benefits

Fuente: [15, 19–24].

Table 2.
Instruments.

4. Other initiatives

Since the beginning of the Pandemic, psychological containment care has been provided through the telephone service, organized at the national level by the Ministry of Health and volunteer psychologists. Additionally, in the Caribbean country, proposals were developed to mitigate the ravages caused by COVID-19, for example, the design and construction of low-cost manual respirators, financed by the National Secretariat of Science, Technology, and Innovation [25]. The performance of civil organizations, non-governmental organizations, and professionals from all areas that kept the country afloat is also praiseworthy. An example is the National Oncology Institute (ION), which, with high biosecurity measures, maintained its operations at 100% capacity. The main religious authorities have also played an essential role during the last two years, transforming their spaces and the way they communicate with their parishioners. It allows an area of secure adherence to their beliefs, certainty about the future, relief for physical losses and emotions, promotes social distancing, and follows the national government's rules. And in the artistic area, the composer Rubén Blades composed a melody called "Panamá" to encourage and support people in the face of the Pandemic [26].

The Panamanian Association of Psychology organized courses, seminars, and interviews to disseminate and train members on the psychological effects of confinement on the general population.

5. Conclusions

Social Psychology is a reference framework that allows explaining through attitudes, social perception, stereotypes, living space, group management, active minorities, the role they play, their locus of control, and behaviors of survivors of the COVID-19 crisis. Alterations in people and their interpersonal relationships were manifested in some psychological disorders identified from this perspective. Some of the results obtained can be included in the following areas:

- The Psychosocial Processes associated with the COVID-19 Pandemic in Panama were diagnosed.
- The capacities of mental health specialists, psychologists, psychiatrists, and educational psychologists were strengthened when working on the COVID-19 crisis through intervention, training, and monitoring of psychosocial processes.
- The human development of the populations that mental health specialists could serve was enhanced.
- The authorities supervised domestic violence due to the confinement and isolation as a sanitary fence by COVID-19 was promoted.
- Micro virtual courses for crisis intervention were developed.
- A directory of mental health professionals trained and trained to care for the psychosocial processes of the adult population in Panama in a situation of confinement due to COVID-19 was prepared.

Acknowledgements

This work was made possible thanks to the support of the Research National System l (SNI) of the Secretaire Nacional de science, Technology e Innovation (Panama).

DOI: http://dx.doi.org/10.5772/intechopen.107845

Author details

Ericka Matus[1,2]* and Lorena Matus[3]

1 Faculty of viosciences an Public Health, Universidad Especializada de las Américas, Panama City, Panama

2 Sistema Nacional de Investigadores (SIN) SENACYT, Panama

3 Departament of Psychology, Universidad Iberoamericana, México City, Mexico

*Address all correspondence to: ericka.matus@udelas.ac.pa; p21218@correo.uia.mx

References

[1] PAHO/WHO. Epidemiological alerts and updates. Novel coronavirus (nCoV). 16 January 2020. Available from: https://www.paho.org/en/epidemiological-alerts-and-updates

[2] PAHO/WHO. Interim Laboratory Biosafety Guidelines for the Handling and Transport of Specimens Associated with the 2019 Novel Coronavirus (2019-nCoV). 2020. Available from: https://iris.paho.org/handle/10665.2/51897

[3] OPS/OMS. 2020. La OMS caracteriza a COVID-19 como una pandemia. Available from: https://www.paho.org/hq/index.php?option=com_content&view=article&id=15756:la-oms-caracteriza-a-COVID-19-como-unapandemia&catid=740&lang=es&Itemid=1926

[4] Worldometer. Coronavirus. 2020. Available from: https://www.worldometers.info/coronavirus/

[5] MINSA. Ministerio de Salud de Panamá. 2020. Available from: http://minsa.gob.pa/coronavirus-COVID19

[6] OMS. Situación de COVID-19. Organización Mundial de la Salud: Región de la OMS de las Américas. República de Panamá; 2022

[7] OMS. 2020. Statement on the meeting of the International Health Regulations Emergency Committee regarding the outbreak of novel coronavirus (2019-nCoV).

[8] Van Zoonen W, Van der Meer T. The importance of source and credibility perception in times of crisis: Crisis communication in a socially mediated era. Journal of Public Relations Research. 2015;**27**(5):371-388. DOI: 10.1080/1062726X.2015.1062382

[9] Moscovici S. Psicología de las minorías activas. Madrid: Morata; 1981

[10] Fromm E. El miedo a la libertad. Buenos Aires: Paidós; 1941

[11] Freud S. El porvenir de una Ilusión. Obras Completas. Libro XXI. Buenos Aires: Amorrortu; 1927

[12] De Paula J, Neto A. Is leadership an ideology? A research project inspired by T. W. Adorno. Revista de Administração Mackenzie. 2017;**18**(1):15-39. DOI: 10.1590/1678-69712017/administracao.v18n1p15-39

[13] Foucault M. Vigilar y castigar. El nacimiento de la prisión. México: Siglo XXI editores; 1975

[14] Scaglia H, García R. Psicología: fenómenos sociales. Eudeba Eudeba: Ciudad Autónoma de Buenos Aires; 2020

[15] Matus E, Matus GL. Escala de actitudes hacia el confinamiento por COVID-19. Propiedades psicométricas. 2020. DOI: 10.5281/zenodo.3840712. Repositorio COVID-9. ZENODO.ORG

[16] Dorantes C. El Proyecto de Investigación en Psicología. De su génesis a la Publicación. Edición electronica ed. México: Universidad Iberoamericana; 2018

[17] Matus E, Molino J, Matus L. Attitudes toward COVID-19 lockdown as a risk predictor in Panama. European Scientific Journal. 2021;**17**(15):1-19

[18] Yamada Y, Ćepulić DB, Coll-Martín T, et al. COVIDiSTRESS global survey dataset on psychological and behavioral consequences of the COVID-19 outbreak. Scientific Data. 2021;**8**:3. DOI: 10.1038/s41597-020-00784-9

[19] Matus E, Matus L, Toriz A, Molino J. Confianza durante la pandemia por COVID-19 en Panamá. European Scientific Journal, ESJ. 2021;**17**(35):51. DOI: 10.19044/esj.2021.v17n35p51

[20] Matus E. Estado de emergencia nacional en Panamá. Periódico nacional: Yo me quedo en casa. La Estrella de Panamá; 2020

[21] Matus E, Matus L, Florez A, Stanziola M, Araguás N, López A, et al. Estrés en Panamá por COVID-19. Revista Cubana de Alternativas en Psicología. 2020;**8**(24):120-135

[22] Matus E, Matus L, Florez A, Tejeira C, López A, Araguas N, et al. Propiedades psicométricas de la escala PSS10-UCLA de estrés percibido por COVID-19 en Panamá. 2020. DOI: 10.5281/zenodo.3951184

[23] Matus E, Matus L, Florez A, Toriz A, Cuevas A, Molino J. Distress about COVID-19 in Panama: Psychometric structure. Journal of Social Sciences. 2021;**17**:169-174

[24] Matus E, Matus L, Toriz A, Molino J. BFI-S applicability in Panama. Investigación y Pensamiento Crítico. 2022;**10**(1):25-31. DOI: 10.37387/ipc.v10i1.273

[25] SENACYT. Presentan avances de Ventiladores por Panamá. Tecnología e Innovación: Secretaría Nacional de Ciencia; 2020

[26] Blades R, Nieto C. Vamos Panamá. 2020. Available from: https://www.bing.com/videos/search?q=Rub%c3%a9n+Blades.+Canci%c3%b3n+vamos+Panam%c3%

Chapter 7

Perspective Chapter: Emerging SARS-CoV-2 Variants of Concern (VOCs) and Their Impact on Transmission Rate, Disease Severity and Breakthrough Infections

Arbind Kumar, Aashish Sharma, Narendra Vijay Tirpude, Yogendra Padwad, Shaifali Sharma and Sanjay Kumar

Abstract

SARS-CoV-2, like all RNA viruses, evolves over time, and genetic mutations have been linked to increased replication fitness and evolvability. SARS-CoV-2 spreads quickly between countries, resulting in new mutations. SARS-CoV-2 genome sequencing reveals that variants emerge through point mutations, insertions, and deletions. Concerns have been raised about the ability of currently approved vaccines to protect against emerging variants. Viral spike protein is a component of many approved vaccine candidates, and mutations in the S-protein may affect transmission dynamics and the risk of immune escape, resulting this pandemic last-longer in populations. Understanding the evolution of the SARS-CoV-2 virus, as well as its potential relationship with transmissibility, infectivity, and disease severity, may help us predict the consequences of future pandemics. SARS-CoV-2 genome studies have identified a few mutations that could potentially alter the transmissibility and pathogenicity of the SARS-CoV-2 virus. At the moment, it is worth mentioning that a few variants have increased the transmissibility of SARS-CoV-2. The Alpha, Beta, Gamma, Delta, Delta+, and omicron variants are designated as variants of concern (VOCs) by the World Health Organisation and have been linked with an increased risk to the community in terms of transmission, hospitalisation, and mortality. This chapter thoroughly discusses the impact of SARS-CoV-2 mutations, mainly VOCs, on public health by mining many published articles.

Keywords: SARS-CoV-2, variant, COVID-19, pandemic, vaccine, transmissibility

1. Introduction

COVID-19 has been declared a pandemic by the World Health Organisation (WHO) on March 11, 2020. For the short time period, the COVID-19 time has passed in a few countries throughout the past 2 years of the pandemic, but there has been a new infection outbreak recorded in a few continents, and it has spread quickly globally, causing new waves in many countries. According to the WHO, as of today, June 22nd, a total of 6,544,553 new infections have been reported worldwide in just 24 hours. All viruses, including SARS-CoV-2, mutate over time, and high mutation rates have been linked to improved replication fitness and evolvability. These characteristics give RNA viruses a high level of adaptability. As a result, RNA viruses adapt quickly to changing environmental conditions [1, 2]. The genomes of RNA viruses, including coronavirus, are prone to mutation in three different ways. The first is due to the low fidelity and proof-reading activity of RNA polymerase, which results in the erroneous incorporation of mutations during replication. The second is due to a recombinational event between two viral lineages, and the third is due to the host RNA editing system. Mutations may be neutral, beneficial, or deleterious. Although the majority of circulating RNA virus mutations are neutral, some may affect viral replication and infectivity [3–5]. The COVID-19 pandemic's longevity could lead to the accumulation of immunologically important mutations in the viral genome that provide the virus an edge in its ability to replicate and survive [6, 7]. In most RNA viruses, RNA polymerase lacks proofreading activity [8, 9]. Mutations in the surface protein can significantly alter viral function and/or interactions with neutralising antibodies. Spike protein receptor-binding domain (RBD) mutations in the SARS-CoV-2 genome are being studied for their potential impact on infectivity and antibody resistance caused by this new variant. This is because the RBD on the S protein of SARS-COV-2 facilitates binding between the S protein and the host angiotensin-converting enzyme 2 (ACE2). S-ACE2 binding allows SARS-CoV-2 to enter the host cell and begin the viral infection process [10, 11]. SARS-CoV-2 infection is only detected in humans, and there have been numerous reports of mutations in the gene that codes for the Spike (S) protein [5, 7, 12, 13]. Since the COVID-19 pandemic disease outbreak, mutations have been reported in 96.5 percent of the SARS-CoV-2 spike protein's amino acid residues [14]. The use of vaccines is the only method for treating the viral pandemic, and several COVID-19 vaccines have been rolled out globally to stop the spread of sickness. However, like other vaccines, these ones are also not 100% effective, and as a result of the SARS-CoV-2 breakthrough infection, vaccine recipients are now being diagnosed with COVID-19. However, despite breakthrough infection, vaccines are still effective in treating serious illnesses linked with COVID-19 [15–17]. A number of variants of SARS-CoV-2 have been reported worldwide since the first reports of pandemics. The World Health Organisation classified some of them as variants of concern because they are extremely contagious and frequently lead to breakthrough infections. VOCs have the ability to neutralise the effects of numerous vaccinations. These are the causes of recent waves and breakthrough infections in various countries. Variants of Concern (VOCs) are an emerging topic of research since they can alter the transmissibility, clinical presentation, and severity of the disease, as well as have an effect on treatment options such as medicines and vaccines.

2. Emergence of variants of concern (VOCs) of SARS-CoV-2

Several variations in the SARS-CoV-2 genome have been reported in the last 2 years of the pandemic. Spike proteins, an outward projection of the SARS-surface, CoV-2's interacted with ACE-2 receptors on host cells, resulting in viral pathogenesis. Since the beginning of the pandemic, the amino acids of spike protein have been mutated, and a large number of variations have emerged. A few variations have been linked to viral replication fitness and survival advantages, which ultimately

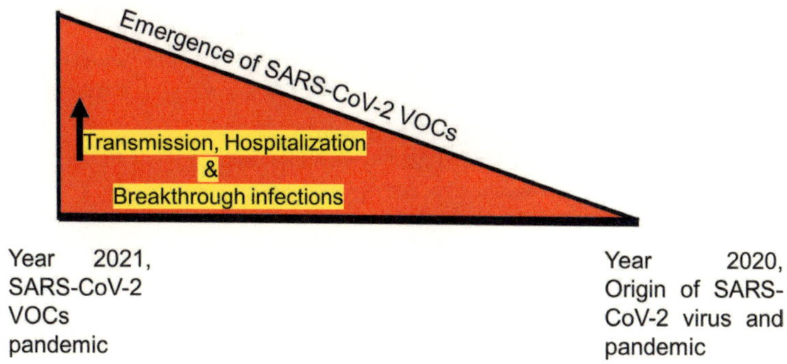

Figure 1.
Schematic representation of emergence of VOCs of SARS-CoV-2 during last 2 years of pandemic and their impact on COVID-19 risk.

increases the risk of disease transmission and severity in the human population (**Figure 1**). Furthermore, a few variants are highly transmissible and less susceptible to vaccine-induced and infection-induced immune responses, causing breakthrough infections. Based on this, the World Health Organisation classified a few SARS-CoV-2 virus variants as Variants of Concern (**Table 1**). This chapter discussed how VOCs have posed health risks to the human population in the last 2 years.

2.1 Impact of the alpha variant (B.1.1.7 & Q lineages) on the severity and spread of the disease

The alpha variant was the first variant of concern for SARS-CoV-2 after the induction of the pandemic in March 2020. The first case of the alpha variant was detected in October 2020 in the United Kingdom and subsequently spread to many countries, causing an outbreak. The WHO labelled the variant as an alpha and in lineage B.1.1.7. The alpha spike protein contains non-synonymous mutations and deletions, including deletions 69–70, 144, N501Y, A570D, D614G, P681H, T716I, S982A, and D1118H, and each mutation has its own biological significance, which increases overall infectivity [29]. The alpha variant spread rapidly in the UK in Oct-Dec 2020 and the most frequently observed mutation was the N501Y mutation in spike protein. The substitution

Strains	Notable mutations in spike protein	Transmission/ Hospitalisation/ICU admission	Breakthrough Infection	First waves in countries	References
Alpha (B.1.1.7 & Q lineages)	N501Y, D614G, P681H	Studies showed that the alpha was linked with a ~ 2 folds increase in hospitalisation and ICU admission risk compared to non-alpha infection	Not reported, a modest anti-CoV-2 antibody neutralisation effect was observed	United Kingdom	[18, 19]
Beta (B.1.351)	K417N, E484K, N501Y, D614G, A701V	Studies showed that ~2.5 folds increased risk of hospitalisation and risk of ICU admission	Prevalence of breakthrough infections increases	South Africa	[20, 21]

Strains	Notable mutations in spike protein	Transmission/ Hospitalisation/ICU admission	Breakthrough Infection	First waves in countries	References
Gamma (P.1.)	K417T, E484K, N501Y, D614G, H655Y	1.4 to 2.2. times more transmission rate and 10–80% more lethal compared to other circulating strains in the prevalent area	Prevalence of breakthrough infections increases	Brazil	[22, 23]
Delta/ Delta+ (B.1.617)	L452R, T478K, D614G, P681R	Very high infection rate, hospitalisation and ICU admission	High rate of breakthrough infections, neutralisation effect on vaccine response	India	[24, 25]
Omicron (BA.1 or B.1.1.529)	K417N, E484A, N440K, T478K, N501Y, Y505H	Infection rate is higher than the delta waves, while the hospitalisation and severity risk were comparatively lower.	Very high rate of re-infection or vaccine breakthrough infections	Affected globally	[26–28]
Descendent lineages					
BA.2	T376A, R408S, D405N				
BA.3	Carry both BA.1 & BA.2 mutations				
BA.4/5	L452R, F486V, and R493Q				

Table 1.
Variant of concerns, notable mutations in SARS-CoV-2 spike and their impact on viral replication fitness and survival advantages over original SARS-CoV-2 virus.

of tyrosine for asparagine at position 501 of spike protein increases its affinity for ACE-2 receptors on host cells. [30], as results increase in transmission rate, which derived the first wave of COVID-19 in many countries. A strain carrying D614G in RBD domains is more infective and resistant to some neutralising antibodies, which has obvious implications for COVID-19 patient recovery [31]. According to studies, the G614 variant has a greater number of functional spikes on its surface than the D614 variant. Furthermore, it has been shown that the D614G mutation stabilises the interaction between the S1 and S2 domains and limits S1 shedding, resulting in increased overall infectivity [32].

2.1.1 Transmission and hospitalisation

It originated in the UK, but the variant was present on all continents within 2 months of its emergence. As of December 2020 [33], B.1.1.7 was the cause of two-thirds of COVID-19 infections in the UK and one-quarter of all cases worldwide as of December 2020 [34]. The emergence of alpha variants resulted in an increase in the transmission rate and hospitalisation of COVID-19 cases, as few studies estimated the infection rate and it was 45–71% higher in the alpha variants than in the original virus [19, 34, 35]. SARS-CoV-2 lineage B.1.1.7 infection was linked to an increased risk of hospitalisation. Bager et al. discovered in 2021 that the hospitalisation rate in alpha variants rises over time. They enrolled 50,958 COVID-19 patients, of whom 30,572 had their SARS-CoV-2 genome sequenced, and followed up with 14 days of hospitalisation data. The Alpha variant infected 34.5 percent of all patients and hospitalised 6.4 percent. 29.4 percent of the hospitalised patients were infected with Alpha, while 70.6 percent were infected with other strains. During the study period, the number of COVID-19 hospitalizations decreased, but the proportion of patients with the Alpha variant increased dramatically, from 3.5 percent in week 1 to 92.1 percent in week 10 [36]. Veneti et al. included 27,753 COVID-19 patients in their study, of whom 23,169 are cases of alpha variant. Study showed that the B.1.1.7 was linked with a 1.9-fold increased risk of hospitalisation and a 1.8-fold increased risk of ICU admission, in comparison to non-alpha strain [37]. Several studies showed that the emergence of the alpha variant was linked to an increase in transmission risk and hospitalisation rate [19, 38].

2.1.2 Vaccine response

According to studies, vaccinated people are less likely to be hospitalised than unvaccinated people. According to Eyre et al., vaccinated individuals infected with alpha variants had a lower transmission and hospitalisation rate [39]. Study of Lopez et al. in UK population infected with alpha variant showed that the one dose of BNT162b2 and ChAdOx1 nCoV-19 (AstraZeneca) vaccine was found to be effective against 48.7% (95% CI, 45.5–51.7) symptomatic alpha variant infection, whereas effectiveness increased to 93.7% (95% CI, 91.6–95.3) and 74.5% (95% CI, 68.4–79.4), respectively, after second dose of administration BNT162b2 and ChAdOx1 nCoV-19 (AstraZeneca) vaccine [40]. A similar study conducted by Chemaitelly et al. showed that the mRNA-1273 vaccines were effective 88.1% (95% CI, 83.7–91.5) after the first dose, whereas it was found to be 100% (95% CI, 91.8–100) after the second dose of administration [41]. Mahase et al. also evaluated the effectiveness of the Novavax vaccine, and it was found to be 85.6% effective against symptomatic COVID-19 with the alpha variant [42].

2.2 Impact of the beta variant (B.1.351) on the severity and spread of the disease

The beta form was first discovered in South Africa, and primarily infected young people with no disease severity risk. This variant was responsible for more than 90% of all cases and the 2nd wave of COVID-19 in South Africa in the last month of 2020 [43], and spread to other African countries, Asia, Australia, and North and Central America [44]. Among several structural and non-structural mutations in beta spike, K417N, E484K, and N501Y are the three critical changes that could give SARS-CoV-2 viral fitness and survival advantages over the circulating strains in the same region where it was common [44].

2.2.1 Transmission and hospitalisation

Studies showed that the beta variant is comparatively highly transmissible than that of earlier circulating strain of SARS-CoV-2. In 2021, Pearson et al. demonstrated that prior exposure only partially protects against beta variant infection, and it has been accounted for about 40% of new SARS-CoV-2 infections compared to only 20% for Alpha variants in the prevalent area. As estimated 501Y.V2 is 1.50 times as transmissible as previously circulating variants [45]. Studies showed that the person infected with beta variant has higher risk for disease severity than the alpha variant. The study of Veneti et al. showed that the B.1.351 was associated with a 2.4-fold increased risk of hospitalisation and a 2.7-fold increased risk of ICU admission compared to non-VOC [20].

2.2.2 Vaccine response and breakthrough infections

Studies showed that the efficacy of vaccines is greatly reduced when dealing with the beta variants. In a study conducted by Garcia-Beltran et al. in 2021, the B.1.351 variant significantly reduced neutralisation even in fully vaccinated individuals with BNT162b2 and mRNA-1273 vaccines, whereas protection for other circulatory strains remained constant during the same period [21]. Wu et al. showed that the B.1.351 reduced the neutralisation efficiency of the mRNA-1273 vaccine but that it was still effective to neutralise the B.1.351 virus in fully vaccinated individuals [46]. Mahase, stated that the Novavax was 60% effective against the B.1.351 variants and 95.6% effective against the original SARS-CoV-2 virus [42].

2.3 Impact of the gamma (P.1 and descendent lineages) on the severity and spread of the disease

The first case of the gamma variant was detected in Tokyo, Japan in Jan-2021 and patients were relocated from the Brazilian Amazon state. The WHO has classified the variant as a gamma and assigned it to lineage P.1. Ten of the non-synonymous defining mutations in the S gene are present in the gamma lineage, which evolved following a period of rapid genetic diversification. Of these changes, three (N501Y, E484K, and K417T) increased favourable stable interaction with the human ACE-2 receptor. This mutation caused an outbreak in the Manaus region of Brazil in December 2020, with gamma variant cases accounting for 42% of all cases [22].

2.3.1 Transmission and hospitalisation

In a study done in Brazil in the year 2021 by Chen and Lu, it was demonstrated that patients with gamma variations have high viral loads that are 10 times higher than those of patients with other lineages. Transmissibility and infectivity were twice higher than the other circulating strains in all age groups. Studies showed that the gamma variant can overcome the immunity developed from earlier infections, increasing the risk of a breakthrough infection. Additionally, the death rate was 10–80% greater in the group infected with the gamma variant [22]. A study by Funk et al. showed that gamma variant patients had significantly higher adjusted odds ratios for hospitalisation (2.6, 95% CI, 1.4–4.8) and ICU admission (2.2, 95% CI, 1.8–2.9) [47].

2.3.2 Vaccine response and breakthroughs infection

Studies revealed that the Gamma variant also had a decrease in anti-RBD antibody neutralisation, and it has been connected to reinfections and breakthrough infections in those who have received vaccinations [48–51]. The Gamma variant was found to reduce the antibody neutralising activity of Pfizer or Moderna vaccines, as the report showed the prevalence of breakthrough infections in fully vaccinated recipients. In a 2021 study on fully vaccinated Gold Miners recipients in French Guiana, Vignier et al. showed that 60% of BNT162b2 vaccine recipients experienced breakthrough infection [52]. Wang et al. also demonstrated that gamma variants had a neutralising effect on multiple monoclonal antibodies and were more resistant to neutralisation by convalescent plasma and vaccinee sera. The gamma variant was estimated to be 3.8–4.8 times more resistant to BNT162b2 or mRNA-1273 vaccine recipients [23, 53].

2.4 Impact of the delta and delta+ (B.1.617) variants on the severity and spread of the disease

The first instance of delta variations was discovered in India, and it was one of the most common SARS-CoV-2 variants that affected the majority of the world. Lineage B.1.617 was assigned to these variations. The L452R, T478K, D614G, and P681R are four of the 17 variations in the Delta variation that are of particular concern, due to their involvement in infectivity and transmission. In comparison to alpha, the infection and transmissibility rates were extremely high. Despite immunisation, this variation resulted in a large number of human deaths. L452R and E484Q is not found in the B.1.617.2 lineage [54, 55]. The B.1.617.2 lineage was first associated with infection in India, and the dominant variant in infection in the UK in 2021. It was highly infectious and spread more rapidly than the original version of the virus. A study conducted by Deng et al. showed that the mutation L425R in the California population resulted in an increase in the binding affinity of the spike protein of SARS-CoV-2 with ACE-2 host receptors, which increased the viral load and 20% transmission rate [56]. Few studies have shown that L452 is not directly linked with the host ACE-2 receptor. This mutation located in the RBD's hydrophobic plaques generates structural alterations that promote binding of spike protein with the ACE-2 receptor [57, 58]. In addition to this, there was 3–6 folds reduction in neutralisation capacity of vaccine elicited sera in experiments with pseudotyped virus (PV) particles [58]. Few studies demonstrated that the D614G mutation in the spike protein promotes viral multiplication in the upper respiratory tract and enhanced transmission rate [59, 60]. The P681R, which is a substitution at position 681, may increase the variant's cell-level infectivity [61, 62]. During outbreak of delta variants worldwide, a new variant was emerged in United Kingdom that carries a novel point mutation' K417N' in delta variant and designated as a delta plus. Lineage AY.1 or B.1.617.2.1 was assigned to this variant. The three most prominent mutation K417N, V70F, and W258L in spike were exclusively present in the Delta Plus variant [63]. Besides this, few other delta variants emerged, Delta-AY.2 in the USA and Delta-Δ144 in Vietnam [64].

2.4.1 Transmission and hospitalisation

During the second wave of the pandemic, COVID-19 patients required more ICU time, oxygen, and non-invasive and invasive ventilatory support. According to estimates, hospital mortality in the second wave was double that of the first [65]. Ong et al. calculated the risk linked with the delta variant by observing the need for oxygen, ICU admission time, and death and found that delta was associated with increased disease severity when compared to non-VOCs [66]. Several studies revealed that a large percentage of vaccine recipients reported breakthrough infection during the delta variant wave [67–71]. Initial studies demonstrated that the delta variant increased the hospitalisation risk in the population, despite the first dosage of vaccination [24, 72, 73]. Non-vaccinated people and those who contacted viruses within 14 days of vaccination were more prone to hospitalisation [74]. A similar study conducted by Twohig et al. showed delta variant infections linked to an increased hospitalisation rate (hazard ratio 226 [95% CI 132–389]) in comparison to alpha variant infections. All age categories experienced an increase in mortality during the Delta wave, with patients under 45 experiencing the most increase in infection (10.5 percent vs. 7.2 percent, p 0.001), compared to pre-Delta wave [24].

2.4.2 Vaccine response and breakthroughs infection

Davis et al. calculated the neutralisation capacity of BNT162b2 (Pfizer/BioNTech) and ChAdOx1 (Oxford/AstraZeneca) vaccines against the SARS-CoV-2 B.1.617.1 and B.1.617.2 lineages. Both B.1.617.1 and B.1.617.2 reduced antibody neutralisation by 4.31 and 5.11-fold in vaccine recipients, respectively. However, the neutralisation response was significantly higher in two doses of BNT162b2 vaccine recipients than in two doses of ChAdOx1 [55]. During a period of high Delta prevalence, Havers et al. found that hospitalisation rates in unvaccinated individuals were more than 10 times higher than in vaccinated recipients [75]. Twohig et al. found that the risk of hospitalisation or emergency care was higher in delta variant patients who were either unvaccinated or received the first dose (dose taken within 21 days) compared to that of alpha variant patients [24]. When compared to unvaccinated individuals, Veneti et al. showed a reduction in hospitalisation risk of 72 percent (95% CI 59–82%) and 76% (95% CI 61–85%) in partially or fully vaccinated individuals after adjusting for gender, age group, country of birth, variant, and underlying comorbidities [37].

2.5 Impact of the omicron (B.1.1.529) variant on the severity and spread of the disease

The omicron (B.1.1.529) variant was first reported in a sample of Botswana on November 11, 2021 and in South Africa on November 24, 2021 (WHO, CDCC). On November 26th, 2021, the WHO classified them as lineage B.1.1.529 and declared them a variant of concern. It contains a large number of variations in the SARS-CoV-2 genome, as more than 60 variations (substitutions/deletions/insertions) in the omicron variant have been reported, some of which are concerning [76]. The spike protein in the Omicron variant has 32–35 mutations, 15 of which are located in the receptor binding domain, which is critical for viral-cell interaction mediated by the ACE-2 receptor. The high variations in spike protein of omicron could be a potential reason for the immune escape and vaccine neutralisation. Few variations shared by earlier SARS-CoV-2 variants have already been reported in immune invasion. The E484 mutation, which is known to be involved in immune escape, has been reported in beta and gamma variants, but the substituted amino acid was lysine in beta and gamma variants, and alanine in omicron variants [63, 77]. The E484A mutation in the Omicron may have been a significant mutation that was also present as E484K in other VOCs. Omicron also shares the most common mutations in spike protein of other variants, including K417N, E484A, N501Y, D614G, and T478K. The K417N mutation, which has previously been reported in beta variants, disrupts the effect of known antibodies. Chen et al. demonstrated that the E484A mutation has a massively disruptive effect on many known antibodies. The combination of K417N and E484A mutations in omicron increases its effectiveness in vaccine neutralisation. Y505H is the third disruptive mutation. It can also disrupt many known antibodies to bind

RBD complexes [78]. Recent genetic research revealed that the omicron continued to evolve, giving rise to a variety of lineages, including BA.1, BA.2, BA.3, BA.4, and BA.5. A few of these sub-lineages have replaced other circulating strains and have emerged as the globally dominant variants, each demonstrating a different pattern of immune escape and transmission rate [28, 79]. Most spike mutations are the same across all sub-lineages. BA.2 shares 12 mutations with BA.1 and has four unique mutations in the receptor binding domain. Apart from, a new NSP6 (A88V) mutation, BA.3 shares the majority of its mutations with BA.1 and BA.2 [80]. The L452R and F486V mutations unique to BA.4/5 or the L452Q mutation specific to BA.2.12.1 play significant roles in immune evasion, resulting in numerous infections and re-infections following vaccine breakthroughs [81]. BA.4 and BA.5 share the same mutant profile in their S proteins, despite showing different spreading trends [28]. The F486V mutation found in BA.4/5 promote immune invasion by evading neutralising antibodies but reduces spike affinities for the viral receptor. The R493Q reversion mutation, on the other hand, restores receptor affinity and, as a result, BA.4/5 fitness [80]. BA.4 differs from BA.5 in that it has several rare mutations, including del 141–143 in NSP1, L11F in ORF7b, and P151S in nucleocapsid protein. A considerable humoral immunity escape could be caused by BA.2.12.1, BA.4 and BA.5 carrying the lineage-specific L452Q/R mutation [82].

2.5.1 Transmission and hospitalisation

Karim and Karim demonstrated that the omicron variant is more infectious than the other variants of concern. As reported, the doubling time of infection rates is comparatively faster than for previously reported VOCs. Omicron infection doubled in 1.2 days, which is faster than the 1.7 and 1.5 days for beta and delta variants, respectively [83]. Mutations in spike's RBD domains (N440K, T478K, and N501Y) may make omicron 10 times more contagious than the original virus and twice as contagious as the delta variant [78, 83]. However, a 2022 study by Nyberg et al. found that the risk of hospitalisation and mortality in omicron was significantly lower than in delta [26]. Like omicron, their sub-lineages appear to be more transmissible. The BA.2 variant is more transmissible and can infect people who have previously been infected with BA.1 [84, 85]. As a result, BA.2 has quickly replaced BA.1 and other circulating strains in many countries, including South Africa, the United Kingdom (UK), and India, and has become the most prevalent strain. However, BA.3 has shown lower fitness and is reported with limited frequency among other variants. During the global pandemic of the BA.2 strain, two new variants emerged, BA.4 and BA.5, which were first reported in South Africa and then detected in many other countries. The BA.4 and BA.5 variants are more transmissible and pathogenic, and they can reinfect previously infected BA.1 and BA.2 patients [79, 86]. According to the Centers for Disease Control and Prevention (CDC), July 2022, Omicron subvariants BA.5 and BA.4 are the predominant strains of SARS-CoV-2 in the United States, accounting for more than 80% of cases, according to the CDC.

2.5.2 Vaccine response/breakthrough infections

Many re-infections and breakthrough infections have been caused by the Omicron variation and its sublineages, which demonstrate enhanced transmissibility and immune invasion from neutralising antibodies produced by prior infection or vaccination [28]. The RBD domain mutations K417N, E484A, and Y505H provide omicron with a strong vaccine breakthrough capability, causing disrupted binding of spike protein with the majority of 132 antibodies [22]. Omicron has been linked to an increased risk of reinfection and breakthrough infection as studies found that the few vaccines did not produce neutralising antibodies against the omicron virus in recipients. The Omicron variant reduced the efficacy of Pfizer-COVID-19 BioNTech's vaccine, but the vaccine still reduced the risk of hospitalisation. A study published in 2021 by Lu et al. revealed that the neutralising ability of BNT162b2 and Coronavac vaccines is much less effective against the Omicron variant than the Beta variant [27]. Hoffmann et al. discovered that the omicron spike conferred 12-to 44-fold lower neutralising antibodies in convalescent patients or BioNTech-Pfizer vaccine (BNT162b2) vaccinated individuals, in comparison to the Delta variant spike [87]. A preliminary laboratory report showed a 25-fold increase in antibody titers against the omicron after the third dose of BNT162b2 administration (https://www.businesswire.com/news/home/20211208005542/en/). Kurhade et al. demonstrated the efficacy of BNT162b2 vaccine against omicron sub-lineages after 1 month of 3 dosages, and found that the vaccine's neutralisation efficacy was 3.6, 4.0, and 6.4-fold lower for the BA.1-, BA.2, and BA.3-spike SARS-CoV-2 s than it was for USA-WA1/2020 (a strain isolated in Jan. 2020), respectively [88]. Xi et al. studies showed that BA.5 had the lowest neutralisation after four dosages of BNT162b2 vaccination, but the efficacy

Strains	Studies vaccine	Tested Populations (location)	Neutralisation (live / pseudotyped virus)	Efficacy of vaccine post booster doses (2nd doses, otherwise specified)	References
Alpha (B.1.1.7 & Q lineages)	BNT162b2 ChAdOx1 nCoV-19 NVX-CoV2373 mRNA-1273	UK UK UK Qatar	Live	93.7% (95% CI, 91.6–95.3) for BNT162b2, post ≥14 days 74.5% for ChAdOx1 post ≥14 days 86.3% (71.3–93.5) for NVX-CoV2373, post ≥7 days 100% (95% CI: 91.8–100.0%) for mRNA-1273, post ≥14 days	[40–42, 90, 91]
Beta (B.1.351)	BNT162b2 ChAdOx1 nCoV-19 mRNA-1273 NVX-CoV2373 BNT162b2 BNT162b2	Canada Qatar South Africa Qatar France	Live	87% (against BNT162b2, ChAdOx1 nCoV-19 and mRNA-1273 vaccines) 96.4% (95% CI 91.9–98.7) for mRNA-1273 post ≥14 days 60% (19.9 to 80.1) for NVX-CoV2373 post ≥7 days 75% (95% CI, 70.5 to 78.9) for BNT162b2, post ≥14 days 49% (14–69) post ≥14 days	[41, 42, 91–94]
Gamma (P.1.)	BNT162b2 mRNA-1273	Canada	Live	88% for BNT162b2, and mRNA-1273 vaccines, post ≥7 days	[92, 95]

Strains	Studies vaccine	Tested Populations (location)	Neutralisation (live / pseudotyped virus)	Efficacy of vaccine post booster doses (2nd doses, otherwise specified)	References
Delta/ Delta+ (B.1.617)	BNT162b2 ChAdOx1 mRNA-1273	UK UK USA Canada	Live	88% (85.3–90.1) for BNT162b2, post ≥14 days 67% (95% CI, 61.3 to 71.8) for ChAdOx1 post ≥14 days 85% after 2 doses post ≥14 days, 93% after 3 doses for mRNA-1273 87–95% for BNT162b2, ChAdOx1 and mRNA vaccine	[40] [90] [92]
Omicron (B.1.1.529)	BNT162b2 mRNA-1273	Canada USA South Africa Canada	live	32 (24–38) after 3rd doses of BNT162b2 (evaluated on days ≤84 days) 65% for two doses on ≥14 days and 86% for three doses of BNT162b2 in US 70% (62–76) for BNT162b2, post ≥14 days 44 (38–49) after 3rd doses (evaluated on ≤84 days) for mRNA-1273	[90, 96, 97]

Table 2.
Tested efficacy of vaccines against VOCs.

against other lineages was increased after booster dosages [89]. Overall, the emergence of VOCs over time decreases the neutralisation efficacy of vaccines, despite booster immunisation. The first VOC alpha had little effect on antibody neutralisation activity in post-vaccination sera (**Table 2**). Neutralisation was reduced even further by new emerging variants and waning with time [90–99], and the newly evolved omicron BA.5 variant has better survival fitness, transmissibility, and neutralisation even after booster immunisation.

3. Concluding remark

The emergence of SARS-CoV-2 signals an emergency for the global health care system. Emerging recent COVID-19 waves and causalities worldwide are due to breakthrough infection among vaccinated or unvaccinated individuals, which demonstrated a reduction in vaccine response in neutralising virus infection, but the hospitalisation rate is significantly lower among those who completed vaccination dosages. The high transmission rate and vaccine breakthrough capability of VOCs, particularly the delta and omicron variants, are the reasons for the community's global spread. During the detla and delta plus waves in India, the situation was critical, and many people were hospitalised and died. Recently emerged Omicron or its sub-lineages have shown multiple re-infections and breakthrough infections due to their high transmissibility and immunological escape from neutralising antibodies produced by prior infections or vaccinations. Vaccines respond differently to each variant of concern. The effectiveness of booster vaccinations is decreasing over time, although it has been enhanced with successive booster doses. The vaccinations are very successful in reducing recipients' risk of developing severe illness due to COVID-19. Overall, despite vaccination efforts, many countries experienced the consequences of omicron variants, and since SARS-CoV-2 tends to mutate and adapt in our community, the emergence of highly transmissible and deadly strains of COVID-19 variants cannot be ruled out. Understanding the origin, transmission, and breakthrough infections of the SARS-CoV-2 variant may allow us to better prepare for future pandemics.

Acknowledgements

Authors dully acknowledge CSIR, New Delhi and Department of Biotechnology, India for providing financial assistance for COVID-19 testing facility [OLP0043].

Conflict of interest

Authors declare no competing interest.

Ethical approval statement

Not applicable.

Author details

Arbind Kumar[1*], Aashish Sharma[1], Narendra Vijay Tirpude[2], Yogendra Padwad[2], Shaifali Sharma[3] and Sanjay Kumar[4*]

1 COVID-19 Testing Facility, CSIR-Institute of Himalayan Bioresource Technology (IHBT), Palampur, India

2 Dietetics and Nutrition Technology Division, CSIR-Institute of Himalayan Bioresource Technology (IHBT), Palampur, India

3 Department of Microbiology, CIVIL Hospital, Palampur, India

4 CSIR-Institute of Himalayan Bioresource Technology (IHBT), Palampur, India

*Address all correspondence to: arbind.tripathi01@gmail.com; surya_prbha@ymail.com and sanjaykumar@ihbt.res.in

References

[1] Duffy S. Why RNA virus mutation so damn high? PLoS Biology. 2018;**16**:e3000003. DOI: 10.1371/journal.pbio.3000003

[2] Fitzsimmonds WJ, Woods RJ, McCrone JT, Woodman A, Amold JJ, Yennawar M, et al. A speed-fidelity trade-off determines then mutation rate and virulence of an RNA virus. PLoS Biology. 2018;**16**:e2006459. DOI: 10.1371/journal.pbio.2006459

[3] Sanjuan R, Domingo-Calap P. Mechanisms of viral mutation. Cellular and Molecular Life Sciences. 2016;**73**:4433-4448. DOI: 10.1007/s00018-016-2299-6

[4] Denison MR, Graham RL, Donaldson EF, Eckerle LD, Baric RS. Coronaviruses. RNA Biology. 2020;**8**:270-279. DOI: 10.4161/rna.8.2.15013

[5] van Dorp L, Richard D, Tan CCS, Shaw LP, Acman M, Balloux F. No evidence for increased transmisibility from recurrent mutations in SARS-CoV-2. Nature Communications. 2020;**11**:1-8. DOI: 10.1101/2020.05.21.108506

[6] Grubaugh ND, Hanage WP, Al R. Making sense of mutation: What D614G means for the COVID-19 pandemic remains unclear. Cell. 2020;**182**:794-795. DOI: 10.1016/j.cell.2020.06.040

[7] Korber B, Fischer WM, Gnanakaran S, Yoon H, Thelier J, Abfalterer W, et al. Tracking changes in SARS-CoV-2 spike : Evidence that D614G increases infectivity of the COVID-19 virus. Cell. 2020;**182**:1. DOI: 10.1016/j.cell.2020.06.043

[8] Wang Q, Wu J, Wang H, Gao Y, Liu Q, Mu A, et al. Structural basis for RNA replication by the SARS-CoV-2 polymerase. Cell. 2020;**182**:417-428. DOI: 10.1016/j.cell.2020.05.034

[9] Pachetti M, Matini B, Benedetti F, Giudici F, Mauro E, Storici P, et al. Emerging SARS-CoV-2 mutation hot spots include a novel RNA-dependent-RNA polymerase variant. Journal of Translational Medicine. 2020;**18**:179. DOI: 10.1186/s12967-020-02344-6

[10] Hoffmann M, Kleine-Weber H, Schroeder S, Krüger N, Herrler T, Erichsen S, et al. SARS-CoV-2 cell entry depends on ACE2 and TMPRSS2 and is blocked by a clinically proven protease inhibitor. Cell. 2020;**181**(2):271-280.e8. DOI: 10.1016/j.cell.2020.02.052

[11] Walls AC, Park YJ, Tortorici MA, Wall A, McGuire AT, Veesler D. Structure, function, and antigenicity of the SARS-CoV-2 spike glycoprotein. Cell. 2020;**181**(2):281-292.e6. DOI: 10.1016/j.cell.2020.02.058

[12] Saha I, Ghosh N, Sharma N, Nandi S. Hotspot mutations in SARS-CoV-2. Frontiers in Genetics. 2021;**12**:753440. DOI: 10.3389/fgene.2021.753440

[13] Sheikh JA, Singh J, Singh H, Jamal S, Khubaib M, Kohli S, et al. Emerging genetic diversity among clinical isolates of SARS-CoV-2: Lessons for today. Infection, Genetics and Evolution. 2020;**84**:104330. DOI: 10.1016/j.meegid.2020.104330

[14] Guruprasad K. Mutations in human SARS-CoV-2 spike proteins, potential drug binding and epitope sites for COVID-19 therapeutics development. Current Research in Structural Biology. 2022;**4**:41-50

[15] Al-Aly Z, Bowe B, Xie Y. Long COVID after breakthrough SARS-CoV-2

infection. Nature Medicine. 2022;**28**(7):1461-1467. DOI: 10.1038/s41591-022-01840-0

[16] Juthani PV, Gupta A, Borges KA, Price CC, Lee AI, Won CH, et al. Hospitalisation among vaccine breakthrough COVID-19 infections. The Lancet Infectious Diseases. 2021;**21**(11):1485-1486. DOI: 10.1016/S1473-3099(21)00558-2

[17] Nixon DF, Ndhlovu LC. Vaccine breakthrough infections with SARS-CoV-2 variants. The New England Journal of Medicine. 2021;**385**(2):e7. DOI: 10.1056/NEJMc2107808

[18] Collier DA, De Marco A, Ferreira IATM, Meng B, Datir RP, Walls AC, et al. Sensitivity of SARS-CoV-2 B.1.1.7 to mRNA vaccine-elicited antibodies. Nature. 2021;**593**:136-141

[19] Curran J, Dol J, Boulos L, Somerville M, McCulloch H, MacDonald M, et al. Transmission characteristics of SARS-CoV-2 variants of concern rapid scoping review. medRxiv. 2021. DOI: 10.1101/2021.04.23.21255515

[20] Veneti L, Seppälä E, Larsdatter Storm M, et al. Increased risk of hospitalisation and intensive care admission associated with reported cases of SARS-CoV-2 variants B.1.1.7 and B.1.351 in Norway, December 2020–May 2021. PLoS One. 2021;**16**(10):e0258513. DOI: 10.1371/journal.pone.0258513

[21] Garcia-Beltran WF, Lam EC, St. Denis K, Nitido AD, Garcia ZH, Hauser BM, et al. Multiple SARS-CoV-2 variants escape neutralization by vaccine-induced humoral immunity. Cell. 2021;**184**(9):2372-2383.e9. DOI: 10.1016/j.cell.2021.03.013

[22] Chen J, Lu H. New challenges to fighting COVID-19: Virus variants, potential vaccines, and development of antivirals. Bioscience Trends. 2021;**15**(2):126-128. DOI: 10.5582/bst.2021.01092

[23] Wang P, Casner RG, Nair MS, Wang M, Yu J, Cerutti G, et al. Increased resistance of SARS-CoV-2 variant P.1 to antibody neutralization. Cell Host & Microbe. 2021;**29**:747-751.e4

[24] Twohig KA, Nyberg T, Zaidi A, Thelwall S, Sinnathamby MA, Aliabadi S, et al. Hospital admission and emergency care attendance risk for SARS-CoV-2 delta (B.1.617.2) compared with alpha (B.1.1.7) variants of concern: A cohort study. The Lancet Infectious Diseases. 2022;**22**(1):35-42. DOI: 10.1016/S1473-3099(21)00475-8

[25] Budhiraja S, Indrayan A, Aggarwal M, et al. Differentials in the characteristics of COVID-19 cases in Wave-1 and Wave-2 admitted to a network of hospitals in North India. MedRxiv. 2021. DOI: 10.1101/2021.06.24.21259438

[26] Nyberg T, Ferguson NM, Nash SG, Webster HH, et al. 2022. Comparative analysis of the risks of hospitalisation and death associated with SARS-CoV-2 omicron (B.1.1.529) and delta (B.1.617.2) variants in England: A cohort study. Lancet. 2022;**399**(10332):1303-1312. DOI: 10.1016/S0140-6736(22)00462-7

[27] Lu L, Mok BW, Chen LL, Chan JM, et al. Neutralization of SARS-CoV-2 omicron variant by sera from BNT162b2 or Coronavac vaccine recipients. Clinical Infectious Diseases. 2021;**2021**:ciab1041. DOI: 10.1093/cid/ciab1041

[28] Xia S, Wang L, Zhu Y, et al. Origin, virological features, immune evasion and intervention of SARS-CoV-2

omicron sublineages. Sig Transduct Target Ther. 2022;**7**:241. DOI: 10.1038/s41392-022-01105-9

[29] Rambaut A, Loman N, Pybus O, Barclay W, Barret J, Corabelli A, et al. Preliminary Genomic Characterization of an emergent SARS-CoV-2 Lineage in the United Kingdom Defined by a Novel Set of Spike Mutation. COVID-19 Genomic Consortium UK (CoG-UK). 2021

[30] Akkiz H. Implications of the novel mutations in the SARS-CoV-2 genome for transmission, disease severity, and the vaccine development. Frontiers in Medicine. 2021;**8**:636532. DOI: 10.3389/fmed.2021.636532

[31] Li Q, Wu J, Nie J, Zhang L, Hao H, Liu S, et al. The impact of mutations in SARS-CoV-2 spike on viral infectivity and antigenicity. Cell. 2020;**182**(5):1284-12e9

[32] Zhang L, Jackson CB, Mou H, Ojha A, Rangarajan ES, Izard T, et al. The D614G mutation in the SARS-CoV-2 spike protein reduces S1 shedding and increases infectivity. bioRxiv. 2020;**11**:6013. DOI: 10.1101/2020.06.12.148726

[33] Conti P, Caraffa A, Gallenga CE, Kritas SK, Frydas I, Younes A, et al. The British variant of the new Coronavirus-19 (Sars-Cov-2) should not create a vaccine problem. Journal of Biological Regulators and Homeostatic Agents. 2021;**35**(1):1-4. DOI: 10.23812/21-3-E

[34] Graham MS, Sudre CH, May A, Antonelli M, Murray B, Varsavsky T, et al. Changes in symptomatology, reinfection, and transmissibility associated with the SARS-CoV-2 variant B.1.1.7: An ecological study. Lancet. Public Health. 2021;**6**(5):e335-e345. DOI: 10.1016/S2468-2667(21)00055-4

[35] Volz E, Mishra S, Chand M, Barrett JC, Johnson R, Geidelberg L, et al. Assessing transmissibility of SARS-CoV-2 lineage B.1.1.7 in England. Nature. 2021;**593**(7858):266-269. DOI: 10.1038/s41586-021-03470-x

[36] Bager P, Wohlfahrt J, Fonager J, et al. Risk of hospitalisation associated with infection with SARS-CoV-2 lineage B.1.1.7 in Denmark: An observational cohort study. Lancet Infectious Diseases. 2021;**21**(11):e341. DOI: 10.1016/S1473-3099(21)00290-5

[37] Veneti L, Valcarcel Salamanca B, Seppälä E, et al. No difference in risk of hospitalisation between reported cases of the SARS-CoV-2 Delta variant and alpha variant in Norway. International Journal of Infectious Diseases. 2022;**115**:178-184. DOI: 10.1016/j.ijid.2021.12.321

[38] Davies NG, Abbott S, Barnard RC, et al. Estimated transmissibility and impact of SARS-CoV-2 lineage B.1.1.7 in England. Science. 2021;**372**(6538):eabg3055. DOI: 10.1126/science.abg3055

[39] Eyre DW, Taylor D, Purver M, Chapman D, Fowler T, Pouwels KB, et al. Effect of Covid-19 vaccination on transmission of alpha and Delta variants. The New England Journal of Medicine. 2022;**386**:744-756. DOI: 10.1056/NEJMoa2116597

[40] Lopez Bernal J, Andrews N, Gower C, Gallagher E, Simmons R, Thelwall S, et al. Effectiveness of Covid-19 vaccines against the B.1.617.2 (Delta) variant. The New England Journal of Medicine. 2021;**385**:585-594

[41] Chemaitelly H, Yassine HM, Benslimane FM, Al Khatib HA, Tang P, Hasan MR, et al. mRNA-1273 COVID-19 vaccine effectiveness against the B.1.1.7 and B.1.351 variants and severe

COVID-19 disease in Qatar. Nature Medicine. 2021;**27**:1614-1621

[42] Mahase E. Covid-19: Novavax vaccine efficacy is 86% against UK variant and 60% against south African variant. BMJ. 2021;**372**:n296

[43] Callaway E, Mallapaty S. Novavax offers first evidence that COVID vaccines protect people against variants. Nature. 2021;**590**(7844):17. DOI: 10.1038/d41586-021-00268-9

[44] Focosi D, Maggi F. Neutralising Antibody Escape of SARS-CoV-2 Spike Protein: Risk Assessment for Antibody-Based Covid-19 Therapeutics and Vaccines. Reviews in Medical Virology;**31**(6):e2231. DOI: 10.1002/rmv.2231

[45] Pearson C, Russell T, Davies NG, Kucharski A, Edmunds W, et al. Estimates of severity and transmissibility of novel South Africa SARS-CoV-2 variant 501Y.V2. 2021. Available from: https://cmmid.github.io/topics/covid19/sa-novel-variant.html

[46] Wu K, Werner AP, Moliva JI, Koch M, Choi A, GBE S-J, et al. mRNA-1273 vaccine induces neutralizing antibodies against spike mutants from global SARS-CoV-2 variants. bioRxiv. 2021. DOI: 10.1101/2021.01.25.427948

[47] Funk T, Pharris A, Spiteri G, Bundle N, Melidou A, et al. COVID study groups. Characteristics of SARS-CoV-2 variants of concern B.1.1.7, B.1.351 or P.1: Data from seven EU/EEA countries, weeks 38/2020 to 10/2021. Euro Surveillance. 2021;**26**(16):2100348. DOI: 10.2807/1560-7917.ES.2021.26.16.2100348

[48] Banho CA, Sacchetto L, Campos GRF, et al. Impact of SARS-CoV-2 gamma lineage introduction and COVID-19 vaccination on the epidemiological landscape of a Brazilian city. Communication & Medicine. 2022;**2**:41. DOI: 10.1038/s43856-022-00108-5

[49] Estofolete CF, Banho CA, Campos GRF, Marques BC, Sacchetto L, Ullmann LS, et al. Case study of two post vaccination SARS-CoV-2 infections with P1 variants in CoronaVac Vaccinees in Brazil. Viruses. 2021;**13**(7):1237. DOI: 10.3390/v13071237

[50] Fabiani M, Margiotti K, Viola A, Mesoraca A, Giorlandino C. Mild symptomatic sars-cov-2 p.1 (b.1.1.28) infection in a fully vaccinated 83-year-old man. Pathogens. 17 May 2021;**10**(5):614. DOI: 10.3390/pathogens10050614

[51] Romano CM, Felix AC, Paula AV, Jesus JG, Andrade PS, Cândido D, et al. SARS-CoV-2 reinfection caused by the P.1 lineage in Araraquara city, Sao Paulo state, Brazil. Revista do Instituto de Medicina Tropical de São Paulo. 2021;**63**(e36). DOI: 10.1590/S1678-9946202163036

[52] Vignier N, Bérot V, Bonnave N, Peugny S, Ballet M, Jacoud E, et al. Breakthrough infections of SARS-CoV-2 gamma variant in fully vaccinated gold miners, French Guiana, 2021. Emerging Infectious Diseases. 2021;**27**(10):2673-2676. DOI: 10.3201/eid2710.211427

[53] Cherian S, Potdar V, Jadhav S, Yadav P, Gupta N, Das M, et al. SARS-CoV-2 spike mutations, L452R, T478K, E484Q and P681R, in the second wave of COVID-19 in Maharashtra, India. Microorganisms. 2021;**9**(7):1542. DOI: 10.3390/microorganisms9071542

[54] Bian L, Gao Q, Gao F, Wang Q, He Q, Wu X, et al. Impact of the Delta variant on vaccine efficacy and response

strategies. Expert Review of Vaccines. 2021;**20**(10):1201-1209. DOI: 10.1080/14760584.2021.1976153

[55] Davis C, Logan N, Tyson G, Orton R, Harvey WT, Perkins JS, et al. COVID-19 Genomics UK (COG-UK) Consortium, Peacock TP, Barclay WS, Cherepanov P, Palmarini M, Murcia PR, Patel AH, Robertson DL, Haughney J, Thomson EC, Willett BJ; COVID-19 DeplOyed VaccinE (DOVE) Cohort Study investigators. Reduced neutralisation of the Delta (B.1.617.2) SARS-CoV-2 variant of concern following vaccination. PLoS Pathog. 2021;**17**(12):e1010022. DOI: 10.1371/journal.ppat.1010022

[56] Deng X et al. Transmission, infectivity, and antibody neutralization of an emerging SARSCoV-2 variant in California carrying a L452R spike protein mutation. medRxiv. 2021. DOI: 10.1101/2021.03.07.21252647

[57] Pascarella S, Ciccozzi M, Zella D, et al. SARS-CoV-2 B.1.617 Indian variants: Are electrostatic potential changes responsible for a higher transmission rate? Journal of Medical Virology. 2021;**jmv.27210**:18. DOI: 10.1002/

[58] Motozono C, Toyoda M, Zahradnik J, et al. SARS-CoV-2 spike L452R variant evades cellular immunity and increases infectivity. Cell Host & Microbe. 2021;**29**(7):1124-1136.e1111

[59] Plante JA, Liu Y, Liu J, et al. Spike mutation D614G alters SARS-CoV-2 fitness. Nature. 2021;**592**:116-121. DOI: 10.1038/s41586-020-2895-3

[60] Hou YJ, Chiba S, Halfmann P, Ehre C, Kuroda M, Dinnon KH 3rd, et al. SARS-CoV-2 D614G variant exhibits efficient replication ex vivo and transmission in vivo. Science. 2020;**370**(6523):1464-1468. DOI: 10.1126/science.abe8499

[61] Lazarevic I, Pravica V, Miljanovic D, Cupic M. Immune evasion of SARS-CoV-2 emerging variants: What have we learnt so far? Viruses. 2021;**13**(7):1192. DOI: 10.3390/v13071192

[62] Lustig Y, Zuckerman N, Nemet I. Neutralizing capacity against Delta (B.1.617.2) and other variants of concern following Comirnaty (BNT162b2, BioNTech/Pfizer) vaccination in health care workers. Israel. Euro Surveillance. 2021;**26**(26):2100557. DOI: 10.2807/1560-7917.ES.2021.26.26.2100557

[63] Kannan S, Ali PSS, Sheeza A. Evolving biothreat of variant SARS-CoV-2–molecular properties, virulence and epidemiology. European Review for Medical and Pharmacological Sciences. 2021;**25**:4405-4412

[64] Liu J, Liu Y, Xia H, Zou J, Weaver SC, Swanson KA, et al. BNT162b2-elicited neutralization of Delta plus, lambda, Mu, B.1.1.519, and theta SARS-CoV-2 variants. NPJ Vaccines. 2022;7(1):41. DOI: 10.1038/s41541-022-00462-4

[65] Khedar RS et al. Greater Covid-19 severity and mortality in hospitalized patients in second (Delta variant) wave compared to the first: Single Centre prospective study in India. medRixv. 2021;**2021**. DOI: 10.1101/2021.09.03.21263091

[66] Ong SWX, Chiew CJ, Ang LW, et al. Clinical and Virological features of severe acute respiratory syndrome coronavirus 2 (SARS-CoV-2) variants of concern: A retrospective cohort study comparing B.1.1.7 (alpha), B.1.351 (Beta), and B.1.617.2 (Delta). Clinical Infectious Diseases. 2022;**75**(1):e1128-e1136. DOI: 10.1093/cid/ciab721

[67] Hacisuleyman E, Hale C, Saito Y, Blachere NE, Bergh M, Conlon EG, et al. Vaccine breakthrough infections with SARS-CoV-2 variants. The New England Journal of Medicine. 2021;**384**:2212-2218

[68] Bergwerk M, Gonen T, Lustig Y, Amit S, Lipsich M, Cohen C, et al. Covid-19 breakthrough infection in vaccinated healthcare workers. The New England Journal of Medicine. 2021;**385**(16):1474-1484. DOI: 10.1056/NEJMoa2109072

[69] Wang R, Chen J, Gao K, Wei-Wei G. Vaccine escape and fast-growing mutations in the United Kingdom, the United States, Singapore, Spain, India and other Covid-19 devastated countries. Genomics. 2021;**113**:2158-2170

[70] Mishra S, Minderman S, Sharma M, Whittaker C, Mellan TA, Wilton T, et al. Changing composition of SARS-CoV-2 lineages and rise of delta variant in England. EClinical Med. 2021;**39**:101064

[71] Rosenberg ES, Holtgrave DR, Dorabawila V, Conroy M, Greene D, Lutterloh E, et al. New Covid-19 cases and hospitalization among adults, by vaccination status- New York, May 3-July 25, 2021. MMWR. Morbidity and Mortality Weekly Report. 2021;**70**:1150-1155

[72] Bager P, Wohlfahrt J, Fonager J, et al. Risk of hospitalisation associated with infection with SARS-CoV-2 lineage B.1.1.7 in Denmark: An observational cohort study. The Lancet Infectious Diseases. 2021;**21**(11):1507-1517. DOI: 10.1016/S1473-3099(21)00290-5

[73] Cevik M, Mishra S. SARS-CoV-2 variants and considerations of inferring causality on disease severity. The Lancet Infectious Diseases. 2021;**21**(11):1472-1474. DOI: 10.1016/S1473-3099(21)00338-8

[74] Bast E, Tang F, Dahn J, Palacio A. Increased risk of hospitalisation and death with the delta variant in the USA. The Lancet Infectious Diseases. 2021;**21**(12):1629-1630. DOI: 10.1016/S1473-3099(21)00685-X

[75] Havers FP, Pham H, Taylor CA, et al. COVID-19-associated hospitalizations among vaccinated and unvaccinated adults ≥18 years—COVID-NET, 13 states, January 1–July 24, 2021. MedRxiv. 2021. DOI: 10.1101/2021.08.27.21262356

[76] He X, Hong W, Pan X, Lu G, Wei X. SARS-CoV-2 Omicron variant: Characteristics and prevention. MedComm. 2021;**2**(4):838-845. DOI: 10.1002/mco2.110

[77] Gong SY, Chatterjee D, Richard J, Prévost J, Tauzin A, Gasser R, et al. Contribution of single mutations to selected SARS-CoV-2 emerging variants spike antigenicity. Virology. 2021;**563**:134-145. DOI: 10.1016/j.virol.2021.09.001

[78] Chen J, Wang R, Gilby NB, Wei GW. Omicron (B.1.1.529): Infectivity, vaccine breakthrough, and antibody resistance. Journal of Chemical Information and Modeling. 2022;**62**(2):412-422

[79] Callaway E. Why does the omicron sub-variant spread faster than the original? Nature. 2022;**602**:556-557

[80] Wang Q et al. Antibody evasion by SARS-CoV-2 omicron subvariants BA.2.12.1, BA.4, and BA.5. Nature. 2022;**608**(7923):603-608. DOI: 10.1038/s41586-022-05053-w

[81] Zhang X et al. SARS-CoV-2 omicron strain exhibits potent capabilities for immune evasion and viral entrance. Signal Transduction and Targeted Therapy. 2021;**6**:430

[82] Cao Y et al. BA.2.12.1, BA.4 and BA.5 escape antibodies elicited by omicron infection. Nature. 2022. DOI: 10.1038/s41586-022-04980-y

[83] Karim SSA, Karim QA. Omicron SARS-CoV-2 variant: A new chapter in the COVID-19 pandemic [published correction appears in lancet. 2022, 399(10320):142]. Lancet. 2021;**398**(10317):2126-2128. DOI: 10.1016/S0140-6736(21)02758-6

[84] Lyngse FP, Kirkeby CT, Denwood M, Christiansen LE, et al. Transmission of sars-cov-2 omicron voc subvariants BA.1 and BA.2: Evidence from danish households. medRxiv. 2022. DOI: 10.1101/2022.01.28.22270044

[85] Stegger M, Edslev SM, Sieber RN, Ingham AC, et al. Occurrence and significance of Omicron BA. 1 infection followed by BA. 2 re-infection. medRxiv. 2022. DOI: 10.1101/2022.02.19.22271112

[86] Kimura I et al. Continued emergence and evolution of omicron in South Africa: New BA.4 and BA.5 lineages. bioRxiv. 2022. DOI: 10.1101/2022.05.26.493539

[87] Hoffmann M, Krüger N, Schulz S, Cossmann A, Rocha C, Kempf A, et al. The omicron variant is highly resistant against antibody-mediated neutralization: Implications for control of the COVID-19 pandemic. Cell. 2022;**185**(3):447-456.e11. DOI: 10.1016/j.cell.2021.12.032

[88] Kurhade C, Zou J, Xia H, et al. Neutralization of omicron BA.1, BA.2, and BA.3 SARS-CoV-2 by 3 doses of BNT162b2 vaccine. Nature Communications. 2022;**13**:3602. DOI: 10.1038/s41467-022-30681-1

[89] Xie X et al. Neutralization of SARS-CoV-2 Omicron sublineages by 4 doses of mRNA vaccine. bioRxiv. DOI: 10.1101/2022.07.29.50205

[90] Lauring AS, Tenforde MW, Chappell JD, et al. Clinical severity of, and effectiveness of mRNA vaccines against, covid-19 from omicron, delta, and alpha SARS-CoV-2 variants in the United States: Prospective observational study. BMJ. 2022;**376**:e069761. DOI: 10.1136/bmj-2021-069761

[91] Heath PT, Galiza EP, Baxter DN, Boffito M, et al. Safety and efficacy of NVX-CoV2373 COVID-19 vaccine. New England Journal of Medicine. 2021;**385**:1172-1183. DOI: 10.1056/NEJMoa2107659

[92] Nasreen S, Chung H, He S, Brown KA, et al. Canadian immunization research network (CIRN) provincial collaborative network (PCN) investigators. Effectiveness of COVID-19 vaccines against symptomatic SARS-CoV-2 infection and severe outcomes with variants of concern in Ontario. Nature Microbiology. 2022;**7**(3):379-385. DOI: 10.1038/s41564-021-01053-0

[93] Abu-Raddad LJ, Chemaitelly H, Butt AA. Effectiveness of the BNT162b2 COVID-19 vaccine against the B.1.1.7 and B.1.351 variants. The New England Journal of Medicine. 2021;**385**:187-189. DOI: 10.1056/NEJMc2104974

[94] Shinde V, Bhikha S, Hoosain Z, Archary M, Bhorat Q, Fairlie L, et al. Efficacy of NVX-CoV2373 Covid-19 vaccine against the B.1.351 variant. The New England Journal of Medicine. 2021;**384**:1899e909

[95] Chung H, He S, Nasreen S, Sundaram ME, et al. Effectiveness of BNT162b2 and mRNA-1273 COVID-19 vaccines against symptomatic SARS-CoV-2 infection and severe COVID-19 outcomes in Ontario,

Canada: Test negative design study. BMJ. 2021;**374**:1943

[96] Grewal R, Kitchen SA, Nguyen L, Buchan SA, Wilson SE, Costa AP, et al. Effectiveness of a fourth dose of covid-19 mRNA vaccine against the omicron variant among long term care residents in Ontario, Canada: Test negative design study. BMJ. 2022;**378**:e071502. DOI: 10.1136/bmj-2022-071502

[97] Collie S, Champion J, Moultrie H, Bekker LG, Gray G. Effectiveness of BNT162b2 vaccine against omicron variant in South Africa. The New England Journal of Medicine. 2022;**386**(5):494-496. DOI: 10.1056/NEJMc2119270

[98] Lefèvre B, Tondeur L, Madec Y, Grant R, Lina B, van der Werf S, et al. Beta SARS-CoV-2 variant and BNT162b2 vaccine effectiveness in long-term care facilities in France. The Lancet Healthy Longevity. 2021;**2**(11):e685-e687. DOI: 10.1016/S2666-7568(21)00230-0

[99] Hayawi K, Shahriar S, Serhani MA, Alashwal H, Masud MM. Vaccine versus variants (3Vs): Are the COVID-19 vaccines effective against the variants? A systematic review. Vaccines (Basel). 2021;**9**(11):1305. DOI: 10.3390/vaccines9111305

Chapter 8

SARS-CoV-2 Variant Surveillance in Genomic Medicine Era

Carmen Cristina Diaconu, Ioana Madalina Pitica, Mihaela Chivu-Economescu, Laura Georgiana Necula, Anca Botezatu, Iulia Virginia Iancu, Ana Iulia Neagu, Elena L. Radu, Lilia Matei, Simona Maria Ruta and Coralia Bleotu

Abstract

In the genomic medicine era, the emergence of SARS-CoV-2 was immediately followed by viral genome sequencing and world-wide sequences sharing. Almost in real-time, based on these sequences, resources were developed and applied around the world, such as molecular diagnostic tests, informed public health decisions, and vaccines. Molecular SARS-CoV-2 variant surveillance was a normal approach in this context yet, considering that the viral genome modification occurs commonly in viral replication process, the challenge is to identify the modifications that significantly affect virulence, transmissibility, reduced effectiveness of vaccines and therapeutics or failure of diagnostic tests. However, assessing the importance of the emergence of new mutations and linking them to epidemiological trend, is still a laborious process and faster phenotypic evaluation approaches, in conjunction with genomic data, are required in order to release timely and efficient control measures.

Keywords: SARS-CoV-2 viral genome, variant surveillance, genomic medicine, molecular diagnostic tests, public health decisions

1. Introduction

In the current COVID-19 pandemic context, with a count of 544 million cases including 6.33 million deaths [1], a worldwide collective effort for observing the SARS-CoV-2 genomic landscape, monitoring the virus mutational rate and the emergence of new variants is noted. As a result of SARS-CoV-2 genome modification, the virus may gain selective advantage regarding transmission and virulence, increase disease severity and eventually, significantly impact public health either by affecting the current vaccine performance or interfering with the current diagnostic and therapeutic strategies [2].

A series of measures have been taken globally for optimal management of the emergence of SARS-CoV-2 variants. World Health Organization (WHO), international health expert networks, and researchers have continuously been monitoring virus evolution by examining the mutations occurring in the SARS-CoV-2 genome.

During an emergency situation in a health care system, the most important actions are the rapid and effective identification of pathogen and epidemiological surveillance to allow disease control reaction. The development of next-generation sequencing (NGS) techniques has led to an enormous amount of genomic sequence data [3]. In COVID-19 genomic era, the accumulation of this considerable amount of genomic data shared in international repositories, such as GISAID EpiCOV, COG-UK, or NCBI, allowed the evaluation of the transmission pattern of viral strains, the impact of each variant, and also the comparison between the available vaccines and the circulating viral variants [4] and it also oriented global public health measures.

At present, two and a half years after the beginning of the pandemic, we can say that given the mutations and recombination of the viral genes, we are facing a different type of SARS-CoV-2 than the one that emerged in China in December 2019. On November 26, 2021, Omicron, B.1.1.529 Pango lineage has emerged, and currently, it represents the circulating variant of concern, still threatening several countries with its sub-lineages.

In this chapter, we summarize the genomic medicine impact on the identification of the new infectious agent that causes COVID-19, on development of molecular tests for diagnostic and surveillance of the emergent variants, describe their importance in managing transmission, preventing failure of diagnostic tests, on sustaining effectiveness of vaccines and therapeutics and eventually, to inform the public health policies.

2. SARS-CoV-2 viral genome – development of molecular tests for diagnostic and surveillance of the emergent variants

One of the first events that led to the diagnosis of Coronavirus disease (COVID-19) following *SARS-CoV-2* infection was the identification of the infectious agent that causes a new disease of unknown origin by characterizing the nucleic acid signature.

The first patient was hospitalized on 12th of December 2019 and on 10th of January a viral genome sequence was already released. The first metagenomic RNA sequencing report of a sample of bronchoalveolar lavage fluid from a patient who was admitted to the Central Hospital of Wuhan on 26th of December 2019 while experiencing a severe respiratory syndrome, identified a new RNA virus strain from the family *Coronaviridae*, which was later named *SARS-CoV-2* (Wuhan-Hu-1, GenBank accession number MN908947) [5]. Confirmation of the results obtained by deep meta-transcriptomic sequencing, regarding the genome sequence of this virus and also its termini, was done by real-time reverse-transcription PCR (rRT – PCR), and this was the beginning of a new era, the era of "COVID-19" because at that time rRT-PCR was routinely used to detect causative viruses from respiratory secretions, but it was not considered a gold standard diagnostic technique. What followed turned this technique into the gold standard in terms of diagnosing COVID-19 disease and SARS-CoV-2 infection [6–9].

The first three determined genomes of the novel coronavirus (SARS-CoV-2), namely: Wuhan/IVDC-HB-01/2019 (GISAID accession ID: EPI_ISL_402119) (HB01), Wuhan/IVDC-HB-04/2019 (EPI_ISL_402120) (HB04), and Wuhan/IVDC-HB-05/2019 (EPI_ISL_402121) (HB05) were compared [10]. The three genomes were almost identical and the findings showed that the SARS-CoV-2

DOI: http://dx.doi.org/10.5772/intechopen.107137

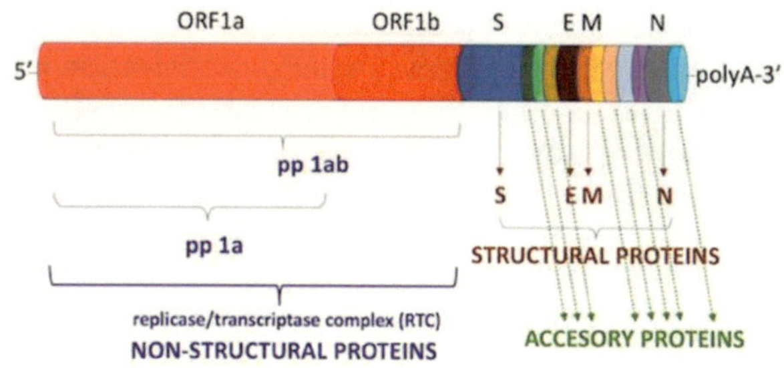

Figure 1.
Schematic diagram of SARS-COV-2 virus genome and most important encoded proteins.

genome, which is approximately 30 kb in size, was a positive sense, single-stranded RNA with a 5′-cap and a 3′-poly-A tail that contained 14 open reading frames (ORFs) encoding 27 proteins (**Figure 1**). The 5′-terminus contains orf1ab and orf1a genes, which encode the polyproteins pp1ab and pp1a. These two polyproteins are further processed by viral proteinases Nsp3 and Nsp5 resulting in 16 nonstructural proteins (Nsps), Nsp1 to Nsp10 and Nsp12 to Nsp16, responsible for viral replication. The 16 nonstructural proteins form a replicase/transcriptase complex (RTC) together. The activity of this complex is dependent on the involvement of viral enzymes Nsp7-Nsp8 primase, the Nsp12 RNA-dependent RNA polymerase (RdRp), the Nsp13 helicase/triphosphatase, the Nsp14 exoribonuclease (the first identified proofreading enzyme encoded by an RNA virus), Nsp15 endonuclease, and Nsp10-Nsp16 N7- and 2′O-methyltransferases. The 3′-terminus encode the four structural proteins spike (S), envelope (E), membrane (M), and nucleocapsid (N) and eight accessory proteins (3a, 3b, p6, 7a, 7b, 8b, 9b, and orf14) [8, 10–13].

After SARS-CoV-2 genome virus sequences were obtained, the similarities and differences between SARS-CoV-2 and other SARS viruses offered the possibility to establish key sequences in the genome for use in diagnosis and surveillance. The release of the first SARS-CoV 2 sequence allowed rapid evaluation of the rRT – PCR techniques for the detection of specific sequences of the SARS-CoV-2 genome and immediately a diagnostic workflow was established [6]. Sequences that offered sensitivity and specificity to the diagnosis were selected, so the detection of a sequence in the E gene provided sensitivity to the test, but not specificity is given the high percentage of similarity with other coronaviruses. The specificity of the test was given by the use of specific primers for certain sequences in genes with less homology to other coronaviruses, as N, S, Orf1ab, and RdRp (located in ORF1ab gene), and in order to increase the sensitivity of the test, the simultaneous detection of several targets have been employed [6, 8].

In addition to rRT-PCR as a standard method for diagnosing SARS-CoV-2 infection, other methods involving the amplification of nucleic acids (NAATs) have been used to detect viral RNA, including digital PCR (dPCR), reverse transcription loop-mediated isothermal amplification (RT-LAMP), and clustered regularly interspaced short palindromic repeats (CRISPR)-based assays. All of that could be a useful tool for surveillance and timely identification of emerging strains. Moreover, NGS has been used since the beginning of the COVID-19 pandemic for the characterization and analysis of viral genetic material and mutation surveillance [8].

There are many studies that evaluated different NAAT strategies for the detection of SARS-CoV-2 and compared their sensitivity and specificity and their conclusion was that rRT-PCRs were significantly more sensitive than other methods [14]. However, for population surveillance, there are need for detection methods that have an increased specificity, are less expensive, and are faster than NGS and rRT-PCR.

dPCR has many advantages over rRT-PCR including higher precision with absolute nucleic acid quantification, it has higher sensitivity and it is not as sensitive to PCR inhibitors or mismatch primer/template. However, this technique has a complicated workflow and depends on expensive instruments and consumables, which results in a higher cost per test [15, 16]. As an important advantage, there are studies that propose using dPCR for SARS-CoV-2 viral load measurement directly from crude lysate without nucleic acid purification [17].

RT-LAMP was previously used for the detection of the Middle East respiratory syndrome coronavirus (MERS-CoV) and severe acute respiratory syndrome coronavirus (SARS-CoV) global outbreaks. RT-LAMP is a reliable and rapid screening test, which can also be used under non-laboratory conditions, but the sensitivity of RT-LAMP is poor, with an important percentage of positive patients remaining undetected [18].

CRISPR-based assays represent a system based on CRISPR-associated endonucleases (Cas), CRISPR-Cas12a, and CRISPR-Cas13a, that recognizes and cleaves nucleic acids in a sequence-specific way. Recently, a CRISPR-based diagnostic platform that combines nucleic acid pre-amplification with CRISPR-Cas enzymology was established for the detection of SARS-CoV-2 RNA. The great advantage is that the detection via fluorescent and colorimetric readouts provides results in less than 1 hour, but even if it is highly sensitive and specific, the multistep nucleic acid amplification process may affect precise target quantification. Additionally, the preparation and testing of reaction components need optimization [19, 20].

Although NAAT techniques have high sensitivity and specificity for the detection of SARS-CoV-2, in the management of the COVID-19 pandemic, a faster detection method was required, which would involve lower costs and also non-laboratory conditions and expertise. These needs have led to the development of rapid tests that detect SARS-CoV-2 viral proteins, intensively used in the detection of other viral and bacterial infections, but which have as a limitation the lower specificity and sensitivity than NAAT-type tests. During the infection with SARS-CoV-2 in the nasopharynx and oropharynx of infected people, high concentrations of S and N protein were detected and because of that, they became ideal candidates for diagnostic targets for the **detection of viral protein** by antigen–antibody (Ag-Ab) reaction. Thus, monoclonal antibodies against viral N and S proteins react with the viral proteins N and/or S present in patients' specimens and this interaction can be easily visualized [21–23]. The major limitations of this technique are that it could generate false negative results for patients with low viral loads, and has lower sensitivity for cycle of quantification >30. The negative results need to be confirmed using molecular tests, particularly when the clinical context is suggestive of SARS-CoV-2 infection.

SARS-CoV-2 has proofreading mechanisms, which make the mutation rate lower compared to other RNA viruses such as HIV and influenza, however, the selection pressure and immune evasion mechanisms have led to mutations that can affect the properties of the virus, thus surveillance of viral evolution is utterly necessary.

Genomic surveillance involves the analysis of similarities and differences between sequences obtained by **viral genome sequencing**.

The development of **NGS** techniques has led to a huge amount of genomic sequence data [3]. As it was shown for emerging infectious diseases, such as SARS, MERS, Zika, and Ebola, **whole-genome sequencing (WGS) metagenomics**

technique offers the possibility to rapidly obtain the full sequence of pathogen genomes, tracing origins, spread and transmission chains of outbreaks, and monitoring the pathogen evolution [24–28].

Metagenomics applications were used for rapid identification and characterization of SARS-CoV-2 and brought critical novel information [5, 29]. The application is simple, cost-effective, and does not require reference sequence for analysis.

In order to obtain complete or nearly complete assemblies of the genome of SARS-CoV-2 clinical samples, shotgun metatranscriptomics – saturation RNA sequencing – has been successfully used. The principle of the method was based on host gene expression monitoring and consists of either enrichment of the poly(A) + RNA fraction, or depletion of host rRNA [30]. Depending on the manufacturer and NGS technology the workflow consists of RNA fragmentation, first- and second-strand cDNA synthesis, and library preparation. Most of the studies were developed on Illumina platforms and the Oxford Nanopore Technology (ONT) [31].

Amplicon-based sequencing approach was developed later, after the enrichment of the knowledge regarding the SARS-CoV-2 genome, as the method is highly specific. The typical workflow consists of first-strand cDNA synthesis followed by genome amplification with multiplex PCRs. The primers used in multiplex PCRs produce a pool of amplicons that cover almost the entire viral genome. Amplicon sequencing is highly specific and robust, but it presents some limitations regarding differences in primer efficiency, amplification across the genome can be biased, with decreased coverage in specific genomic regions and/or 3′ and 5' UTRs regions are not targeted leading to an incomplete assembly [30]. For library preparation, several commercial and noncommercial protocols are available, and libraries can be sequenced on benchtop platforms (i.e., Illumina NextSeq and Miseq; Ion torrent platforms, etc.) [30].

Hybrid capture-enrichment sequencing is similar to amplicon-based sequencing that allows to target regions of a genome and enrich through hybridization to specific biotinylated probes. This approach was initially developed for exome sequencing [32]. Libraries obtained can be sequenced on benchtop platforms (Illumina NextSeq and MiSeq, Ion torrent, etc.). Hybrid capture-enrichment method uses a larger number of fragments/probes, providing more complete profiling of the target sequences and more robust to genomic variability [33].

Direct RNA sequencing is relatively recent approach in sequencing technologies that do not require RNA revers-transcription and allow the direct determination of the sequence of single nucleic acid molecules, without amplification [34]. This technology provides longer reads than regular NGS methods, but with higher error rates [35]. However, this method can provide the sequence of a single mature and precursor transcripts, and information about complex transcriptional patterns, which accompany coronavirus infection (recombination, alternative transcript maturation, rare transcriptional isoforms, etc.) [12].

The global effort of NGS for SARS-CoV-2 in COVID-19 pandemics generated a massive number of reads that had to be analyzed organized and stored in international databases with global access. Basically, the NGS data analysis involves several essential steps: quality control of the NGS data, removal of host/rRNA data, reads assembly, taxonomic classification, and virus genome verification [36].

2.1 SARS-CoV-2 genome data analysis

The assembly of the SARS-CoV-2 genome is a quite straightforward process, as the viral genome is small and does not contain any large repetitive sequence. The main method for the assembly of NGS data that provides a complete and accurate representation of the genome (highly contiguous and accurate assemblies) is based on Overlap Layout Consensus, de Bruijn graphs, or, in general, reference-based assembly [37]. SARS-CoV-2 sequencing with a 30x coverage is generally considered sufficient to generate high-quality assembly [30]. The coverage is dependent on the sequencing platform and on the sequencing strategy, however, data obtained from targeted-enrichment-based library preparation methods (hybrid capture and amplicon sequencing) provide a sufficient viral genomic read.

The first step of bioinformatics workflow is to establish the quality of the reads. Fastq files are processed for subsequent analyses as follows: removing the adapter sequences and filtering low-quality/complexity reads, error correction, etc. [36].

Metagenomics sequencing protocols provide uniform coverage, but the number of viral reads depends on the viral load of the sample and may contain reads, derived from viral sub-genomic RNAs and replication intermediates [38]. For metagenomics reads assembly-efficient software tools are currently available [39].

In order to obtain an accurate representation of the genomic sequence of a SARS-CoV-2 strain, de-novo assembly method could be used, but there were also available, less sensitive methods, such as reference-guided assembly algorithms [40, 41].

2.2 SARS-CoV-2 genome verification and classification

Taxonomic classification is the following step after the reads are assembled into contigs. The quality of contigs can be evaluated by read mapping. The reliable contigs with unassembled overlaps are fused to form longer viral contigs using contig assembly tools (e.g., SEQMAN and Geneious).

2.3 SARS-CoV-2 phylogenetic analyses

The best-known portals for the real-time monitoring of the evolution SARS-CoV-2 strains are Nextstrain [42] and the HyPhy COVID-19 [43]. These systems provide real-time information of on worldwide distribution of different clades and lineages of SARS-CoV-2 (Nexstrain), and detailed phylogenetic analyses of SARS-CoV-2 protein-coding genes (Hyphy).

2.4 SARS-CoV-2 genomic data deposition and exploratory access

At present, the GISAID [44] with EpiCov portal represents the most widely used repository of SARS-CoV-2 genomic data. Along with sequencing data, metadata are provided including the type of sample, the sequencing technology and protocol, patient status (e.g. hospitalized or released), vaccination, etc.

Exploratory access is available from the three most popular portals for SARS-CoV-2 genome data: COG-UK [45], GISAID EpiCoV [44], and the NCBI [46].

Technical advances in NGS and bioinformatics have permitted a fast identification of causative agent of COVID-19, tracking its global spread and confirming the genomic modifications when they occurred. Current bioinformatics resources are multiple, but big datasets pose challenges for data storage and analysis and a solution must be found not only for the control of the current COVID-19 pandemic but for future outbreaks response.

Although NGS is a very precise tool, allowing the detection of each mutation in a sample (thus being considered the gold standard in tracking the viral variants), it has a few drawbacks regarding the price, the duration, and the accessibility [47–49].

To overcome these limitations, other genotyping strategies have been developed [50]: Multiplex PCR tests that use either TaqMan probes or molecular beacon probes, identify and monitor specific SARS-CoV-2 variants, and, even if they target preselected known mutations, they are more rapid, cheaper options, and could easily be deployed in settings with limited resources as an alternative to genome sequencing methods [47, 51].

New appeared mutations had an important effect on the detection sensitivity of RT-PCR that could be reduced if the mutations were located where probes and primers bind [52]. Because of this, commercial variants of kits that detected several genes that included the RdRp and Orf1ab genes in addition to the S and N genes were used and commercial multiplexing tests for tracking mutations in the population, for the surveillance and sequencing prioritization were rapidly developed.

The occurrence of the mutations in the S gene led to S gene target failure or so-called S gene dropout, which generated false negative RT-PCR results. This test failure, however, turned later in new pre-screening rRT-PCR assays that analyzed simultaneous detection of del-HV69/70 and N501Y in order to distinguish between B.1.1.7 and B1.351 lineages or have been used as a marker of B.1.1.529 variant [51, 53].

A TaqMan SNP genotyping test, recently developed by a Taiwanese team [50], targets nine mutations in receptor-binding domain of the spike protein of SARS-CoV-2 (delH69/V70, K417T, K417N, L452R, E484K, E484Q, N501Y, P681H, and P681R), and it is designed to simultaneously detect five important variants (Alpha, Beta, Gamma, Delta, and Omicron).

Molecular diagnostic companies are closely tracking data collected from laboratories all over the world in order to develop commercial multiplex genotyping kits that identify and screen variants as new significant functional mutations emerge.

3. Emergence of SARS-CoV-2 variants – genotype to phenotype analysis and global public health effects

A series of measures have been taken globally for optimal management of the emergence of SARS-CoV-2 variants. A global system has been established to detect SARS-CoV-2 lineages and to assess the potential risk for the circulating viral variants. For effective surveillance and viral characterization worldwide, it was essential to better describe the recently emerging variants and to establish a joint nomenclature.

Considering the large amount of collected data generated by sequencing, WHO experts after consultation with the Technical Advisory Group on SARS-CoV-2 Virus Evolution (TAG-VE) establish the current nomenclature in use when referring to SARS-CoV-2 variants [54]. Thus, for each identified lineage, it was assigned a Greek alphabet letter (e.g., Alpha, Beta, Delta, or Omicron) and when choosing the working terminology for SARS-CoV-2 variants, it was considered the current terminology adopted by well-known open-source databases that performed phylogenetic analysis. Such examples are **PANGOLIN** – The Phylogenetic Assignment of Named Global Outbreak Lineages [55]; **Nextstrain** [56] or **GISAID** – The Global Initiative on Sharing All Influenza Data [57]. At the same time, the term "index virus" was established when referring to the SARS-CoV-2 genome characterized at the beginning of the pandemic (December 2019) in the situation of the first cases reported [58]. Considering the rapid evolution of the virus from a mutational point of view, the present nomenclature may undergo changes.

Specific viral variants that pose a risk to public health have been named, are considered a priority in monitoring, and are categorized using the following working terms:

- Variants of Interest (VOIs)
- Variants of Concern (VOCs)
- VOC lineages under monitoring (VOC-LUM).
- Variants under monitoring (VUM)

Variant of Interest (VOI) - a SARS-CoV-2 variant presenting a certain genetic constellation that is predicted to cause changes in virus properties impacting its transmissibility, virulence, the diagnostic and treatment methods, the severity of the disease, and immune system escape. It is also acknowledged to be responsible for high community spread, prevalence in multiple clusters or many countries, or hint of an emerging risk to global public health. At present, there are no circulating VOIs [58].

Among the circulating VOIs reported in the past [58, 59] (presented chronologically with spike mutation of interest and using the WHO and Pango lineage terminology) are:

- **Eta (B.1.525/VOI: 17-Mar-2021)**- E484K, D614G, Q677H;
- **Theta (P.3/VOI: 24-Mar-2021)**- E484K, N501Y, D614G, P681H;
- **Iota (B.1.526/VOI: 24-Mar-2021)**- E484K, D614G, A701V;
- **Kappa (B.1.617.1/VOI: 4-April-2021)**- L452R, E484Q, D614G, P681R;
- **Lambda (C.37/VOI: 14-Jun-2021)**- L452Q, F490S, D614G;
- **Mu (B.1.621/VOI: 30-Aug-2021)**- R346K, E484K, N501Y, D614G, P681H.

According, to WHO a **Variant of Concern (VOC)** is defined as a viral variant that meets the criteria for a VOI and in addition correlates with a higher degree of virulence and transmission or a change in COVID-19 epidemiology or clinical presentation, or a decrease in the effectiveness of currently available public health measures or of diagnostics, therapeutics, or vaccines [58].

Current VOC is **Omicron lineage (B.1.1.529/VOC: 26-Nov-2021)** including sublineages **BA.1, BA.2, BA.3, BA.4, BA.5,** and **XE** (**BA.1/BA.2** circulating recombinant) that WHO recommend to be monitored by public health authorities as distinct lineages.

The mutational profiles in spike sequence in Omicron sub-lineages are listed below:

- **BA.1** - A67V, Δ69–70, T95I, G142D, Δ143–145, N211I, Δ212, ins215EPE, G339D, S371L, S373P, S375F, K417N, N440K, G446S, S477N, T478K, E484A, Q493R, G496S, Q498R, N501Y, Y505H, T547K, D614G, H655Y, N679K, P681H, N764K, D796Y, N856K, Q954H, N969K, L981F;

- **BA.2** - G142D, N211I, Δ212, V213G, G339D, S371F, S373P, S375F, T376A, D405N, R408S, K417N, N440K, S477N, T478K, E484A, Q493R, Q498R, N501Y, Y505H, D614G, H655Y, N679K, P681H, N764K, D796Y, Q954H, N969K;

- **BA.3** - A67V, Δ69–70, Δ143–145, N211I, Δ212, G339D, S371F, S373P, S375F, D405N, K417N, N440K, G446S, S477N, T478K, E484A, Q493R, Q498R, N501Y, Y505H, D614G, H655Y, N679K, P681H, D796Y, Q954H, N969K;

- **BA.4** -L452R, F486V, R493Q;

- **BA.5** - L452R, F486V, R493Q.

From the collected data, a higher transmission is observed also accompanied by a lower severity for the Omicron BA.1 and BA.2 variants with BA.2 displaying a dominant transmission in the EU/EEA countries. On the other hand, for the BA.4 and BA.5 there is not enough evidence regarding the impact of these variants on transmission rate or severity [59].

VOCs circulating in the past include:

- **Alpha (B.1.1.7/VOC: 18-Dec-2020)** - N501Y, D614G, P681H;

- **Beta (B.1.351/VOC: 18-Dec-2020)** - K417N, E484K, N501Y, D614G, A701V;

- **Gamma (P.1/VOC: 11-Jan-2021)** - K417T, E484K, N501Y, D614G, H655Y;

- **Delta (B.1.617.2/VOC: 11-May-2021)** - L452R, T478K, D614G, P681R.

VOC lineages under monitoring (VOC-LUM) are characterized as variants that, from a phylogenetic point of view, belong to VOCs, which are currently circulating, nevertheless compared to the circulating VOCs exhibit some genetic alterations that show better transmission and also present amino acids changes that might explain the epidemiologic modifications compared to circulating variants [58].

Currently, all **VOC-LUMs** are Omicron sublineages being under surveillance. Thus, the **BA.4 and BA.5** sublineages from a phylogenetic point of view belong to the same circulating VOC, presenting the same mutations profile for S (**BA.2-like** + del69/70, L452R, F486V, Q493) and also displaying two Nsp4 reversions: L438 and ORF6:D61. On the other hand, these two VOC-LUMs vary from each other through mutations outside spike, thus BA.4 shows the following additional mutations: ORF7b:L11F, N: P151S while BA.5 exhibits D3N mutation in M gene. **BA.2.12.1** is another current VOC-LUM belonging to BA.2 sublineage and which shares the same S mutational pattern plus L452Q and S704F. **BA.2.9.1** and **BA.2.13** come from BA.2 sublineage with which they share S mutational profile and also L452M additional mutation, while **BA.2.9.1** displays other genomic mutations outside of S, respectively, in N gene (P67S, S412I) and in ORF3a:H78Y [58].

It is very important to keep these lineages and their modifications under close observation in key sites or hotspots, in order to detect in real-time a divergence from the generating VOC and a possible new risk to global public health.

Variants under monitoring (VUM) are defined as variants that are suspected to pose future risk but with unclear evidence of phenotypic or epidemiological impact which requires enhanced monitoring. Currently, there is no variant under monitoring.

In the generation of SARS-CoV-2 variants, two processes, replication and recombination, have major implications. The SARS-CoV-2 replication process requires an RNA-dependent RNA polymerase (RdRp) that is prone to an error leading to the replication-associated changes. Due to the proofreading process assured by the virus-encoded 3′ exonuclease, nsp14, the mutation rate remains in the low range if we consider the magnitude of the SARS-CoV-2 extension [60].

The factors that may impact SARS-CoV-2 replication, error rate accumulation, and the variants selection include wildlife reservoirs (permissive host species and species-specific adaptation in different hosts) [61], biochemical characteristics of different infected cell types generating a heterogeneous mix of viral proteins [62], and population-level immunity driving selection of these variants [63]. Recombination can occur in a cell coinfected with more than one virus variant through discontinuous transcription of SARS-CoV-2 genomes via 'strand switching' by the viral RdRp or through breakage and rejoining of genomes based on homology regions to form chimeric genomes [63, 64].

Careful monitoring of new SARS-CoV-2 variants must reduce transmission rate, pathogenicity, and resistance to immune responses. This refers especially to molecules involved in cell entry and those that provide antigenicity.

The characteristics of SARS-CoV-2 variants are determined by the structural spike (S) protein cleaved in infected cells by a cellular protease, furin, yielding two subunits, S1 and S2. The S1 subunit binds the receptor ACE2 and the S2 subunit anchors the S protein to the membrane and mediates membrane fusion [65, 66].

In order to identify SARS-CoV-2 genome hotspots, a phylogenetic analysis of the virus is required. This analysis enables detection of the occurrence of variants that may present concern [67]. Until now numerous SARS-CoV-2 genome hotspots have been recognized. Being considered an important SARS-CoV-2 hotspot, spike genomic sequence is frequently altered (various substitutions/deletions) causing modifications in the protein sequence that ultimately may have a significant impact on virus evolution and can cause major difficulties in pandemic management. Consequently, certain mutations in spike protein can determine an increase in infectivity and also a more severe disease, while on the other hand can affect the therapeutic effectiveness [68].

During the early evolution of SARS-CoV-2, the **D614G** substitution in the receptor-binding domain (RBD) on Spike is considered to be one of the earliest S hotspots being detected in almost all previously circulating VOCs (Alpha, Beta, Delta, Gamma) as well in the current circulated VOC Omicron [69]. The mutation, originated from genetic drift and obtained a selective advantage [70, 71], being detected first in Europe in January 2020 and accounting for 98% of the SARS-CoV-2 spread in September 2021 [72]. In these variants, replacing the aspartic acid with glycine at position 614 of the spike protein induced structural change that increased binding affinity to ACE2 and virus entry [73], associated with increases in transmissibility (*in vivo* infectivity) but without affecting the severity of disease [71, 74].

Another recognized S hotspot is considered to be N501Y substitution also in RBD region, shared by Alpha, Beta, and Gamma lineages from previous VOCs. N501Y is known to promote viral replication through increasing affinity between the receptor-binding domain (RBD) and ACE2 and to facilitate the antibody escape [75]. P681H augments viral infectivity being located in the furin cleavage site [75], and delH69/V70 detected in Alpha and Omicron VOCs, was associated with disease severity and long-term infection [76].

Interfering also with antibody escape and thus being associated with vaccination failure were another two hotspots found in RBD region namely E484K and K417N/T substitutions. E484K is found in Beta, Gamma, Delta, and Omicron VOCs while K417N/T is only in Beta and Gamma [77]. Hoter and Naim analyzed the biosynthetic forms and glycosylation of intracellular and secreted forms of double mutants L452R and E484Q (Indian B.1.617 variant) in comparison with E484K and N501Y (B.1.351 and P.1 variant) and observed that the double mutants L452R and E484Q were comparatively highly secreted, associated with a strong interaction with ACE2 in the human lung Calu3 cells [78]. L452R and T478K hotspots, identified in Delta variant, were associated with an increased ACE2 binding and also with antibody escape, which led to an increase in virulence [79, 80].

Compared with wild-type Wuhan-1 bearing D614G, the **Delta (B.1.617.2)** was six-fold less sensitive to serum neutralizing antibodies from previously infected individuals, and eight-fold less sensitive to vaccine-elicited antibodies, lower in ChAdOx1 vaccinees than in BNT162b2 vaccinees [81]. The B.1.617.2 variant proved to be highly fusogenic and notably more pathogenic than its parental virus due to the highly conserved P681R mutation in the spike protein facilitating cleavage of the spike protein and enhancing viral fusogenicity [82].

It is crucially important to determine spike mutations that affect antigenic profiles and the level of cross-protection provided by prior infection with other viruses. The immunogenic regions of the spike refer especially to the spike receptor-binding domain (RBD) because ~90% of the serum neutralizing antibodies from SARS-CoV-2 infected individuals target this region [83–85]. But, also, the N-terminal domain (NTD) of the S protein is targeted [86–89].

4. SARS-CoV-2 vaccine development in COVID-19 genomic era

A major advantage in reducing the COVID-19 pandemic was the development of vaccines against SARS-CoV-2 since all the approved COVID-19 vaccines, although based on the initial SARS CoV-2 strain, continue to preserve efficacy against hospitalization and death, especially after administration of a booster dose [90]. Until the appearance of Omicron, all variants had a convergent evolution pattern [91], selecting similar mutations in particularly vulnerable genomic sites and clustering in similar serotypes. Omicron is highly antigenically divergent from the other VOCs [92] and is characterized by a continuous antigenic drift, giving rise to several sublineages, with limited cross-antigenicity. The most recently selected sub-lineages, designated as variants of concern (BA4, BA5) have higher neutralization escape capacity [93], and vaccination efficacy seems to decrease, although not significantly, even in terms of protection against severe forms of the disease.

Currently, according to the WHO, more than 150 vaccines are in clinical development and almost 200 are in preclinical development [94]. Reported studies demonstrated that the benefits of COVID-19 vaccination compensate for the risks that involve rare but serious adverse effects [95]. For example, a study focused on the administration of almost two million first doses of the vaccine Pfizer-BioNTech vaccine in the US reported only 21 cases of anaphylaxis after administration, with no fatalities reported [96].

COVID-19 vaccines developed so far and tested or approved for clinical trials can be classified into inactivated vaccine, live attenuated, viral vector-based vaccine, RNA, DNA, protein subunit, and virus-like particle (VLP) vaccines [97].

Inactivated vaccines are obtained from a virus multiplied on cell cultures and then chemically inactivated. This system can sustain stably expressed, conformationally native antigenic epitopes [98]. The advantages of inactivated vaccines include the capacity of the vaccine to induce an immune response that results in production of antibodies against many epitopes of the SARS-CoV-2, including S protein, N protein, and E protein [99]. On the other hand, the vaccine is well tolerated, the adverse reactions reported are rare, without reported deaths, and the study and development of this type of vaccine are relatively complete [100]. The disadvantages arise mainly from the fact that the living virus must be manipulated in a biosafety level-3 laboratory at least and there is a limitation in vaccine production that depends on viral productivity [97].

Viral vector-based vaccine is also considered a classic vaccine since this medical technology was introduced in 1972 by Jackson et al., and uses a secondary virus as a transient gene expression vector. Nonreplicating viral vector-based vaccine, the most commonly utilized, uses viral vectors deficient in replication, to deliver a specific antigen to the host cell in order to induce immunity against the desired antigen. The vector used in the viral vector-based vaccine developed against SARS-CoV-2 infection is adenovirus [101]. Administration of this type of vaccine against SARS-CoV-2 infection seems to induce rapid and complex antibody responses as well as cellular immune responses by activation of Th1 cell responses [102]. Comparing to inactivated vaccines the production of viral vector vaccines is safer as there is no need to manipulate live SARS-CoV-2. However, in the case of adenovirus-based viral vector vaccines, rare but severe reactions have been reported, especially thrombocytopenia, sustaining the need of monitoring platelet levels. The mechanism that triggers these effects is mainly the development of pathological anti-platelet factor 4 (PF4) antibodies, as result of vaccine administration that activates platelets and the coagulation system. Also, the immunogenicity of these vaccines can be reduced in some people that present neutralizing antibodies against several adenoviruses [103].

Live attenuated vaccines are developed by a recoding of the virus genome, being a well-known method of immunization against pathogens. Thus, the virus is attenuated by *in vitro* or *in vivo* passage or reverse-genetic mutagenesis, resulting in a weakly pathogenic that is also able to mimic the live virus infection. Usually, this type of vaccine can produce a durable immune response, but the apparition of secondary mutations that can cause reversion into virus wild-type strains, especially in the case of RNA viruses is considered a disadvantage for this type of vaccine [99, 104, 105].

DNA vaccines use a sequential transcription-to-translation process that sustain the production in host cells of a viral antigen that is encoded by a recombinant DNA plasmid, inducing neutralizing antibodies [105]. DNA vaccines present a higher stability compared with mRNA vaccines, the production risk of DNA vaccines is relatively low and does not require the presence of an infectious agent. On the other hand, the immunogenicity of the DNA vaccine is low and the efficacy depends on the injection method [97].

mRNA-based vaccines comprise mRNA molecules that encode viral protein antigens and the main problem of this type of vaccine is removed by utilization of nanoparticle delivery carriers that overcome mRNA instability. Moreover, these nanoparticles are adjuvants to sustain the activation of the immune response. The method to obtain these vaccines is based on the *in vitro* transcription process for obtaining mRNA and the technology is quite developed today to allow obtaining large doses in a short time for any pathogen [106]. Due to the high vaccination rate with this type of vaccine, it can be clearly demonstrated that SARS-CoV-2 mRNA-based vaccination induces a persistent germinal center B cell response and Th1 cell responses, which allows the development of strong humoral immunity [107]. The main disadvantages are the reported adverse reactions, especially myocarditis and the necessity to preserve the vaccines at low temperatures to avoid mRNA degradation [108].

Protein subunit vaccines use key viral proteins or peptides that can be obtain *in vitro* using bacteria, yeast, or mammalian cells [99]. COVID-19 protein subunit vaccine can induce Th1 cell responses and a high titer of neutralizing antibodies but due to the large molecular weight, the *in vitro* synthesis rate of the viral S protein is relatively low [97].

Virus-like particle vaccines use viral capsid proteins or replication-defective virus particles without the viral genomes but the technology for obtaining this type of vaccine is more complex [109].

Although studies to date show that the administration of COVID-19 vaccines may reduce the risk of symptomatic infection and decrease mortality, a decline in virus-neutralizing activity with the emergence of new variants has been reported. Therefore, the strong contagious activity of Alpha and Delta variants and the powerful immune escape ability of Beta and Gamma variants were outclassed by the capacity of the Omicron variant to evade the immunity induced by the COVID-19 vaccines [97]. For example, the efficacy of BNT162b2 COVID-19 vaccine (Pfizer BioNTech) against SARS-CoV-2 VOCs starts at almost 90% in the case of B.1.1.7 (Alpha) [110] and decreases (in some reports) to about 35% in the case of B.1.1.529 (Omicron) [111].

Several studies have shown that breakthrough infections including Omicron VOC increase the breadth of the immune response in vaccinated persons [112]. As such, Omicron-specific vaccine candidates have been developed by several pharmaceutical companies and might be administered as booster doses for the recipients of a primary vaccination scheme or for persons already infected with previously circulating variants. In recent press releases, both Pfizer and Moderna [113, 114] announced that a second booster with Omicron-adapted vaccine candidates (either in a monovalent or bivalent formulation with the classic vaccine) increased significantly the magnitude of the immune response against the Omicron sublineages. It is hoped that such broad responses will be preserved for a longer period of time, as shown by data from trials with a previous version of a Moderna vaccine candidate developed against Beta-another highly immune evasive variant. Presently, administration of an Omicron-specific vaccine in unvaccinated persons is not recommended, due to insufficient data on the level of cross-protection against unrelated variants [115].

Future vaccination strategies are envisioned, aimed at finding better administration regimens (using extended intervals between doses, increased antigen concentrations, heterologous prime-boost schemes), or better vaccine formulations (multivalent vaccines, encoding the Spike protein of multiple VOCs, pan-coronavirus vaccines, and mucosal vaccines, administered intra-nasally).

5. Antiviral treatment development and emergent SARS-CoV-2 variants

The development of direct antiviral drugs was rather slow, direct medication being replaced by vaccines in the treatment of COVID-19. However direct antiviral treatment proved to be effective, indifferent to the mutations that have accumulated while SARS-CoV-2 variants have emerged. Currently, the main therapeutic strategies are directed toward (a) direct inhibition of the viral entry, (b) inhibition of viral replication, and (c) immunomodulatory treatment to block the cytokine release storm that underlies COVID-19 severe evolution [116].

5.1 Direct inhibition of the viral entry

In the first category, there are several anti-spike protein monoclonal antibodies (MAB) such as bebtelovimab, sotrovimab, casirivimab and imdevimab, bamlanivimab and etesevimab used for the treatment of mild-to-moderate COVID-19 in adults and pediatric patients (12 years of age and older weighing at least 40 kg). Additionally, tixagevimab and cilgavimab were authorized for emergency use as pre-exposure prophylaxis for prevention of COVID-19 in adults and pediatric individuals. However, in the context of high frequency of the Omicron BA.2 sub-variant, authorizations for all of these monoclonal antibodies were revoked, except for Bebtelovimab that has a broad neutralizing activity, unaffected by the most common mutations present in all of the known variants of concern of SARS-CoV-2, including the Omicron subvariants BA1/BA2 [117, 118].

The administration of MABs has several significant drawbacks, including the need for intravenous administration in healthcare units by qualified healthcare personnel who have access to emergency medications to treat severe reactions, including anaphylaxis. Common side effects include hypersensitivity, with anaphylaxis and infusion-related reactions, nausea, vomiting, pruritus, and rash. Among advantages, we can count no drug-drug interactions.

This strategy can be used against the receptor binding domain only as long as no mutations in the spike glycoprotein occur. One possible way around this problem would be administration of several MAB antibodies that could simultaneously bind to different parts of the receptor binding domain of the SARS-CoV-2 spike protein.

5.2 Inhibition of viral replication

To date, several antivirals received conditional authorizations for usage in the interest of public health because they address an unmet medical need and the benefit of immediate availability outweighs the risk from less comprehensive data than normally required (**Table 1**) [119]. The oldest is remdesivir, a drug that has to be intravenously administrated, with plenty of adverse effects, which drastically reduce its utility, conditioning its administration by hospitalization. The newest molnupiravir and nirmatrelvir – ritonavir are both oral antivirals, less expensive, with huge advantage that they can be administered in patients isolated at home. However, the treatment has to be started early, and Paxlovid came with several drug–drug interactions that can complicate its use in patients taking other medications. Moreover, there is a concern about molnupiravir regarding a potential impairment of bone and cartilage growth, being restricted for usage in children [120].

Molnupiravir is a slightly modified small-molecule drug developed from a ribonucleoside known as NHC (β-d-N^4-hydroxycytidine) by a research team at Emory University in Atlanta, Georgia. Intended initially to enter clinical trials against influenza, tested it as a treatment for COVID-19 by Ridgeback Biotherapeutics Company, which partnered later with Merck in May 2020, for large-scale clinical trials [121].

After oral administration, molnupiravir breaks down to form NHC that is further phosphorylated to NHC triphosphate. Under this form, NHC is linked by SARS-CoV-2 RNA-dependent RNA polymerase (RdRP) and used for RNA chain elongation during viral replication instead of guanosine or adenosine. This leads to an accumulation of errors in the viral genome that ultimately render the virus noninfectious and unable to replicate [122–124].

Compound	Molnupiravir	Nirmatrelvir - Ritonavir	Remdesivir
Brand name:	Lagevrio	Paxlovid	Veklury
Market authorization:	Merck Sharp and Dohme (UK) Limited	Pfizer Limited	Gilead Sciences, Inc
Alternative names:	MK MK-4482, EIDD-2801	PF-07321332	GS-5734
Pharmacological classification	inhibitor of the viral RNA-dependent RNA polymerase (RdRp)	Mpro viral protease inhibitor	inhibitor of the viral RNA-dependent RNA polymerase (RdRp)
Indications:	Treatment of mild-to-moderate COVID-19 in adults with symptom onset within 5 days from diagnosis with risk for developing severe illness.	Treatment of mild-to-moderate COVID-19 patients aged 12 years and older, with risk for progression to severe COVID-19, without need for supplemental oxygen.	Treatment of mild-to-moderate COVID-19 patients with symptom onset within the previous 7 days, with at least one risk factor for disease progression (age ≥ 60 years, obesity, or certain coexisting medical conditions)
Dose:	800 mg every 12 hours for 5 days	300 mg nirmatrelvir with 100 mg ritonavir, every 12 hours for 5 days	200 mg on day one, followed by 100 mg daily for up to 9 additional days

Table 1.
Anti-viral drugs currently used for COVID-19 therapy.

Efficacy and safety were evaluated in phase 3 double-blind, randomized, placebo-controlled trial MOVe-OUT clinical trials [NCT04575597] on unvaccinated and seronegative subjects, with final results published on February 10, 2022, reporting a relative risk reduction of 30% for hospitalization or death at 29 days [122]. Moreover, new results in evaluating virological outcomes presented at the 2022 European Congress of Clinical Microbiology and Infectious Diseases (ECCMID) (Abstract #4514) showed that molnupiravir was associated with more rapid elimination of infectious viruses than placebo. Thus, at 3 and 5 days of treatment, no infectious virus was detected in patients who received LAGEVRIO compared with 21.8%, and 2.2% respective, of patients who received placebo [125]. The risk for adverse effects was 30% with molnupiravir vs. 33% with placebo. The most common adverse effects reported were diarrhea (3%) and nausea (2%) classified as mild or moderate. Also, no drug–drug interactions have been identified [122].

Molnupiravir received an Emergency Use Authorization (EUA) issued by the Food and Drug Administration (FDA) on December 23, 2021 for LAGEVRIO as treatment of mild-to-moderate COVID-19 in adults with positive results of direct SARS-CoV-2 viral testing, who are at high-risk for progression to severe COVID-19, including hospitalization or death [126]. Also, received authorization in the United Kingdom (U.K.) for molnupiravir (MK-4482, EIDD-2801), and currently is under review for authorization by European Medicines Agency (EMA).

Nirmatrelvir – Ritonavir (Paxlovid) is a combination of two drugs, ritonavir (a pharmacokinetic enhancer) and newly developed protease inhibitor nirmatrelvir

(PF-07321332), a structure-based potent inhibitor of SARS-CoV-2 3-chymotrypsin–like cysteine protease enzyme (Mpro) [127]. Mpro protease is involved in processing viral polyproteins into functional units, and since essential to viral replication. Within the absence of recognized human analog, Mpro is an attractive antiviral target across a wide spectrum of coronaviruses. Nirmatrelvir is administrated with ritonavir, an inhibitor of cytochrome P450 (CYP) 3A4, that blocks the metabolism of nirmatrelvir increasing and maintaining its plasma concentration approximately five to six times higher than the in vitro 90% effective concentration [127, 128].

Evidence for efficacy and safety comes from a phase 2–3 double-blind, randomized, and controlled trial, which enrolled unvaccinated, non-hospitalized adults with high risk for progression to severe COVID-19. Subjects that were treated within 3 days after symptom onset with 300 mg of nirmatrelvir plus 100 mg of ritonavir had an 89% lower risk of progression to severe COVID-19 than placebo group [NCT04960202]. The risk for adverse effects was 22.6% with nirmatrelvir plus ritonavir vs 23.9% with placebo. The most common adverse effects were dysgeusia (5.6%) and diarrhea (3.1%) [129].

Paxlovid is associated with several drug–drug interactions that could complicate its use in the community due to ritonavir association that inhibits CTP3A and therefore may increase plasma concentration of drugs that may be associated with serious, life-threatening events (e.g., colchicine, clozapine, diazepam, simvastatin, etc.). Conversely, products that may increase the metabolism of nirmatrelvir/ritonavir and reduce their concentrations may be associated with a loss of antiviral effect (e.g., rifampicin, carbamazepine) [130]. Thus, a careful assessment of patients' medication is needed before administrating Paxlovid. A web tool developed by the University of Liverpool, which monitors drug interactions with current anti-COVID-19 therapies, may be helpful [131].

Nirmatrelvir – Ritonavir received a EUA issued by the FDA on December 22, 2021, for PAXLOVID for the treatment of mild-to-moderate COVID-19 in adults and pediatric patients (12 years of age and older weighing at least 40 kg) with high risk for progression to severe COVID-19 [132]. It is also authorized for use in European Union [133] since January 2022, under a conditional marketing authorization.

Both molnupiravir and nirmatrelvir, effectively inhibited viral replication of the Delta variant and the Omicron variant however, slight differences in antiviral response among wild-type, Delta, and Omicron variants were observed [134].

Remdesivir is a broad-spectrum antiviral medication administered via intravenous injection. The compound is a prodrug whose metabolizing leads to the release of a nucleoside analog GS-441524 monophosphate with subsequent biotransformation into GS-441524 triphosphate. Under this form, it acts as an inhibitor of the viral RNA-dependent RNA polymerase (RdRp) with potent activity against an array of RNA virus families including Filoviridae, Paramyxoviridae, Pneumoviridae, and Orthocoronavirinae [135]. Various studies have documented its inhibitory activity against SARS-CoV-1, Middle East respiratory syndrome (MERS-CoV), and SARS-CoV-2 in vitro [136, 137].

Data on its efficacy on COVID-19 infected patients came from ACTT-1 clinical trial [NCT04280705], which showed that remdesivir treatment shorten recovery times in hospitalized patients with COVID-19 (median recovery time of 10 days (95% confidence interval [CI], 9 to 11), in remdesivir treated patients as compared with 15 days (95% CI, 13 to 18) among those who received placebo) [138] and reduces chances of hospitalization or death with 87% for patients at high risk of severe disease [139].

The most common adverse effects that occurred in 5% of patients treated with remdesivir were respiratory failure, decreased glomerular filtration rate with increased creatinine in the blood, decreased lymphocyte and hemoglobin counts, anemia, and increased blood sugar levels [138]. Also, 5% of patients experienced nausea, headache, and cough.

In October 2020, remdesivir received the first FDA EUA as a treatment for COVID-19, which was extended in April 2022, for the first time for pediatric patients under 12 years of age including those who are older than 28 days, weighing at least 3 kg [140]. Also, in July 2020 received a conditional marketing authorization from EMA.

Remdesivir showed similar antiviral activity against the wild-type virus and the VOCs Alpha, Beta, Gamma, Delta, and Omicron variants. These findings are justified by the fact that the target proteins of these antivirals, viral RNA dependent RNA polymerase, and the viral main protease Mpro, respectively, are highly conserved. These results indicate that is a high probability that VOC that might emerge in the future will remain susceptible to antivirals that do not target the spike protein [141].

5.3 Immunomodulatory treatment

Many of the complications associated with COVID-19 are due to an augmented host immune response, which contributes to the increased severity of COVID-19 and death. Several immunomodulatory drugs can be administered in-hospital to severely ill patients to reduce inflammation and prevent a cytokine storm. These include corticosteroids, monoclonal antibodies that block the IL-6 receptor (tocilizumab, sarilomab, and siltuximab), monoclonal antibodies that block the IL-1 beta receptor (anakinra), and selective Janus kinase 1 and 2 inhibitors (JAK1 and 2) (baricitinib and ruxolitinib).

Immunomodulatory treatment leads to an improvement in clinical outcome. Among positive results, a decrease in hospitalization lengths, duration of mechanical ventilation, and mortality with 8.7% in the critically ill, and 6.7% in patients with severe COVID-19, are the most notable ones. Coadministration with anti-viral such as remdesivir, improved the clinical outcome, reducing the number of patients who experience progression to severe respiratory failure or death [142].

However, reported side effects are major. For example, anakinra treatment induces a decrease in hematological parameters, headache, diarrhea, an increase of liver function tests, and hyperglycemia [143]. Treatment with tocilizumab also caused neutropenia with severe infections, thrombocytopenia, and increased the liver enzyme levels. Moreover, several cases of bowel perforation were also reported [144, 145].

Another strategy that has been used in COVID-19 treatment included the use of COVID-19 convalescent plasma or ultrapotent antibodies isolated from SARS-CoV-2 elite neutralizers. These are individuals that displayed a highly potent neutralizing response with IgG 50% inhibitory concentration (IC50) values of <20 μg/mL. The ultrapotent antibodies are directed against conserved viral epitopes with broad spectrum activity against ancestral variant and the variant that emerged lately: B.1.1.7, B.1.351, B.1.429, B.1.617, and B.1.617.2 variants [146].

Convalescent plasma administration is nevertheless limited to high-titer products. It was associated with allergic and anaphylactic reactions febrile nonhemolytic reactions, hemolytic reactions, metabolic complications, transfusion-transmitted infections, and thrombotic events. Moreover, there is a theoretical risk of antibody-mediated enhancement of infection and suppressed long-term immunity [147].

Currently, due to the intense studies carried out during the SARS-CoV-2 pandemic, several treatment modalities are available for COVID-19. There are both molecules that block the virus from entering the cell, and molecules that interfere with and block viral replication. In addition, there are immunological modulators that can prevent severe development and even death. These therapeutic strategies are supported by prophylactic ones (e. g. vaccines), all in conjunction with aim of avoiding the disruption of social and economic calm.

6. The impact of genomics on public health decisions

The emergence of SARS-CoV-2 in December 2019 triggered an unprecedented cascade of public health measures aiming at delaying the virus introduction in specific countries; prevention or limitation of viral transmission in the community; rapid tracing, identification, and isolation of contacts; and sheltering of the most vulnerable populations. These measures benefited from almost real-time surveillance of viral spread using genomic characterization.

At the beginning of the pandemic, the rapid development of sensitive real-time PCR tests was facilitated by the immediate sharing of genome sequence data. This allowed the implementation of national NAAT-based testing programs and supported the rapid diagnosis of infection, followed by preventive measures of contact tracing and isolation and quarantine – a policy known as TETRIS or TTI or TTIQ - test, track, isolate (and quarantine).

Whole genome sequencing has identified independent introduction of SARS-COV-2 from international travels, followed by local transmission clusters in individuals with no previous travel history, triggering interdictions of mass gathering and stay-at-home orders in many European countries [148, 149]. Further on, large nationwide programs of routine genetic sequencing implemented by several countries across all continents allowed for the rapid identification of new viral variants, further labeled as variants of interest (VOIs) and variants of concern (VOCs). The COG-UK consortium has identified the emergence of B.1.1.7/Alpha VOC at the end of 2020, a finding that triggered a reinstatement of lock-down in the UK [150].

Mathematical modeling of many epidemiological and social parameters were important pieces in the complicated scenarios of policymaking, as they sometimes furnished reliable predictions on the shape, amplitude, and severity of the pandemic. These parameters were adapted each time a new variant of concern was identified. In addition, genomic sequencing revealed specific mutations in the circulating viral strains that allowed rapid testing for variant monitoring – such as S target failure in a specific PCR test in the case of the Alpha VOC (B.1.1.7), due to deletion at positions 69 and 70 of the spike protein (delH69/V70). These data were conducted for a fast implementation of this biomarker in the SARS-CoV-2 community PCR testing program of Public Health England in the early autumn months of 2021 [151]. Whole genome sequencing allowed a rapid warning of the global community when variants of concern emerged and further monitoring of their dissemination and displacement of previously circulating variants. The availability of free giant repositories for whole viral genomes such as GISAID, sometimes with associated epidemiological and clinical metadata, enabled a fast follow-up of the viral spread, and thorough characterization of the variants' transmissibility and pathogenicity. For example, the genetic surveillance network in South Africa has rapidly spotted the Beta variant (B.1.351. identified in October 2020) harboring mutations associated with immune evasiveness) and the highly-mutated Omicron variant (B.1.1.529; first identified in November, 2021) [152, 153]. This information was used to back up reinforcements or relaxations of some of the most drastic public health measures, such as lockdowns, border control, closing working places and schools, social distancing, mobility restrictions, and obligatory green passes. For example, accumulating genomic information on the spread of the highly transmissible, yet low pathogenicity Omicron variant triggered a progressive abandonment of the "zero COVID" policy with compulsory curfews, testing and strict mobility control initially adopted by a series of Eastern-Asian countries [154].

The importance of genomics for public health is underlined by the unexpected emergence of the Omicron variant, attributed either to (a) a continuous, baseline circulation of a slowly changing ancillary strain in a region with low genomic surveillance; (b) persistent infections with prolonged viral shedding and high variability in immunosuppressed persons; and (c) spill out from an unknown animal reservoir [155]. To prevent a similar episode, genomic informed public health measures must be upscaled, including:

- The establishment of an extended global network of pathogen surveillance pursuing a "one health" policy at the human-animal interface
- The use of portable nanopore DNA sequencers for rapid outbreak monitoring in low resource settings
- Early viral detection and characterization using wastewater surveillance systems. Cryptic SARS-CoV-2 lineages, previously unreported by sequencing of symptomatic human cases of SARS CoV-2 infections, harboring common mutations with the Omicron variant and partially resistant to neutralizing antibodies from vaccinated and especially from previously infected patients have been detected in New York City wastewater in 2021 [156].

Genomic data can inform public health policies by:

- Identifying the source of initial clusters of cases in particular settings (health care settings, long-term care facilities, travel vehicles-airplanes, and cruises ships) or in the community, by linkage of the genomic data to demographic, epidemiological, and clinical data sets [157]
- Analyzing super-spreading events to identify human behaviors that are more prone to viral transmission [158]
- Monitoring the viral variability and assessing their potential impact on the community by associating new genotypic features with changes in the antigenicity, infectivity, pathogenicity, and susceptibility to available antivirals and vaccines.
- Adaptation of the vaccine composition to ensure the production of the most efficient vaccines in a timely manner [159].

7. Conclusions

The rapid development of diagnostic tools and COVID-19 vaccines was possible due to the characterization of viral genome and of the structure of the main viral immunogen-the spike glycoprotein.

Surveillance of the emergent variants and assessing their potential impact on the community by genotype to phenotype analysis may control reduction of the effectiveness of available antivirals and vaccines. COVID-19 vaccines developed to date proved to be highly active against hospitalizations and death across all ages, and their large-scale deployment in the middle and high-income countries, has decreased the pressure on the medical system and helped in reopening the economy.

Currently available antiviral therapies prove to be reasonably effective regardless of viral variants and their development should be an important strategy together with vaccination strategy improvement.

With the emergence of viral variants more antigenically distant from the vaccine strains, the utility of adaptation of the vaccine composition, either by adding a variant specific version or by developing a pan-coronavirus vaccine become an important point on the public health agenda.

Acknowledgements

This work was supported by a grant from EU Horizon 2020 Research and Innovation Program, PERISCOPE: Pan European Response to the Impacts of COVID-19 and future Pandemics and Epidemics under grant agreement no. 101016233, H2020-SC1-PHE-CORONAVIRUS-2020-2-RTD (support for C.C. Diaconu), and grants from the Romanian Ministry of Research, Innovation, and Digitization, CNCS-UEFISCDI, PN-III-P1-1.1-PD-2021-0825 and PN-III-P2-2.1-PED-2021-4131.

Conflict of interest

The authors declare no conflict of interest.

Author details

Carmen Cristina Diaconu[1*], Ioana Madalina Pitica[1], Mihaela Chivu-Economescu[1], Laura Georgiana Necula[1], Anca Botezatu[1], Iulia Virginia Iancu[1], Ana Iulia Neagu[1], Elena L. Radu[1,2], Lilia Matei[1], Simona Maria Ruta[1,3] and Coralia Bleotu[1]

1 Stefan S. Nicolau Institute of Virology, Romanian Academy, Bucharest, Romania

2 Institute for Water Quality and Resource Management, TU Wien, Vienna, Austria

3 Faculty of Medicine, Carol Davila University of Medicine and Pharmacy, Bucharest, Romania

*Address all correspondence to: ccdiaconu@yahoo.com; carmen.diaconu@virology.ro

References

[1] Coronavirus Disease. Statistics. New Cases and Deaths. 2022. Available from: https://www.google.com/search?sxsrf=ALeKk03CS16RzZv2-d4WNLT2UeCH7MSOMA:1589689664696&q=covid+19+case+count+worldwide. [Accessed: June 26, 2022]

[2] Thakur S, Sasi S, Pillai SG, Nag A, Shukla D, Singhal R, et al. SARS-CoV-2 mutations and their impact on diagnostics, therapeutics and vaccines. Frontiers in Medicine (Lausanne). 2022;**9**:815389. DOI: 10.3389/fmed.2022.815389

[3] Suwinski P, Ong C, Ling MHT, Poh YM, Khan AM, Ong HS. Advancing personalized medicine through the application of whole exome sequencing and big data analytics. Frontiers in Genetics. 2019;**10**:49. DOI: 10.3389/fgene.2019.00049

[4] Chen Z, Azman A, Chen X, Zou J, Tian Y, et al. Global landscape of SARS-CoV-2 genomic surveillance and data sharing. Nature Genetics. 2022;**54**:499-507. DOI: 10.1038/s41588-022-01033-y

[5] Wu F, Zhao S, Yu B, Chen YM, Wang W, Song ZG, et al. A new coronavirus associated with human respiratory disease in China. Nature. 2020;**579**:265-269. DOI: 10.1038/s41586-020-2008-3

[6] Corman VM, Landt O, Kaiser M, Molenkamp R, Meijer A, Chu DK, et al. Detection of 2019 Novel coronavirus (2019-nCoV) by real-time RT-PCR. Euro Surveillance 2020;25. DOI: 10.2807/1560-7917.ES.2020.25.3.2000045

[7] Zimmerman PA, King CL, Ghannoum M, Bonomo RA, Procop GW. Molecular diagnosis of SARS-CoV-2: Assessing and interpreting nucleic acid and antigen tests. Pathogens and Immunity. 2021;**6**:135-156. DOI: 10.20411/pai.v6i1.422

[8] Habibzadeh P, Mofatteh M, Silawi M, Ghavami S, Faghihi MA. Molecular diagnostic assays for COVID-19: An overview. Critical Reviews in Clinical Laboratory Sciences. 2021;**58**:385-398. DOI: 10.1080/10408363.2021.1884640

[9] CDC. CDC's Diagnostic Test for COVID-19 Only and Supplies. USA: CDC; 2020. Available from: https://www.cdc.gov/coronavirus/2019-ncov/lab/virus-requests.html. [Accessed: May 31, 2022]

[10] Wu A, Peng Y, Huang B, Ding X, Wang X, Niu P, et al. Genome composition and divergence of the novel coronavirus (2019-nCoV) originating in China. Cell Host & Microbe. 2020;**27**:325-328. DOI: 10.1016/j.chom.2020.02.001

[11] Naqvi AAT, Fatima K, Mohammad T, Fatima U, Singh IK, Singh A, et al. Insights into SARS-CoV-2 genome, structure, evolution, pathogenesis and therapies: Structural genomics approach. Biochimica et Biophysica Acta - Molecular Basis of Disease. 2020;**1866**:165878. DOI: 10.1016/j.bbadis.2020.165878

[12] Kim D, Lee JY, Yang JS, Kim JW, Kim VN, Chang H. The architecture of SARS-CoV-2 transcriptome. Cell. 2020;**181**:914-921 e10. DOI: 10.1016/j.cell.2020.04.011

[13] Feng W, Newbigging AM, Le C, Pang B, Peng H, Cao Y, et al. Molecular diagnosis of COVID-19: Challenges and research needs. Analytical Chemistry.

2020;**92**:10196-10209. DOI: 10.1021/acs.analchem.0c02060

[14] Mustafa Hellou M, Gorska A, Mazzaferri F, Cremonini E, Gentilotti E, De Nardo P, et al. Nucleic acid amplification tests on respiratory samples for the diagnosis of coronavirus infections: A systematic review and meta-analysis. Clinical Microbiology and Infection. 2021;**27**:341-351. DOI: 10.1016/j.cmi.2020.11.002

[15] Hindson CM, Chevillet JR, Briggs HA, Gallichotte EN, Ruf IK, Hindson BJ, et al. Absolute quantification by droplet digital PCR versus analog real-time PCR. Nature Methods. 2013;**10**:1003-1005. DOI: 10.1038/nmeth.2633

[16] Kuypers J, Jerome KR. Applications of digital PCR for clinical microbiology. Journal of Clinical Microbiology. 2017;**55**:1621-1628. DOI: 10.1128/JCM.00211-17

[17] Vasudevan HN, Xu P, Servellita V, Miller S, Liu L, Gopez A, et al. Digital droplet PCR accurately quantifies SARS-CoV-2 viral load from crude lysate without nucleic acid purification. Scientific Reports. 2021;**11**:780. DOI: 10.1038/s41598-020-80715-1

[18] Pu R, Liu S, Ren X, Shi D, Ba Y, Huo Y, et al. The screening value of RT-LAMP and RT-PCR in the diagnosis of COVID-19: Systematic review and meta-analysis. Journal of Virological Methods. 2022;**300**:114392. DOI: 10.1016/j.jviromet.2021.114392

[19] Patchsung M, Jantarug K, Pattama A, Aphicho K, Suraritdechachai S, Meesawat P, et al. Clinical validation of a Cas13-based assay for the detection of SARS-CoV-2 RNA. Nature Biomedical Engineering. 2020;**4**:1140-1149. DOI: 10.1038/s41551-020-00603-x

[20] Kellner MJ, Koob JG, Gootenberg JS, Abudayyeh OO, Zhang F. SHERLOCK: Nucleic acid detection with CRISPR nucleases. Nature Protocols. 2019;**14**:2986-3012. DOI: 10.1038/s41596-019-0210-2

[21] Barrera-Avalos C, Luraschi R, Vallejos-Vidal E, Mella-Torres A, Hernandez F, Figueroa M, et al. The rapid antigen detection test for SARS-CoV-2 underestimates the identification of COVID-19 positive cases and compromises the diagnosis of the SARS-CoV-2 (K417N/T, E484K, and N501Y) variants. Frontiers in Public Health. 2021;**9**:780801. DOI: 10.3389/fpubh.2021.780801

[22] Khandker SS, Nik Hashim NHH, Deris ZZ, Shueb RH, Islam MA. Diagnostic accuracy of rapid antigen test kits for detecting SARS-CoV-2: A systematic review and Meta-analysis of 17,171 suspected COVID-19 patients. Journal of Clinical Medicine. 2021;**10**:1-19. DOI: 10.3390/jcm10163493

[23] Salcedo N, Reddy A, Gomez AR, Bosch I, Herrera BB. Monoclonal antibody pairs against SARS-CoV-2 for rapid antigen test development. PLoS Neglected Tropical Diseases. 2022;**16**:e0010311. DOI: 10.1371/journal.pntd.0010311

[24] de Wit E, van Doremalen N, Falzarano D, Munster VJ. SARS and MERS: Recent insights into emerging coronaviruses. Nature Reviews. Microbiology. 2016;**14**:523-534. DOI: 10.1038/nrmicro.2016.81

[25] Kamelian K, Montoya V, Olmstead A, Dong W, Harrigan R, Morshed M, et al. Phylogenetic surveillance of travel-related Zika virus infections through whole-genome sequencing methods. Scientific Reports. 2019;**9**:16433. DOI: 10.1038/s41598-019-52613-8

[26] Shrivastava S, Puri V, Dilley KA, Ngouajio E, Shifflett J, Oldfield LM, et al. Whole genome sequencing, variant analysis, phylogenetics, and deep sequencing of Zika virus strains. Scientific Reports. 2018;**8**:15843. DOI: 10.1038/s41598-018-34147-7

[27] Kugelman JR, Wiley MR, Mate S, Ladner JT, Beitzel B, Fakoli L, et al. Monitoring of Ebola virus Makona evolution through establishment of advanced genomic capability in Liberia. Emerging Infectious Diseases. 2015;**21**:1135-1143. DOI: 10.3201/eid2107.150522

[28] Quick J, Loman NJ, Duraffour S, Simpson JT, Severi E, Cowley L, et al. Real-time, portable genome sequencing for Ebola surveillance. Nature. 2016;**530**:228-232. DOI: 10.1038/nature16996

[29] Chen L, Liu W, Zhang Q, Xu K, Ye G, Wu W, et al. RNA based mNGS approach identifies a novel human coronavirus from two individual pneumonia cases in 2019 Wuhan outbreak. Emerging Microbes & Infections. 2020;**9**:313-319. DOI: 10.1080/22221751.2020.1725399

[30] Chiara M, D'Erchia AM, Gissi C, Manzari C, Parisi A, Resta N, et al. Next generation sequencing of SARS-CoV-2 genomes: Challenges, applications and opportunities. Briefings in Bioinformatics. 2021;**22**:616-630. DOI: 10.1093/bib/bbaa297

[31] Chan JF, Yuan S, Kok KH, To KK, Chu H, Yang J, et al. A familial cluster of pneumonia associated with the 2019 novel coronavirus indicating person-to-person transmission: A study of a family cluster. Lancet. 2020;**395**:514-523. DOI: 10.1016/S0140-6736(20)30154-9

[32] Albert TJ, Molla MN, Muzny DM, Nazareth L, Wheeler D, Song X, et al. Direct selection of human genomic loci by microarray hybridization. Nature Methods. 2007;**4**:903-905. DOI: 10.1038/nmeth1111

[33] Maurano MT, Ramaswami S, Zappile P, Dimartino D, Boytard L, Ribeiro-Dos-Santos AM, et al. Sequencing identifies multiple early introductions of SARS-CoV-2 to the new York City region. Genome Research. 2020;**30**:1781-1788. DOI: 10.1101/gr.266676.120

[34] Vacca D, Fiannaca A, Tramuto F, Cancila V, La Paglia L, Mazzucco W, et al. Direct RNA Nanopore sequencing of SARS-CoV-2 extracted from critical material from swabs. Life (Basel). 2022;**12**:1-13. DOI: 10.3390/life12010069

[35] Amarasinghe SL, Su S, Dong X, Zappia L, Ritchie ME, Gouil Q. Opportunities and challenges in long-read sequencing data analysis. Genome Biology. 2020;**21**:30. DOI: 10.1186/s13059-020-1935-5

[36] Hu T, Li J, Zhou H, Li C, Holmes EC, Shi W. Bioinformatics resources for SARS-CoV-2 discovery and surveillance. Briefings in Bioinformatics. 2021;**22**:631-641. DOI: 10.1093/bib/bbaa386

[37] Wee Y, Bhyan SB, Liu Y, Lu J, Li X, Zhao M. The bioinformatics tools for the genome assembly and analysis based on third-generation sequencing. Briefings in Functional Genomics. 2019;**18**:1-12. DOI: 10.1093/bfgp/ely037

[38] Doddapaneni H, Cregeen SJ, Sucgang R, Meng Q, Qin X, Avadhanula V, et al. Oligonucleotide capture sequencing of the SARS-CoV-2 genome and subgenomic fragments from COVID-19 individuals. bioRxiv. 2020. 29 p. DOI: 10.1101/2020.07.27.223495 [Preprint]

[39] Vollmers J, Wiegand S, Kaster AK. Comparing and evaluating metagenome assembly tools from a Microbiologist's perspective - not only size matters! PLoS One. 2017;**12**:e0169662. DOI: 10.1371/journal.pone.0169662

[40] Simpson JT, Pop M. The theory and practice of genome sequence assembly. Annual Review of Genomics and Human Genetics. 2015;**16**:153-172. DOI: 10.1146/annurev-genom-090314-050032

[41] Dominguez Del Angel V, Hjerde E, Sterck L, Capella-Gutierrez S, Notredame C, Vinnere Pettersson O, et al. Ten steps to get started in genome assembly and annotation. F1000Res. 2018;7:1-24. DOI: 10.12688/f1000research.13598.1

[42] Hadfield J, Megill C, Bell SM, Huddleston J, Potter B, Callender C, et al. Nextstrain: Real-time tracking of pathogen evolution. Bioinformatics. 2018;**34**:4121-4123. DOI: 10.1093/bioinformatics/bty407

[43] Pond SL, Frost SD, Muse SV. HyPhy: Hypothesis testing using phylogenies. Bioinformatics. 2005;**21**:676-679. DOI: 10.1093/bioinformatics/bti079

[44] Shu Y, McCauley J. GISAID: Global initiative on sharing all influenza data - from vision to reality. Euro Surveillance. 2017;**22**:1-3. DOI: 10.2807/1560-7917.ES.2017.22.13.30494

[45] Meredith LW, Hamilton WL, Warne B, Houldcroft CJ, Hosmillo M, Jahun AS, et al. Rapid implementation of SARS-CoV-2 sequencing to investigate cases of health-care associated COVID-19: A prospective genomic surveillance study. The Lancet Infectious Diseases. 2020;**20**:1263-1272. DOI: 10.1016/S1473-3099(20)30562-4

[46] Brister JR, Ako-Adjei D, Bao Y, Blinkova O. NCBI viral genomes resource. Nucleic Acids Research. 2015;**43**:D571-D577. DOI: 10.1093/nar/gku1207

[47] Dikdan RJ, Marras SAE, Field AP, Brownlee A, Cironi A, Hill DA, et al. Multiplex PCR assays for identifying all major severe acute respiratory syndrome coronavirus 2 variants. The Journal of Molecular Diagnostics. 2022;**24**:309-319. DOI: 10.1016/j.jmoldx.2022.01.004

[48] John G, Sahajpal NS, Mondal AK, Ananth S, Williams C, Chaubey A, et al. Next-generation sequencing (NGS) in COVID-19: A tool for SARS-CoV-2 diagnosis, monitoring new strains and Phylodynamic Modeling in molecular epidemiology. Current Issues in Molecular Biology. 2021;**43**:845-867. DOI: 10.3390/cimb43020061

[49] Fu JYL, Chong YM, Sam IC, Chan YF. SARS-CoV-2 multiplex RT-PCR to detect variants of concern (VOCs) in Malaysia, between January to may 2021. Journal of Virological Methods. 2022;**301**:114462. DOI: 10.1016/j.jviromet.2022.114462

[50] Chung HY, Jian MJ, Chang CK, Lin JC, Yeh KM, Chen CW, et al. Emergency SARS-CoV-2 variants of concern: Novel multiplex real-time RT-PCR assay for rapid detection and surveillance. Microbiology Spectrum. 2022;**10**:e0251321. DOI: 10.1128/spectrum.02513-21

[51] Zhen W, Berry GJ. Development of a new multiplex real-time RT-PCR assay for severe acute respiratory syndrome coronavirus 2 (SARS-CoV-2) detection. The Journal of Molecular Diagnostics. 2020;**22**:1367-1372. DOI: 10.1016/j.jmoldx.2020.09.004

[52] Khateeb J, Li Y, Zhang H. Emerging SARS-CoV-2 variants of concern and potential intervention approaches.

Critical Care. 2021;**25**:244. DOI: 10.1186/s13054-021-03662-x

[53] Nörz D, Grunwald M, Olearo F, Fischer N, Aepfelbacher M, Pfefferle S, et al. Evaluation of a fully automated high-throughput SARS-CoV-2 multiplex qPCR assay with build-in screening functionality for DelHV69/70- and N501Y variants such as B.1.1.7. Journal of Clinical Virology. 2020;**141**:104894, 1-4. DOI: 10.1016/j.jcv.2021.104894

[54] WHO. Terms of Reference for the Technical Advisory Group on SARS-CoV-2 Virus Evolution (TAG-VE). 2021. Available from: https://www.who.int/publications/m/item/terms-of-reference-for-the-technical-advisory-group-on-sars-cov-2-virus-evolution-(tag-ve). [Accessed: June 23, 2022]

[55] PANGO. 2022. Available from: https://cov-lineages.org/index.html#global_reports. [Accessed: June 23, 2022]

[56] Nextstrain. 2022. Available from: https://nextstrain.org [Accessed: June 23, 2022]

[57] GISAID. 2022. Available from: https://www.gisaid.org/hcov19-variants/. [Accessed: June 23, 2022]

[58] WHO. Tracking SARS-CoV-2 Variants. 2022. Available from: https://www.who.int/en/activities/tracking-SARS-CoV-2-variants/. [Accessed: June 24, 2022]

[59] ECDC. SARS-CoV-2 Variants of Concern as of 9 June 2022. 2022. Available from: https://www.ecdc.europa.eu/en/covid-19/variants-concern. [Accessed: June 24, 2022]

[60] Amoutzias GD, Nikolaidis M, Tryfonopoulou E, Chlichlia K, Markoulatos P, Oliver SG. The remarkable evolutionary plasticity of coronaviruses by mutation and recombination: Insights for the COVID-19 pandemic and the future evolutionary paths of SARS-CoV-2. Viruses. 2022;**14**:78

[61] MacLean OA, Lytras S, Weaver S, Singer JB, Boni MF, Lemey P, et al. Natural selection in the evolution of SARS-CoV-2 in bats created a generalist virus and highly capable human pathogen. PLOS Biology. 2021;**19**:e3001115. DOI: 10.1371/journal.pbio.3001115

[62] Amicone M, Borges V, Alves MJ, Isidro J, Zé-Zé L, Duarte S, et al. Mutation rate of SARS-CoV-2 and emergence of mutators during experimental evolution. Evolution, Medicine, and Public Health. 2022;**10**:142-155. DOI: 10.1093/emph/eoac010

[63] Banerjee A, Mossman K, Grandvaux N. Molecular determinants of SARS-CoV-2 variants. Trends in Microbiology. 2021;**29**:871-873. DOI: 10.1016/j.tim.2021.07.002

[64] Pollett S, Conte MA, Sanborn M, Jarman RG, Lidl GM, Modjarrad K, et al. A comparative recombination analysis of human coronaviruses and implications for the SARS-CoV-2 pandemic. Scientific Reports. 2021;**11**:17365. DOI: 10.1038/s41598-021-96626-8

[65] Yamasoba D, Kimura I, Nasser H, Morioka Y, Nao N, Ito J, et al. Virological characteristics of the SARS-CoV-2 omicron BA.2 spike. Cell. 2022;**185**:2103-2115 e19. DOI: 10.1016/j.cell.2022.04.035

[66] Jackson CB, Farzan M, Chen B, Choe H. Mechanisms of SARS-CoV-2 entry into cells. Nature Reviews. Molecular Cell Biology. 2022;**23**:3-20. DOI: 10.1038/s41580-021-00418-x

[67] Saha I, Ghosh N, Sharma N, Nandi S. Hotspot mutations in SARS-CoV-2.

Frontiers in Genetics. 2021;**12**:1-16. DOI: 10.3389/fgene.2021.753440

[68] Rahbar MR, Jahangiri A, Khalili S, Zarei M, Mehrabani-Zeinabad K, Khalesi B, et al. Hotspots for mutations in the SARS-CoV-2 spike glycoprotein: A correspondence analysis. Scientific Reports. 2021;**11**:23622. DOI: 10.1038/s41598-021-01655-y

[69] Zhang L, Jackson CB, Mou H, Ojha A, Peng H, Quinlan BD, et al. SARS-CoV-2 spike-protein D614G mutation increases virion spike density and infectivity. Nature Communications. 2020;**11**:6013. DOI: 10.1038/s41467-020-19808-4

[70] Grubaugh ND, Hanage WP, Rasmussen AL. Making sense of mutation: What D614G means for the COVID-19 pandemic remains unclear. Cell. 2020;**182**:794-795. DOI: 10.1016/j.cell.2020.06.040

[71] Volz E, Hill V, McCrone JT, Price A, Jorgensen D, O'Toole A, et al. Evaluating the effects of SARS-CoV-2 spike mutation D614G on transmissibility and pathogenicity. Cell. 2021;**184**:64-75 e11. DOI: 10.1016/j.cell.2020.11.020

[72] Al Kaabi N, Zhang Y, Xia S, Yang Y, Al Qahtani MM, Abdulrazzaq N, et al. Effect of 2 inactivated SARS-CoV-2 vaccines on symptomatic COVID-19 infection in adults: A randomized clinical trial. Journal of the American Medical Association. 2021;**326**:35-45. DOI: 10.1001/jama.2021.8565

[73] Yurkovetskiy L, Wang X, Pascal KE, Tomkins-Tinch C, Nyalile TP, Wang Y, et al. Structural and functional analysis of the D614G SARS-CoV-2 spike protein variant. Cell. 2020;**183**:739-751 e8. DOI: 10.1016/j.cell.2020.09.032

[74] Zhang Y, Zhang H, Zhang W. SARS-CoV-2 variants, immune escape, and countermeasures. Frontiers in Medicine. 2022;**16**:196-207. DOI: 10.1007/s11684-021-0906-x

[75] Harvey WT, Carabelli AM, Jackson B, Gupta RK, Thomson EC, Harrison EM, et al. SARS-CoV-2 variants, spike mutations and immune escape. Nature Reviews Microbiology. 2021;**19**:409-424. DOI: 10.1038/s41579-021-00573-0

[76] Meng B, Kemp SA, Papa G, Datir R, Ferreira I, Marelli S, et al. Recurrent emergence of SARS-CoV-2 spike deletion H69/V70 and its role in the alpha variant B.1.1.7. Cell Reports. 2021;**35**:109292. DOI: 10.1016/j.celrep.2021.109292

[77] Thakur S, Sasi S, Pillai SG, Nag A, Shukla D, Singhal R, et al. SARS-CoV-2 mutations and their impact on diagnostics. Therapeutics and Vaccines. Frontiers in Medicine. 2022;**9**:1-16. DOI: 10.3389/fmed.2022.815389

[78] Hoter A, Naim HY. Biochemical characterization of SARS-CoV-2 spike RBD mutations and their impact on ACE2 receptor binding. Frontiers in Molecular Biosciences. 2022;**9**:893843. DOI: 10.3389/fmolb.2022.893843

[79] Tchesnokova V, Kulasekara H, Larson L, Bowers V, Rechkina E, Kisiela D, et al. Acquisition of the L452R mutation in the ACE2-binding Interface of spike protein triggers recent massive expansion of SARS-CoV-2 variants. Journal of Clinical Microbiology. 2021;**59**:e00921-e00921. DOI: 10.1128/JCM.00921-21

[80] Di Giacomo S, Mercatelli D, Rakhimov A, Giorgi FM. Preliminary report on severe acute respiratory syndrome coronavirus 2 (SARS-CoV-2) spike mutation T478K. Journal of Medical Virology. 2021;**93**:5638-5643. DOI: 10.1002/jmv.27062

[81] Mlcochova P, Kemp SA, Dhar MS, Papa G, Meng B, Ferreira I, et al. SARS-CoV-2 B.1.617.2 Delta variant replication and immune evasion. Nature. 2021;**599**:114-119. DOI: 10.1038/s41586-021-03944-y

[82] Saito A, Irie T, Suzuki R, Maemura T, Nasser H, Uriu K, et al. Enhanced fusogenicity and pathogenicity of SARS-CoV-2 Delta P681R mutation. Nature. 2022;**602**:300-306. DOI: 10.1038/s41586-021-04266-9

[83] Piccoli L, Park YJ, Tortorici MA, Czudnochowski N, Walls AC, Beltramello M, et al. Mapping neutralizing and Immunodominant sites on the SARS-CoV-2 spike receptor-binding domain by structure-guided high-resolution serology. Cell. 2020;**183**:1024-1042 e21. DOI: 10.1016/j.cell.2020.09.037

[84] Zeng X, Li L, Lin J, Li X, Liu B, Kong Y, et al. Isolation of a human monoclonal antibody specific for the receptor binding domain of SARS-CoV-2 using a competitive phage biopanning strategy. Antibody Therapeutics. 2020;**3**:95-100. DOI: 10.1093/abt/tbaa008

[85] Brouwer PJM, Caniels TG, van der Straten K, Snitselaar JL, Aldon Y, Bangaru S, et al. Potent neutralizing antibodies from COVID-19 patients define multiple targets of vulnerability. Science. 2020;**369**:643-650. DOI: 10.1126/science.abc5902

[86] Cerutti G, Guo Y, Zhou T, Gorman J, Lee M, Rapp M, et al. Potent SARS-CoV-2 neutralizing antibodies directed against spike N-terminal domain target a single supersite. Cell Host & Microbe. 2021;**29**:819-833 e7. DOI: 10.1016/j.chom.2021.03.005

[87] Chi X, Yan R, Zhang J, Zhang G, Zhang Y, Hao M, et al. A neutralizing human antibody binds to the N-terminal domain of the spike protein of SARS-CoV-2. Science. 2020;**369**:650-655. DOI: 10.1126/science.abc6952

[88] Wang N, Sun Y, Feng R, Wang Y, Guo Y, Zhang L, et al. Structure-based development of human antibody cocktails against SARS-CoV-2. Cell Research. 2021;**31**:101-103. DOI: 10.1038/s41422-020-00446-w

[89] Barnes CO, West AP Jr, Huey-Tubman KE, Hoffmann MAG, Sharaf NG, Hoffman PR, et al. Structures of human antibodies bound to SARS-CoV-2 spike reveal common epitopes and recurrent features of antibodies. Cell. 2020;**182**:828-842 e16. DOI: 10.1016/j.cell.2020.06.025

[90] Andrews N, Stowe J, Kirsebom F, Toffa S, Sachdeva R, Gower C, et al. Effectiveness of COVID-19 booster vaccines against COVID-19-related symptoms, hospitalization and death in England. Nature Medicine. 2022;**28**:831-837. DOI: 10.1038/s41591-022-01699-1

[91] Burioni R, Topol EJ. Has SARS-CoV-2 reached peak fitness? Nature Medicine. 2021;**27**:1323-1324. DOI: 10.1038/s41591-021-01421-7

[92] Simon-Loriere E, Schwartz O. Towards SARS-CoV-2 serotypes? Nature Reviews Microbiology. 2022;**20**:187-188. DOI: 10.1038/s41579-022-00708-x

[93] Hachmann NP, Miller J, A-rY C, Ventura JD, Yu J, Rowe M, et al. Neutralization escape by SARS-CoV-2 omicron subvariants BA.2.12.1, BA.4, and BA.5. New England Journal of Medicine. 2022;**387**:86-88. DOI: 10.1056/NEJMc2206576

[94] WHO. COVID-19 Vaccine Tracker and Landscape. 2022. Available from: https://www.who.int/publications/m/

item/draft-landscape-of-covid-19-candidate-vaccines [Accessed: June 28, 2022]

[95] Fiolet T, Kherabi Y, MacDonald C-J, Ghosn J, Peiffer-Smadja N. Comparing COVID-19 vaccines for their characteristics, efficacy and effectiveness against SARS-CoV-2 and variants of concern: A narrative review. Clinical Microbiology and Infection. 2022;**28**:202-221. DOI: 10.1016/j.cmi.2021.10.005

[96] CDC. Allergic reactions including anaphylaxis after receipt of the first dose of Pfizer-BioNTech COVID-19 vaccine - United States, December 14-23, 2020. MMWR. Morbidity and Mortality Weekly Report. 2021;**70**:46-51. DOI: 10.15585/mmwr.mm7002e1

[97] Li M, Wang H, Tian L, Pang Z, Yang Q, Huang T, et al. COVID-19 vaccine development: milestones, lessons and prospects. Signal Transduction and Targeted Therapy. 2022;**7**:146. DOI: 10.1038/s41392-022-00996-y

[98] Creech CB, Walker SC, Samuels RJ. SARS-CoV-2 Vaccines. Journal of the American Medical Association. 2021;**325**:1318-1320. DOI: 10.1001/jama.2021.3199

[99] Dai L, Gao GF. Viral targets for vaccines against COVID-19. Nature Reviews Immunology. 2021;**21**:73-82. DOI: 10.1038/s41577-020-00480-0

[100] Xia S, Zhang Y, Wang Y, Wang H, Yang Y, Gao GF, et al. Safety and immunogenicity of an inactivated SARS-CoV-2 vaccine, BBIBP-CorV: A randomised, double-blind, placebo-controlled, phase 1/2 trial. The Lancet Infectious Diseases. 2021;**21**:39-51. DOI: 10.1016/S1473-3099(20)30831-8

[101] Vanaparthy R, Mohan G, Vasireddy D, Atluri P. Review of COVID-19 viral vector-based vaccines and COVID-19 variants. Le Infezioni in Medicina. 2021;**29**:328

[102] Folegatti PM, Ewer KJ, Aley PK, Angus B, Becker S, Belij-Rammerstorfer S, et al. Safety and immunogenicity of the ChAdOx1 nCoV-19 vaccine against SARS-CoV-2: A preliminary report of a phase 1/2, single-blind, randomised controlled trial. The Lancet. 2020;**396**:467-478. DOI: 10.1016/S0140-6736(20)31604-4

[103] Pavord S, Hunt BJ, Horner D, Bewley S, Karpusheff J. Vaccine induced immune thrombocytopenia and thrombosis: Summary of NICE guidance. BMJ. 2021;**375**:n2195. DOI: 10.1136/bmj.n2195

[104] Trimpert J, Dietert K, Firsching TC, Ebert N, Thi Nhu Thao T, Vladimirova D, et al. Development of safe and highly protective live-attenuated SARS-CoV-2 vaccine candidates by genome recoding. Cell Reports. 2021;**36**:1-19. DOI: 10.1016/j.celrep.2021.109493

[105] Motamedi H, Ari MM, Dashtbin S, Fathollahi M, Hossainpour H, Alvandi A, et al. An update review of globally reported SARS-CoV-2 vaccines in preclinical and clinical stages. International Immunopharmacology. 2021;**96**:107763. DOI: 10.1016/j.intimp.2021.107763

[106] Fathizadeh H, Afshar S, Masoudi MR, Gholizadeh P, Asgharzadeh M, Ganbarov K, et al. SARS-CoV-2 (Covid-19) vaccines structure, mechanisms and effectiveness: A review. International Journal of Biological Macromolecules. 2021;**188**:740-750. DOI: 10.1016/j.ijbiomac.2021.08.076

[107] Turner JS, O'Halloran JA, Kalaidina E, Kim W, Schmitz AJ, Zhou

JQ, et al. SARS-CoV-2 mRNA vaccines induce persistent human germinal centre responses. Nature. 2021;**596**:109-113. DOI: 10.1038/s41586-021-03738-2

[108] Rosner CM, Genovese L, Tehrani BN, Atkins M, Bakhshi H, Chaudhri S, et al. Myocarditis temporally associated with COVID-19 vaccination. Circulation. 2021;**144**:502-505. DOI: 10.1161/CIRCULATIONAHA.121.055891

[109] Kim C, Kim J-D, Seo S-U. Nanoparticle and virus-like particle vaccine approaches against SARS-CoV-2. Journal of Microbiology. 2022;**60**:335-346. DOI: 10.1007/s12275-022-1608-z

[110] Abu-Raddad LJ, Chemaitelly H, Butt AA. Effectiveness of the BNT162b2 Covid-19 vaccine against the B.1.1.7 and B.1.351 variants. New England Journal of Medicine. 2021;**385**:187-189. DOI: 10.1056/NEJMc2104974

[111] Gruell H, Vanshylla K, Tober-Lau P, Hillus D, Schommers P, Lehmann C, et al. mRNA booster immunization elicits potent neutralizing serum activity against the SARS-CoV-2 omicron variant. Nature Medicine. 2022;**28**:477-480. DOI: 10.1038/s41591-021-01676-0

[112] Lechmere T, Snell LB, Graham C, Seow J, Shalim ZA, Charalampous T, et al. Broad neutralization of SARS-CoV-2 variants, including omicron, following breakthrough infection with Delta in COVID-19-vaccinated individuals. MBio. 2022;**13**:e03798-e03721. DOI: 10.1128/mbio.03798-21

[113] Pfizer. Pfizer and BioNTech Announce Omicron-Adapted COVID-19 Vaccine Candidates Demonstrate High Immune Response against Omicron. 2022. Available from: https://www.pfizer.com/news/press-release/press-release-detail/pfizer-and-biontech-announce-omicron-adapted-covid-19. [Accessed: June 26, 2022]

[114] Moderna. Moderna Announces Omicron-Containing Bivalent Booster Candidate mRNA-1273.214 Demonstrates Superior Antibody Response against Omicron. 2022. Available from: https://investors.modernatx.com/news/news-details/2022/Moderna-Announces-Omicron-Containing-Bivalent-Booster-Candidate-mRNA-1273.214-Demonstrates-Superior-Antibody-Response-Against-Omicron/default.aspx. [Accessed: June 26, 2022]

[115] WHO. Interim Statement on the Composition of Current COVID-19 Vaccines. 2022. Available from: https://www.who.int/news/item/17-06-2022-interim-statement-on--the-composition-of-current-COVID-19-vaccines. [Accessed: June 25, 2022]

[116] Lupașcu RE, Ilie MI, Velescu BȘ, Udeanu DI, Sultana C, Ruță S, et al. COVID-19-current Therapeutical approaches and future perspectives. PRO. 2022;**10**:1053

[117] US Food&Drug Administration. Emergency Use Authorization. 2022. Available from: https://www.fda.gov/emergency-preparedness-and-response/mcm-legal-regulatory-and-policy-framework/emergency-use-authorization#coviddrugs. [Accessed: May 28, 2022]

[118] Westendorf K, Žentelis S, Wang L, Foster D, Vaillancourt P, Wiggin M, et al. LY-CoV1404 (bebtelovimab) potently neutralizes SARS-CoV-2 variants. Cell Reports. 2022;**39**:1-17. DOI: 10.1016/j.celrep.2022.110812

[119] European Medicines Agency. Conditional Marketing Authorization. 2022. Available from: https://www.

ema.europa.eu/en/human-regulatory/marketing-authorisation/conditional-marketing-authorisation. [Accessed: May 28, 2022]

[120] LiverTox: Clinical and Research Information on Drug-Induced Liver Injury. Bethesda (MD): National Institute of Diabetes and Digestive and Kidney Diseases; 2012

[121] Merck and Ridgeback Bio Collaborate to Advance Development of Novel Antiviral Candidate, EIDD-2801. USA: Business Wire; 2022

[122] Jayk Bernal A, Gomes da Silva MM, Musungaie DB, Kovalchuk E, Gonzalez A, Delos Reyes V, et al. Molnupiravir for Oral treatment of Covid-19 in nonhospitalized patients. The New England Journal of Medicine. 2022;**386**:509-520. DOI: 10.1056/NEJMoa2116044

[123] Sheahan TP, Sims AC, Zhou S, Graham RL, Pruijssers AJ, Agostini ML, et al. An orally bioavailable broad-spectrum antiviral inhibits SARS-CoV-2 in human airway epithelial cell cultures and multiple coronaviruses in mice. Science Translational Medicine. 2020;**12**:1-20. DOI: 10.1126/scitranslmed.abb5883

[124] Urakova N, Kuznetsova V, Crossman DK, Sokratian A, Guthrie DB, Kolykhalov AA, et al. beta-d-N (4)-Hydroxycytidine is a potent anti-alphavirus compound that induces a high level of mutations in the viral genome. Journal of Virology. 2018;**92**: 1-22. DOI: 10.1128/JVI.01965-17

[125] Merck. Merck and Ridgeback to Present Data Demonstrating that Treatment with LAGEVRIO™ (Molnupiravir) Was Associated with more Rapid Elimination of Infectious SARS-CoV-2 than Placebo. 2022. Available from: https://www.merck.com/news/merck-and-ridgeback-to-present-data-demonstrating-that-treatment-with-lagevrio-molnupiravir-was-associated-with-more-rapid-elimination-of-infectious-sars-cov-2-than-placebo/. [Accessed: May 28, 2022]

[126] US Food & Drug Administration. Emergency Use Authorization 108. 2022. Available from: https://www.fda.gov/media/155053/download. [Accessed: May 28, 2022]

[127] Owen DR, Allerton CMN, Anderson AS, Aschenbrenner L, Avery M, Berritt S, et al. An oral SARS-CoV-2 M(pro) inhibitor clinical candidate for the treatment of COVID-19. Science. 2021;**374**:1586-1593. DOI: 10.1126/science.abl4784

[128] Sevrioukova IF, Poulos TL. Structure and mechanism of the complex between cytochrome P4503A4 and ritonavir. Proceedings of the National Academy of Sciences of the United States of America. 2010;**107**:18422-18427. DOI: 10.1073/pnas.1010693107

[129] Hammond J, Leister-Tebbe H, Gardner A, Abreu P, Bao W, Wisemandle W, et al. Oral Nirmatrelvir for high-risk, nonhospitalized adults with Covid-19. The New England Journal of Medicine. 2022;**386**:1397-1408. DOI: 10.1056/NEJMoa2118542

[130] European Medicines Agency. Paxlovid, INN-PF-07321332 + Ritonavir. Summary of Product Characteristics. 2022. Available from: https://www.ema.europa.eu/en/documents/product-information/paxlovid-epar-product-information_en.pdf. [Accessed: May 29, 2022]

[131] Marzolini C, Kuritzkes DR, Marra F, Boyle A, Gibbons S, Flexner C, et al. Prescribing Nirmatrelvir-ritonavir: How to recognize and manage

drug-drug interactions. Annals of Internal Medicine. 2022;**175**:744-746. DOI: 10.7326/m22-0281

[132] US Food & Drug Administration. Emergency Use Authorization 105 2022. Available from: https://www.fda.gov/media/155049/download. [Accessed: May 29, 2022]

[133] European Medicines Agency. Paxlovid. 2022. Available from: https://www.ema.europa.eu/en/medicines/human/EPAR/paxlovid. [Accessed: May 29, 2022]

[134] Li P, Wang Y, Lavrijsen M, Lamers MM, de Vries AC, Rottier RJ, et al. SARS-CoV-2 omicron variant is highly sensitive to molnupiravir, nirmatrelvir, and the combination. Cell Research. 2022;**32**:322-324. DOI: 10.1038/s41422-022-00618-w

[135] Brown AJ, Won JJ, Graham RL, Dinnon KH 3rd, Sims AC, Feng JY, et al. Broad spectrum antiviral remdesivir inhibits human endemic and zoonotic deltacoronaviruses with a highly divergent RNA dependent RNA polymerase. Antiviral Research. 2019;**169**:104541. DOI: 10.1016/j.antiviral.2019.104541

[136] Sheahan TP, Sims AC, Leist SR, Schäfer A, Won J, Brown AJ, et al. Comparative therapeutic efficacy of remdesivir and combination lopinavir, ritonavir, and interferon beta against MERS-CoV. Nature Communications. 2020;**11**:222. DOI: 10.1038/s41467-019-13940-6

[137] Agostini ML, Andres EL, Sims AC, Graham RL, Sheahan TP, Lu X, et al. Coronavirus susceptibility to the antiviral Remdesivir (GS-5734) is mediated by the viral polymerase and the proofreading exoribonuclease. MBio. 2018;**9**:1-15. DOI: 10.1128/mBio.00221-18

[138] Beigel JH, Tomashek KM, Dodd LE, Mehta AK, Zingman BS, Kalil AC, et al. Remdesivir for the treatment of Covid-19 - final report. The New England Journal of Medicine. 2020;**383**:1813-1826. DOI: 10.1056/NEJMoa2007764

[139] Gottlieb RL, Vaca CE, Paredes R, Mera J, Webb BJ, Perez G, et al. Early Remdesivir to prevent progression to severe Covid-19 in outpatients. The New England Journal of Medicine. 2022;**386**:305-315. DOI: 10.1056/NEJMoa2116846

[140] US Food & Drug Administration. FDA NEWS RELEASE: FDA Takes Actions to Expand Use of Treatment for Outpatients with Mild-to-Moderate COVID-19. 2022. Available from: https://www.fda.gov/news-events/press-announcements/fda-takes-actions-expand-use-treatment-outpatients-mild-moderate-covid-19. [Accessed: May 30, 2022]

[141] Vangeel L, Chiu W, De Jonghe S, Maes P, Slechten B, Raymenants J, et al. Remdesivir, Molnupiravir and Nirmatrelvir remain active against SARS-CoV-2 omicron and other variants of concern. Antiviral Research. 2022;**198**:105252. DOI: 10.1016/j.antiviral.2022.105252

[142] Kalil AC, Patterson TF, Mehta AK, Tomashek KM, Wolfe CR, Ghazaryan V, et al. Baricitinib plus Remdesivir for hospitalized adults with Covid-19. The New England Journal of Medicine. 2021;**384**:795-807. DOI: 10.1056/NEJMoa2031994

[143] Kyriazopoulou E, Poulakou G, Milionis H, Metallidis S, Adamis G, Tsiakos K, et al. Early treatment of COVID-19 with anakinra guided by soluble urokinase plasminogen receptor plasma levels: A double-blind, randomized controlled phase 3 trial.

Nature Medicine. 2021;**27**:1752-1760. DOI: 10.1038/s41591-021-01499-z

[144] Vikse J, Henry BM. Tocilizumab in COVID-19: Beware the risk of intestinal perforation. International Journal of Antimicrobial Agents. 2020;**56**:106009. DOI: 10.1016/j.ijantimicag.2020.106009

[145] Bruce-Hickman D, Sajeed SM, Pang YH, Seow CS, Chen W, Gulati KM. Bowel ulceration following tocilizumab administration in a COVID-19 patient. BMJ Open Gastroenterology. 2020;**7**:1-5. DOI: 10.1136/bmjgast-2020-000484

[146] Vanshylla K, Fan C, Wunsch M, Poopalasingam N, Meijers M, Kreer C, et al. Discovery of ultrapotent broadly neutralizing antibodies from SARS-CoV-2 elite neutralizers. Cell Host & Microbe. 2022;**30**:69-82.e10. DOI: 10.1016/j.chom.2021.12.010

[147] National Institutes of Health (NIH). COVID-19 Treatment Guidelines. 2022. Available from: https://www.covid19treatmentguidelines.nih.gov/therapies/anti-sars-cov-2-antibody-products/convalescent-plasma/. [Accessed: May 30, 2022]

[148] López MG, Chiner-Oms Á, García de Viedma D, Ruiz-Rodriguez P, Bracho MA, Cancino-Muñoz I, et al. The first wave of the COVID-19 epidemic in Spain was associated with early introductions and fast spread of a dominating genetic variant. Nature Genetics. 2021;**53**:1405-1414. DOI: 10.1038/s41588-021-00936-6

[149] Oude Munnink BB, Nieuwenhuijse DF, Stein M, O'Toole Á, Haverkate M, Mollers M, et al. Rapid SARS-CoV-2 whole-genome sequencing and analysis for informed public health decision-making in the Netherlands. Nature Medicine. 2020;**26**:1405-1410. DOI: 10.1038/s41591-020-0997-y

[150] Vöhringer HS, Sanderson T, Sinnott M, De Maio N, Nguyen T, Goater R, et al. Genomic reconstruction of the SARS-CoV-2 epidemic in England. Nature. 2021;**600**:506-511. DOI: 10.1038/s41586-021-04069-y

[151] Volz E, Mishra S, Chand M, Barrett JC, Johnson R, Geidelberg L, et al. Assessing transmissibility of SARS-CoV-2 lineage B.1.1.7 in England. Nature. 2021;**593**:266-269. DOI: 10.1038/s41586-021-03470-x

[152] Tegally H, Wilkinson E, Giovanetti M, Iranzadeh A, Fonseca V, Giandhari J, et al. Detection of a SARS-CoV-2 variant of concern in South Africa. Nature. 2021;**592**:438-443. DOI: 10.1038/s41586-021-03402-9

[153] Viana R, Moyo S, Amoako DG, Tegally H, Scheepers C, Althaus CL, et al. Rapid epidemic expansion of the SARS-CoV-2 omicron variant in southern Africa. Nature. 2022;**603**:679-686. DOI: 10.1038/s41586-022-04411-y

[154] Cai J, Deng X, Yang J, Sun K, Liu H, Chen Z, et al. Modeling transmission of SARS-CoV-2 omicron in China. Nature Medicine. 2022;**28**:1468-1475. DOI: 10.1038/s41591-022-01855-7

[155] Telenti A, Hodcroft EB, Robertson DL. The evolution and biology of SARS-CoV-2 variants. Cold Spring Harbor Perspectives in Medicine. 2022;**12**:1-24. DOI: 10.1101/cshperspect.a041390

[156] Smyth DS, Trujillo M, Gregory DA, Cheung K, Gao A, Graham M, et al. Tracking cryptic SARS-CoV-2 lineages detected in NYC wastewater. Nature Communications. 2022;**13**:635, 1-9. DOI: 10.1038/s41467-022-28246-3

[157] Colijn C, Earn DJ, Dushoff J, Ogden NH, Li M, Knox N, et al. The need

for linked genomic surveillance of SARS-CoV-2. Canada Communicable Disease Report. 2022;**48**:131-139. DOI: 10.14745/ccdr.v48i04a03

[158] Koopsen J, van Ewijk CE, Bavalia R, Cornelissen A, Bruisten SM, de Gee F, et al. Epidemiologic and genomic analysis of SARS-CoV-2 Delta variant Superspreading event in nightclub, the Netherlands, June 2021. Emerging Infectious Diseases. 2022;**28**:1012-1016. DOI: 10.3201/eid2805.212019

[159] WHO. Interim Statement on COVID-19 Vaccines in the Context of the Circulation of the Omicron SARS-CoV-2 Variant from the WHO Technical Advisory Group on COVID-19 Vaccine Composition (TAG-CO-VAC). 2022. Available from: https://www.who.int/news/item/11-01-2022-interim-statement-on-covid-19-vaccines-in-the-context-of-the-circulation-of-the-omicron-sars-cov-2-variant-from-the-who-technical-advisory-group-on-covid-19-vaccine-composition. [Accessed: June 26, 2022]

Section 2

Diagnosis and Treatment

Chapter 9

Advances in Diagnosis and Treatment for SARS-CoV-2 Variants

Naheed Akhter, Sadia Sana, Muhammad Adnan Ahsan, Zafaar Siddique, Abu Huraira and Somara Sana

Abstract

The COVID-19 pandemic's epidemiological and clinical characteristics have been affected in recent months by the introduction of SARS-CoV-2 variants with unique spikes of protein alterations. These variations can lessen the protection provided by suppressing monoclonal antibodies and vaccines, as well as enhance the frequencies of transmission of the virus and/or the risk of contracting the disease. Due to these mutations, SARS-CoV-2 may be able to proliferate despite increasing levels of vaccination coverage while preserving and enhancing its reproduction efficiency. This is one of the main strategies in tackling the COVID-19 epidemics, the accessibility of precise and trustworthy biomarkers for the SARS-CoV-2 genetic material and also its nucleic acids is important to investigate the disease in suspect communities, start making diagnoses and management in symptomatic or asymptomatic persons, and evaluate authorization of the pathogen after infection. Quantitative reverse transcriptase polymerase chain reaction (qRT-PCR) for virus nucleic acid identification is still the most effective method for such uses due to its sensitivity, quickness, high-throughput sequencing capacity, and trustworthiness. It is essential to update the primer and probe sequences to maintain the recognition of recently emerging variations. Concerning viral variations could develop that are dangerously resistant to the immunization induced by the present vaccinations in coronavirus disease 2019. Additionally, the significance of effective public health interventions and vaccination programs will grow if some variations of concern exhibit an increased risk of transmission or toxicity. The international reaction must've been immediate and established in science. These results supported ongoing efforts to prevent and identify infection, as well as to describe mutations in vaccine recipients, and they suggest a potential risk of illness following effective immunization and transmission of pathogens with a mutant viral.

Keywords: coronavirus 2 (SARS-CoV-2), DNA testing, RT-PCR test, diagnosis, treatment, ADAR enzyme

1. Introduction

According to the World Health Organization (WHO), incidences of pneumonia with an unknown cause were reported in many locations in late 2019 and early 2020 [1]. This pneumonia's pathogen was recognized as severe acute respiratory syndrome coronavirus 2 (SARS-CoV-2) [2] and was given the label coronavirus infectious disease (COVID-19).

SARS-CoV-2 infections affected more than 83 million known COVID-19 patients by the end of 2020, but significant progress had been achieved with the approval and implementation of vaccines and antibody treatments. These treatments target the infectious spike protein, although the advent of vigorous variations puts their effectiveness in danger (**Figure 1**) [3].

These fears have prompted an increase in viral DNA testing and sequencing in infected patients in terms of understanding the risk of transmission, virulence, and potential of variants to avoid modern vaccinations. The number of viral variants in New York City has risen alarmingly. As of March 30, 2021, the B.1.1.7 variant, first discovered in Great Britain (UK) for 26.2% of all the cases of coronavirus disease, and the B.1.526 variant, initially discovered in New York City, contributed to even more than 72% of cases, which were newly admitted (in 42.9%) [3]. The ability of variations to circumvent vaccine-induced immunity and cause asymptomatic infection (and thus viral transmission) or disease is of particular concern. Both repercussions are significant and must be evaluated separately.

Reliable laboratory testing is one of the top priorities for facilitating public actions. A reliable test is now the most efficient method for detecting patients in a large community, especially asymptomatic illnesses, identifying transmission pathways and hosts, evaluating the success of therapeutic options, and determining infection's eradication. As one of the most important instruments for monitoring, isolating, as well as diagnosing COVID-19 pandemics, each country should priorities investing in cutting-edge techniques and offering economic incentives for the implementation and verification of accurate COVID-19 diagnostics. To

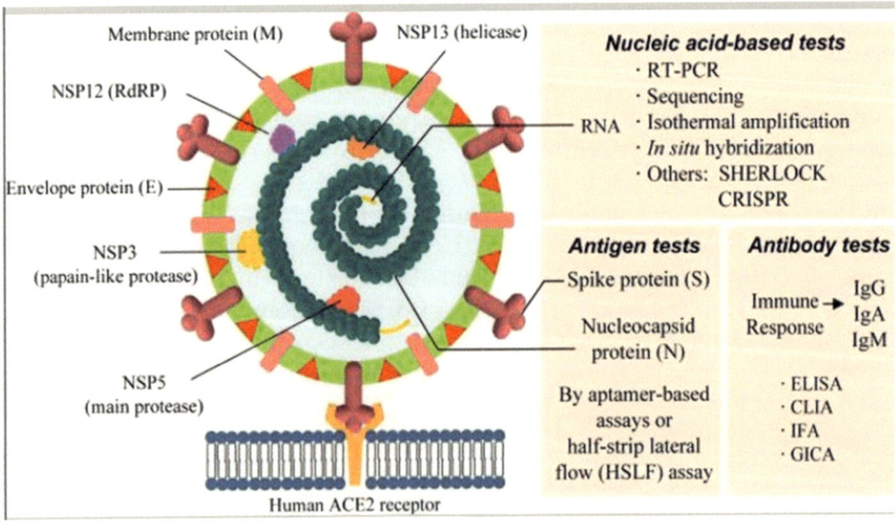

Figure 1.
Structure of the SARS-CoV-19 variants.

present, most existing examinations typically meet the expectations of mass testing examination, personal diagnosis, or variation detection; however, capability varies significantly between countries, regions, and races, mainly to socioeconomic inequalities. Because the pathogen of COVID-19 is recognized, as well as the genome, transmission channels, and host antigen for viral attachment, there are two types of tests presently offered: For the identification of viral antigens or host antibodies, there are two types of diagnostics: (1) nucleic-acid-based tests and (2) serology-based tests. Serological techniques identify antibodies found within blood serum and infectious antigens within tissues, discharge fluids, or eliminations by persons who have current or previous infections, whereas nucleic acid tests immediately investigate for viruses RNA via the throat and nose swabs taken from patients [4].

Many common areas in the SARS-CoV-2 genomes were selected as effective objectives for sample preparation in several PCR techniques, and they are used in the majority of COVID-19 molecular diagnoses around the world. According to the WHO [5], at least two targets should be used in clinical practice to avoid SARS-CoV-2 genetic mutation and cross-multiplication with the other COVID-19 viruses. For the construction of primers and probes, three portions that have been preserved (the E, N, and ORF1ab genes) are commonly chosen as standard objectives. Furthermore, sequencing the viral DNA aids in the detection of novel coronavirus variants that emerge over time. Newly developed portable or quantitative sequence alignment techniques, as opposed to classical sequence alignment methods, which are typically highly expensive, may offer accurate elevated diagnostics throughout pandemics.

1.1 Epidemiology of SARS-CoV-2 variants

Coronaviruses have a nuclease enzyme that reduces the likelihood of replication failure in vitro by 15–20 times, resulting in a 10-fold reduced risk of virus mutation in vivo than influenza [6]. When variations with mutated genes infected the same victim [7], however, they gather alterations and produce greater variety through the recombination mechanism. SARS-CoV-2 [8] is considered to have formed as a result of recombination between different SARS-related coronaviruses, and recombination is still occurring among propagating SARS-CoV-2 variants [9], showing the challenges in detecting it based on the similarities among most sequences. As evidenced by the prevalence of C to U changes in specific dinucleotide situations, SARS-CoV-2 diversity is further supported by host-mediated transcriptional control by APOBEC and ADAR enzymes [10, 11].

Although that was initially thought that decreasing immunity would have been the reason for people's frequent reinfection with symptomatic widely accepted COVID-19 viruses [12], recent research suggests that genetic variation could also play a significant role in the absence of lengthy resistance after COVID-19 virus outbreaks [13]. HCoV-229E and HCoV-OC43 sequence data demonstrate a ladder-like phylogenetic evaluation topology over a 30-year period, which has been maintained with the incidence of novel variants going to spread through the global population at a slower rate than seasonal influenza, with pathogens separated from one point and time frequently evading neutralization by blood plasma from individuals infected numerous decades prior [14].

SARS-CoV-2 is thought to evolve at a rate between about $4*10^{-4}$ and $2*10^{-3}$ variations per codon per annum [15–17]. Even though the probability of synonymous variations influencing SARS-CoV-2 morphologic features must be discounted, zero reviews of this concept happening inside the SARS-CoV-2 spikes genotype have been found. As a result, we refer to an NH_2 mutation from the Wuhan-Hu-1 known sequences (GenBank accession: NC 045512.2) as a mutation in this Review.

Because new lineages are sometimes separated from some nucleotides, the classification of emerging SARS-CoV-2 genotypes based on organic evolution has proven difficult [18]. Because the majority of mutations have been identified in a variety of countries, and the number of viruses undergoing sequencing varies substantially between countries, geographical classification has proven difficult. The NextStrain and Phylogenetic Assignment of Named Global Outbreak (PANGO) genealogy [19] systems have been developed for control and prevention. The Phylogenetic Assignment of Named Global Outbreak genealogy approach is more popular and provides greater specificity. Sub-lineages are indicated by an alphabetical beginning as well as termination containing two to three digits interspersed with periods (such as B.1.1.7). However, because the method only supports three levels of hierarchy, the variant's parental relationship cannot be established by adding a new genealogy ending. The linkage of a virus may not always correlate to the changes in its components. For example, a virus may acquire new genetic alterations related to its physiological function without ever being associated with a recent linkage.

The very first evidence of SARS-CoV-2 genetic development evolutionary changes appeared in early 2020 when a unique viral variant with the spike variant D614G arose and spread rapidly to a prevalence of over 100% by June 2020 [20, 21]. By the end of 2020 and early 2021, plenty of variants with long-term mutations (most notably D614G) had been discovered, mostly but not exclusively in the spikes protein. B.1.1.7, a fast-growing species in England connected with an extremely large number of genetic changes, was reported on the virological.org conversation forum27 in December 2020. The first therapeutic specimen of this kind was obtained in late September 2020 in England, according to retrospective analysis.

Two further fast expanding links with significant amounts of genetic variations were found in South Africa within a month [16] and Brazil [22]. The frequency of the B.1.351 variant jumped from 11percentage points in October to 87% in December [23] in South Africa. The P.1 variety was detected in Manaus, Brazil, a town with a 75% infection rate in October 2020, but a spike in new cases began in November 2020 [24, 25]. Following that, the prevalence of a novel variant (B.1.617.2) increased from 2 percentage points around February 2021 to 87% in May 2021 in Maharashtra, India, which, like the rest of the country, experienced a significant increase in the number of cases [26]. Since then, the B.1.617.2 variety has expanded over a number of countries [27] and has shown to be much greater spreadable than that of the B.1.1.7 variant. It has a higher risk of causing disease than prior viral variation (**Figure 2**) [28].

Variants of concern (VOCs) are those that have spread widely and shown evidence of being more transmissible, causing more severe disease, and/or reducing neutralization by immunoglobulin produced during prior infection or vaccination, according to the World Health Organization (WHO), the US Centers for Disease Control and Prevention (CDC), and the COVID-19 Genome sequencing UK Consortium (COG-UK) [29]. Those that have not quite expanded as broadly include alterations comparable to those found in VOCs are of particular relevance (VOIs). On May 31, 2021, the WHO began using the Greek alphabet to classify VOCs and VOIs, with the current VOC classifications being Alpha (B.1.1.7), Beta (B.1.351), Gamma (P.1), and Delta (D.1) (B.1.617.2).

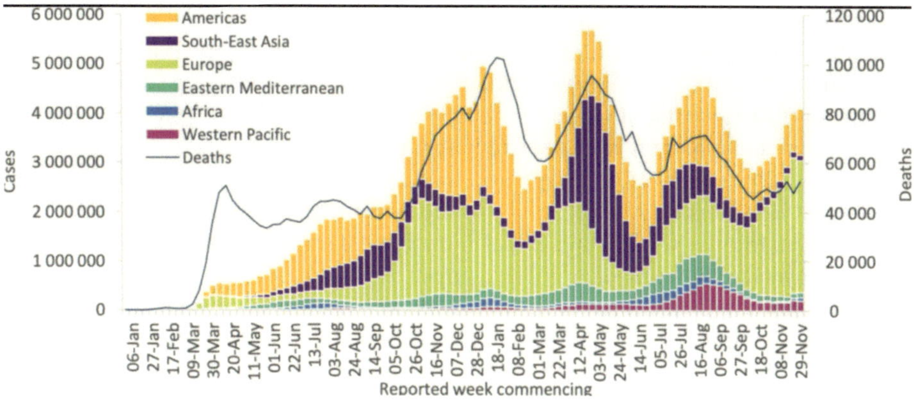

Figure 2.
Epidemiology of COVID-19 variants cases.

1.2 Diagnostic capability

1. Nuclear-acid-based testing of SARS-CoV-2 variants

2. Protein-based testing of SARS-CoV-2 variants

1.2.1 Nuclear acid based testing of SARS-CoV-2 variants

1.2.1.1 Detection of mutated variants with standard RT-PCR

As it multiplies, the virus's genome is continually changing. New SARS-CoV-2 pandemic events could be triggered by new variants containing genetic mutations. Because most PCR primers were built using solitary virions in their early stages [30], notably the standard genetic material (SARS-CoV-2, NC 045512.2) [31], just a genetic variation during a first evolution sequence could result in reduced RT-PCR test amplification efficiency and false-negative detection results [32]. Studies of genotyping samples reported to GenBank and GISAID indicated that variations in the ORF1ab region were most common in Germany and China [33].

Another analysis relies on 31,421 SARS-CoV-2 genomic specimens and discovered that the majority of alterations were with the objective of several N genome primers and probes [34], which could alter the accuracy of PCR amplification in RT-PCR tests that probe the N genome. Variations in the N genome have been observed to interfere with detection in some cases [35]. All objectives of the US CDC-recommended COVID-19 diagnosis primers had mutations, while the targets of N genome primers and probes used throughout Japan, Thailand, and China had various mutations in distinct clusters, suggesting that the N gene may not have been a reliable target for RT-PCR kits and that these N gene-based kits should be reported periodically for a rising alpha, beta, gamma, delta variants [35].

1.2.1.2 Sequencing for diagnosis of SARA-CoV-2 variants

When compared with real time-PCR, virus genotype had the limitations of being more expensive, requiring more analysis of given information, and having lesser medical efficiency, making it inappropriate for massive population detection. However, utilizing metagenomics RNA sequencing techniques [31], the first genetic arrangement of SARS-CoV-2 was obtained. A study by the WHO and China found that during the beginning of December 2019 to the middle of February 2020, Illumina and Nanopore technologies were used to identify and sequence 104 SARS-CoV-2 variants [36]. More than 1000 comparable variants have since been published in the GISAID and GenBank databases, and the genomic and proteomics of SARS-CoV-2 have also been found [37]. The benefit of homologous recombination identification is that it allows for the tracking of viral changes by gathering data on recent variants. The viral genome is sequenced for the detection and classification of novel coronavirus variants throughout time [36]. Random changes in the genetic coding accrue with the speed of about 2/month when the virus multiplies and expands, according to data from closely watching viral development [38]. The latest mutant (changed) coronaviruses had been discovered, such as alpha (B.1.1.7), beta (B.1.351), gamma (P.1), and delta (B.1.617.2), which could result in the virus spreading considerably faster [39].

High-throughput approaches or portable fast sequence arrangement technologies had already been designed as distinguishing equipment for COVID-19 due to increased demand. Nanopore target sequencing (NTS) is appealing for clinical testing since it is fast, accessible, and efficient. In 1 h of sequencing [40], an NTS technique sequencing viral areas can identify very few as 10 viral copies/mL. These recently developed portable or quantifiable technologies, in comparison to classic sequencing techniques, which are typically expensive, may give accurate elevated diagnostics during epidemics. In the United Kingdom, NTS is being used in a projected genetic monitoring effort to create real-time genetic monitoring of SARS-CoV-2 [41], allowing sample-to-report in less than 24 hours. The use of genetic and epidemiologic analyses together speeds up the detection of possible transmission events and aids in the implementation of prompt control and prevention measures. When NTS is utilized to examine for reductions and different mutations in the SARS-CoV-2 gene in patients who have been infected with the virus, a putative pathogenic mechanism may be uncovered [42]. Furthermore, a novel molecular testing method relying on Sanger sequence techniques was capable to identify SARS-CoV-2 Genetic code (RNA) from viruses suspended components in the transmissible channel, RNA extraction could be skipped altogether without sacrificing performance at a testing flow rate of more than 1,000,000 tests per day [43], meaning that RNA extraction may be omitted fully without sacrificing performance. Natural variations in large populations could be tracked at general genomic ranges or specific regions over time or within a geographic location with this capability, allowing the locations and provenance of mutations to be identified once the quantitative capability is in place (**Figure 3**).

1.2.2 Protein-based testing of SARS-CoV-2 variants

1. Antibody testing

2. Antigen testing

1.2.2.1 Antibody testing

As a growing number of people around the world prefer to keep a maximum distance from every person and remain at their houses, the concentration of pandemic protection and management has moved to comprehensive serological antibody

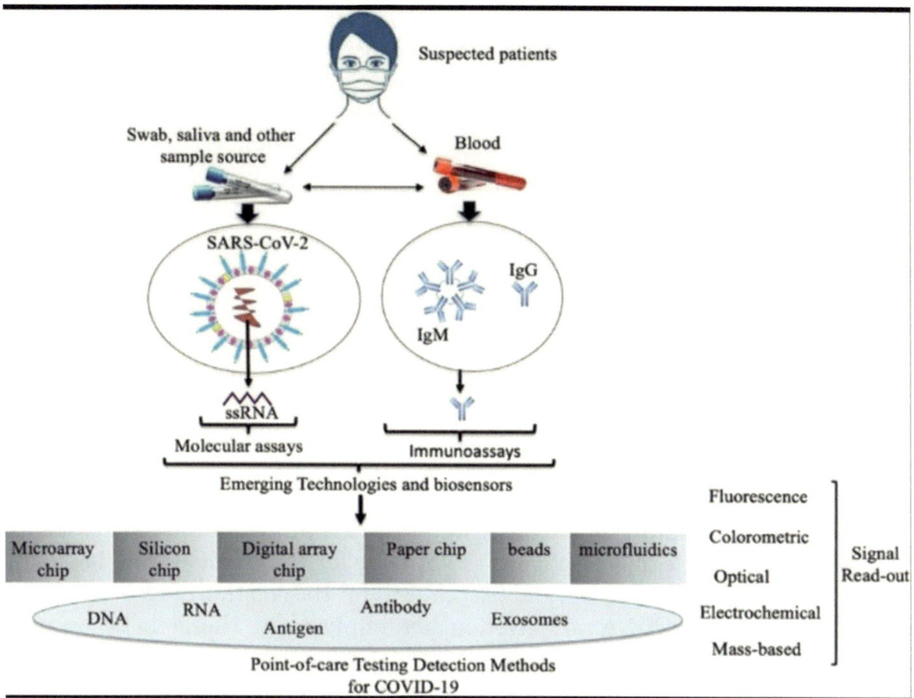

Figure 3.
Type of diagnostic method.

diagnostics of community to supervise infectious disease condition, vaccine effectiveness, immune defense perseverance, and high-titer neutralizing antibody monitoring and selection. These diagnostics, including the enzyme-linked immunochromatographic analysis (ELISA), chemiluminescent immunoassay (CLIA), immunofluorescent test (IFA), and colloidal gold immune chromatographic test (GICA), are lying on the detection of SARS-CoV-2 via IgM and/or IgG antibodies in blood plasma or biological fluids specimen. Several months before the first case was identified, one study looked for SARS-CoV-2 special antibody in 959 patients taken acquired from a prospective lung cancerous tumor testing between healthy people [44]. According to tests, SARS-CoV-2 disorders were found in about 11.6% of a native community before COVID-19 was discovered. Antibody tests are useful in community exposure research to determine the speed of exposure during a special pandemic episode in an area, as well as to determine regardless of where neutraliziable antibodies are progressing in people who were attacked by the COVID-19 virus, as well as the period and titer modified into neutralizing antibodies with the time. Since many types of vaccinations preventing SARS-CoV-2 disease are provided to the public, it is crucial to monitor neutralizing antibody production after immunization.

1.2.2.2 Antigen testing

N protein and S protein are now primary immunogens in SARS-CoV 2, and antibodies to such two proteins can survive up to 30 weeks in SARS patients' serum [45]. A new antigen-based ensures quick diagnostic test had high specificity and sensitivity during the first week between many patients diagnosed and specimens with greater primary infection [46], whereas a quick procedure relies upon a fluorescence immunologic chromatography screening test detecting N protein had effectiveness just in the first stage of the disease. N protein was identified in a gargle liquid specimen from a COVID-19-effective person [47], according to mass spectrometry analysis. In 73.6% of COVID-19 patients, a fluorescence immunological chromatography analysis identified N protein in a urine specimen. S protein is more useful for monitoring during the recovery phase because of its late development [48], and a supersensitive antigen screening for S protein is easily done with a microplate reader [49].

With popular approaches, the SARS-CoV-2 coronavirus nucleocapsid antigen-identifying half-strip lateral flow (HSLF) analysis has been created, which has higher therapeutic effectiveness than classic serology techniques, with an LOD of 3.03 ng/mL [50] for publically present Genscript N protein. With an LOD of 0.1 ng/mL for synthesized spikes antigen of SARS-CoV-2 [51], a unique nanozyme-based chemiluminescent paper test may be performed by using a lens of a standard mobile.

A particular nucleotide gene encoding opposite to N protein seems to have identical features to recognize the objective as an antibody for antigen detection; however, it may have superior effectiveness and best choices for the creation of tests for other purposes. A particular ssDNA transcription factor linked with N protein had been recommended as a reliable and efficient probe for the identification of SARS-CoV-2 using a SELEX screening strategy [52]. Another investigation found four DNA microarrays with a sensitivity of less than 5 nM that form a sandwich-type interaction with the N protein with an LOD of 1 ng/mL78. When compared with using simply antibodies in ELISA with LODs ranging from 50 to 100 ng/mL [53], the LOD of aptamer-based approaches was significantly lesser than that of standard immune screening inside a short turn-around time (TAT) having remarkable consistency and renewability [54]. As a result, in terms of diagnostic accuracy and biosensor conjugation flexibility, aptamer-based antigen recognition might well be superior to antibody-based detection of antibodies [52].

Finally, fast antigen detection has a sensitivity 1000 times lower than virus incubation and 10^3 times smaller than RT-PCR [55]. According to previous studies, the effectiveness of the rapid diagnostic test is only around 30% of that of nucleic acid screening [56], implying this antigen screening is not a fast technique but could be utilized as verification or analysis for a special patient specimen.

1.3 Vaccination and its effectiveness

1.3.1 Examining the efficacy of existing vaccines against variants

While current immunizations are being administered, therapeutic information can be collected not just from preplanned controlled research [57], but also through clinical experiments comparing immunizations versus placebo, one vaccination against the other, or various immunization schedules (e.g., various doses, different counts of doses, and time duration between doses).

In areas where vaccine supply or delivery capacity is limited, trying to make the first vaccine dosage accessible to several of the test group on just a randomly selected basis can give valuable important knowledge about effectiveness against significant variants rather than enabling management plans to evaluate the sequence wherein individuals are fully immunized. This is particularly true if the number of individuals who are randomly assigned is high enough to support the measurement of "hard" endpoints like hospitalization or serious disease.

In simple controlled studies conducted during vaccine deployment, the roles of scientists, vaccines, and vaccinators are deployed.

If a huge randomized was used during vaccination installation to compare the impact of parental secondary doses with that of postponed secondary shots, any changes in efficacy may be accurately measured not just too generally but possibly concerning such genetic variation. In some populations, public health programs may include random assignment of vaccination dates or locations, and those who become suitable for vaccination may be assigned randomly to appointments with a longer or shorter gap between vaccinations. This technique could permit hundreds of thousands of people to be randomly assigned vaccines at little or no expense to the immunization program and with little or no disruption to current vaccination capability. Whether any immunizations had been discovered to be capable of preventing COVID-19 even after an encounter with SARS-CoV-2, modest, controlled trials of post-exposure prophylaxis might provide crucial insights into vaccination effectiveness (or comparative efficiency) versus different strains.

Bias exists throughout all nonrandomized epidemiological research seeking to establish vaccine efficiency. In regions where differences are co-circulating, including several but hardly all of the community members have received vaccinations, epidemiological data specifically planned to show the dispersion of highly contagious genetic variants between instances in immunized and unvaccinated people may generate reasonably effective forecasts of comparative vaccine efficacy against various variations. If the level of vaccines is related to the relative frequency of alterations between sites, such research must take prospective interference into account. Recent disease patients' epidemiological investigations may show a lack of defense against problematic variations.

To examine the effects of concern variants on vaccination effectiveness and duration, new methodologic methods are still needed. Almost complete genotyping of isolates from specified sentinel areas could eliminate bias in the sample chosen for sequencing in vaccination sensitivity studies against variations of concern. Samples from unassigned vaccination receptors with emerging diseases and identical non-vaccinated subjects can be utilized to evaluate the impact of specific genomic characteristics on vaccine effectiveness. Important insights regarding the importance of particular viral properties could be gained using such methodologies in trials or research published after vaccine deployment, and these insights could propagate to an enhanced selection of the variants in the development of a mutated vaccine.

It's unclear how reliable any immunological sign could be like a "correlate of protection." The impact of vaccines on these biomarkers could enable regulatory action for novel candidate vaccines if such biomarkers proved to be a reliable assumption of vaccine effects on frequency of outbreak infections. However, there are some drawbacks, such as the possibility that immunological correlates of prevention are dependent on vaccine-specific variables, virus variants, and COVID-19 research exit points.

1.3.2 Examining the efficacy of new and modified vaccines for variants

Although there will be an unwillingness to dispatch vaccination lies on recent sequence data until there is perfect proof that earliest vaccination having failed [57], there would also an unwillingness to permit a sustained flow of vaccine-resistant variant while fresh immunizations or adapted vaccination are now established if that could be avoided. Because vaccine-resistant variations are certain to occur, now is necessary to schedule the creation of modified vaccinations that can defend against them. The impact of vaccine alteration on vaccine production and rollout timelines should be considered during planning.

Adapted vaccines (i.e., vaccines that deliver a fresh pathogen through with a vaccine, which have proven for being extremely effective against traditionally circulatory highly contagious variations) must be tested for their ability to evoke immune function in both people who have never had an immune reaction to SARS-CoV-2 and people who have already been vaccinated. Variations in the in vitro eradication of systemic pathogens by immunization antibodies do not always imply decreased efficiency. Even neutralization reactions should not be used to indicate vaccination effectiveness, large variations may be sufficient to justify regulatory decisions. For example, after receiving a customized vaccination, testing size of the immune reaction between greater than one mutation of concern might be evaluated to the immunological response against the prototypes virus after receiving the initial, confirmed vaccine. Analyzing neutralizing reactions to multiple different variations of concern as well as the prototype virus may assist in deciding whether more than one vaccine (or, eventually, a powerful and versatile vaccine) is required.

In regulatory changes discussions and WHO recommendations, it has been agreed that large, traditional clinical terminal trials are unlikely to be required to launch modified vaccinations against variations of concern. Because discrepancies in immune response analyses can make direct comparisons difficult, According to the FDA, animal specimen should be utilized to provide additional proof of the efficacy of customized vaccinations against variations of concern (**Figure 4**) [58].

Even if some vaccines are administered that are medically beneficial, greater would be required to combat the global epidemic. Latest vaccines against new viral variations may be more beneficial than prior vaccinations, and they may be given in a standard injection, be non-injectable, circumvent cold-chain restrictions, or have enhanced manufacturing scalability. International antigenic composition recommendations should be used in the development of modified or entirely new vaccines.

By using randomization, analyzing impacts not just on immunologic as well as on clinical endpoints and using placebo controls when ethically appropriate [59], such as in communities where vaccine supply is limited or subpopulations where the possibility of advancement to dangerous infections is very low [60], new vaccine trials can still give accurate and easily understandable results in an efficient manner.

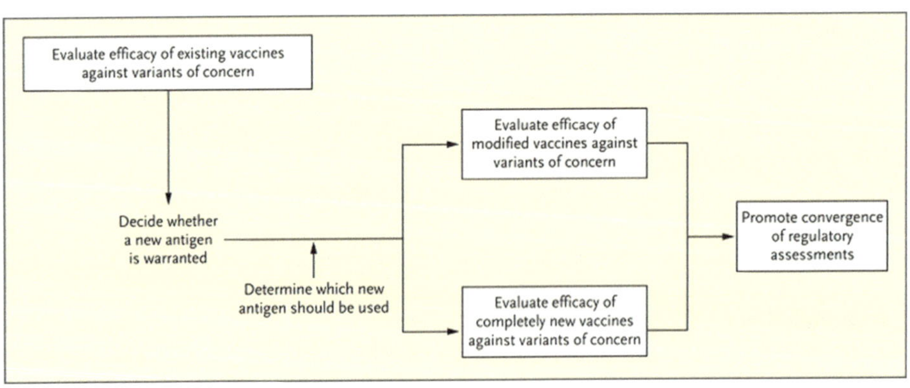

Figure 4.
A framework for evaluating vaccines against variants of concern.

Randomized trials involve more planning, but they avoid undiscovered research strategy differences from affecting research results when possible [61]. Multiple analyses, along with the evaluation of the impact of viral variation on vaccination effectiveness, and virus sequencing in persons having an outbreak infectious disease may support this theory (during or after trials). In randomized, controlled research, such sequencing likewise provides neutral details regarding variant-specific efficiency. Countries that take part in this kind of study can evaluate vaccine efficacy against regionally predominant virus strains and should have immediate access to investigational vaccinations if they have been proved to be safe and effective. In regions in which placebo-controlled experiments of novel vaccines aren't acceptable, the inclusion of an effective comparison could nevertheless yield important results [62]. The authenticity of a nonrandomized experiment wherein an effective comparator vaccination is used like the supervision depends upon the ability of prior active comparator vaccine research providing researchers with recognition accuracy into the effective comparator vaccine's effectiveness against virion variants that are currently present in the trial's communities.

Following the introduction of modified or entirely new vaccines to resolve new variants, the process could be restarted by screening for even more variants that may demand additional modifications in the vaccine antigen sequencing. Multiple varieties may propagate in the same area, therefore development and deployment plans should accommodate for this possibility. It would also be beneficial to do research in which one vaccine is supplemented with a subsequent dose of another.

2. Conclusion

The worldwide COVID-19 epidemic has been the greatest catastrophic infectious disorder into human historical life in the form of disease rates and death rates and strongly affected regions facing the high hospitalization rate and death rates still now, despite continued immunization for large populations. The appearance and outbreak of novel variants in more than 20 nations have resulted in a large increase in the number of infections and faster transmission in the affected areas. Mutated variants provide some new issues in diagnosing nucleic acid identification and the efficiency of presently offered mRNA-based, recombinant, or neutralized vaccines, such as false negativity. Due to the reemergence of community-acquired transmission in China as a result of people traveling abroad or commodities being imported, large-scale population screening has been implemented. As a result, society and small-scale pandemics have been effectively controlled. Detecting pathogenic factors, such as non-symptomatic people, infectious people with this virus, or infectious commodities, has thus become a useful tool for limiting population spread.

As previously discussed, RT-PCR seems to be the most precise as well as a rapid method for inspection and diagnosing in a huge population, whereas viral genotyping has been the most successful way for tracking contagious causes, tracking genetic changes, and defining genomic different kinds with reduced capability for particular people. The use of RT-PCR to determine infection rate is useful for tracking illness progression, therapy effectiveness, and diagnosis.

New variants of significance can originate and propagate swiftly in any area of the world, and recurrent alterations have been observed in variants of significance reported in different regions of the globe. Modifications of vaccination sequence patterns to satisfy the requirements of one state could have consequences in other countries. As a result, vaccine research, vaccine development, and vaccine deployment should be considered global endeavors, with organizations that are facing the WHO assisting in the global distribution of benefits.

Coordination is necessary in order to determine the need for the latest or improved vaccinations and advance research knowledge about the risks presented by emerging variations and the linkages between genetic differences and immunological escape, To determine which variants of significance warrant attention, a clear and timely scientific discussion is required. Criteria are performed to evaluate the compatibility of existing vaccinations and the potential effect of developing variants on vaccinations and to support guidelines for the improvement and development of changed and new vaccines, as well as the scheduling of their implementation. This technique can expand on the global platform that the WHO utilizes on a regular basis to coordinate antigen selection in influenza vaccinations.

Author details

Naheed Akhter[1], Sadia Sana[1*], Muhammad Adnan Ahsan[1], Zafaar Siddique[2], Abu Huraira[1] and Somara Sana[3]

1 College of Allied Health Professionals Government College University Faisalabad, Pakistan

2 Faculty of Allied Health Sciences, University Institute of Radiological Sciences and Medical Imaging Technology, The University of Lahore, Pakistan

3 Saleema Siddique Maternity Home Kalar Khar Chowk, District Chakwal, Pakistan

*Address all correspondence to: sadiasana203@gmail.com

References

[1] Zhou P, Yang X-L, Wang X-G, Hu B, Zhang L, Zhang W, et al. A pneumonia outbreak associated with a new coronavirus of probable bat origin. Nature. 2020;**579**(7798):270-273

[2] Han GZ. Pangolins harbor SARS-CoV-2-related coronaviruses. Trends in Microbiology. 1 Jul 2020;**28**(7):515-517

[3] Hacisuleyman E, Hale C, Saito Y, Blachere NE, Bergh M, Conlon EG, et al. Vaccine breakthrough infections with SARS-CoV-2 variants. New England Journal of Medicine. 2021;**384**(23):2212-2218

[4] Esbin MN, Whitney ON, Chong S, Maurer A, Darzacq X, Tjian R. Overcoming the bottleneck to widespread testing: A rapid review of nucleic acid testing approaches for COVID-19 detection. RNA. 2020;**26**(7):771-783

[5] Guan WJ, Ni ZY, Hu Y, Liang WH, Ou CQ, He JX, et al. Clinical characteristics of coronavirus disease 2019 in China. New England Journal of Medicine. 30 Apr 2020;382(18):1708-1720

[6] Eckerle LD, Becker MM, Halpin RA, Li K, Venter E, Lu X, et al. Infidelity of SARS-CoV Nsp14-exonuclease mutant virus replication is revealed by complete genome sequencing. PLoS Pathogens. 2010;**6**(5):e1000896

[7] Gribble J, Stevens LJ, Agostini ML, Anderson-Daniels J, Chappell JD, Lu X, et al. The coronavirus proofreading exoribonuclease mediates extensive viral recombination. PLoS Pathogens. 2021;**17**(1):e1009226

[8] Boni MF, Lemey P, Jiang X, Lam TT-Y, Perry BW, Castoe TA, et al. Evolutionary origins of the SARS-CoV-2 arbovirus lineage responsible for the COVID-19 pandemic. Nature Microbiology. 2020;**5**(11):1408-1417

[9] Korber B, Fischer WM, Gnanakaran S, Yoon H, Theiler J, Abfalterer W, et al. Tracking changes in SARS-CoV-2 spike: Evidence that D614G increases infectivity of the COVID-19 virus. Cell. 2020;**182**(4):812-27.e19

[10] Simmonds P. Rampant C→ U hypermutation in the genomes of SARS-CoV-2 and other coronaviruses: Causes and consequences for their short-and long-term evolutionary trajectories. Msphere. 2020;**5**(3):e00408-e00420

[11] van Dorp L, Richard D, Tan C, Shaw LP, Acman M, Balloux F. No evidence for increased transmissibility from recurrent mutations in SARS-CoV-2. Nature Communications. 2020;**11**(1):1-8

[12] Edridge AW, Kaczorowska J, Hoste AC, Bakker M, Klein M, Loans K, et al. Seasonal coronavirus protective immunity is short-lasting. Nature Medicine. 2020;**26**(11):1691-1693

[13] Kistler KE, Bedford T. Evidence for adaptive evolution in the receptor-binding domain of seasonal coronaviruses OC43 and 229e. eLife. 2021;**10**:e64509

[14] Eguia RT, Crawford KH, Stevens-Ayers T, Kelnhofer-Millevolte L, Greninger AL, Englund JA, et al. A human coronavirus evolves antigenically to escape antibody immunity. PLoS Pathogens. 2021;**17**(4):e1009453

[15] Candido DS, Claro IM, De Jesus JG, Souza WM, Moreira FR, Dellicour S,

et al. Evolution and epidemic spread of SARS-CoV-2 in Brazil. Science. 2020;**369**(6508):1255-1260

[16] Tegally H, Wilkinson E, Giovanetti M, Iranzadeh A, Fonseca V, Giandhari J, et al. Detection of a SARS-CoV-2 variant of concern in South Africa. Nature. 2021;**592**(7854):438-443

[17] Pereson MJ, Mojsiejczuk L, Martínez AP, Flichman DM, Garcia GH, Di Lello FA. Phylogenetic analysis of SARS-CoV-2 in the first few months since its emergence. Journal of Medical Virology. 2021;**93**(3):1722-1731

[18] Moravian C, Pond SK, Marini S, Magalis BR, Vandamme A-M, Dellicour S, et al. Sampling bias and incorrect rooting make phylogenetic network tracing of SARS-COV-2 infections unreliable. Proceedings of the National Academy of Sciences. 2020;**117**(23):12522-12523

[19] Rambaut A, Holmes EC, O'Toole Á, Hill V, McCrone JT, Ruis C, et al. A dynamic nomenclature proposal for SARS-CoV-2 lineages to assist genomic epidemiology. Nature Microbiology. 2020;**5**(11):1403-1407

[20] Dearlove B, Lewitus E, Bai H, Li Y, Reeves DB, Joyce MG, et al. A SARS-CoV-2 vaccine candidate would likely match all currently circulating variants. Proceedings of the National Academy of Sciences. 2020;**117**(38):23652-23662

[21] Martin DP, Weaver S, Tegally H, San JE, Shank SD, Wilkinson E, et al. The emergence and ongoing convergent evolution of the SARS-CoV-2 N501Y lineages. Cell. 30 Sep 2021;**184**(20):5189-5200

[22] Faria NR, Mellan TA, Whittaker C, Claro IM, Candido DDS, Mishra S, et al. Genomics and epidemiology of the P. 1 SARS-CoV-2 lineage in Manaus, Brazil. Science. 2021;**372**(6544):815-821

[23] Abdool Karim SS, de Oliveira T. New SARS-CoV-2 variants—Clinical, public health, and vaccine implications. New England Journal of Medicine. 2021;**384**(19):1866-1868

[24] Buss LF, Prete CA Jr, Abraham CM, Mendrone A Jr, Salomon T, de Almeida-Neto C, et al. Three-quarters attack rate of SARS-CoV-2 in the Brazilian Amazon during a largely unmitigated epidemic. Science. 2021;**371**(6526):288-292

[25] Sabino EC, Buss LF, Carvalho MP, Prete CA, Crispim MA, Fraiji NA, et al. Resurgence of COVID-19 in Manaus, Brazil, despite high seroprevalence. The Lancet. 2021;**397**(10273):452-455

[26] Gupta N, Kaur H, Yadav PD, Mukhopadhyay L, Sahay RR, Kumar A, et al. Clinical characterization and genomic analysis of samples from COVID-19 breakthrough infections during the second wave among the various states of India. Viruses. 7 Sep 2021;**13**(9):1782

[27] Lucas C, Vogels CB, Yildirim I, Rothman JE, Lu P, Monteiro V, et al. Impact of circulating SARS-CoV-2 variants on mRNA vaccine-induced immunity. Nature. Dec 2021;**600**(7889):523-529

[28] Challen R, Dyson L, Overton CE, Guzman-Rincon LM, Hill EM, Stage HB, et al. Early epidemiological signatures of novel SARS-CoV-2 variants: establishment of B. 1.617. 2 in England. Medrxiv. 2021

[29] COVID T. An integrated national scale SARS-CoV-2 genomic surveillance network. The Lancet Microbe. 2020;**1**(3):e99

[30] Chan JF-W, Yip CC-Y, To KK-W, Tang TH-C, Wong SC-Y, Leung K-H, et al. Improved molecular diagnosis of COVID-19 by the novel, highly sensitive, and specific COVID-19-RdRp/Hel real-time reverse transcription-PCR assay validated in vitro and with clinical specimens. Journal of Clinical Microbiology. 2020;**58**(5):e00310-e00320

[31] Wu F, Zhao S, Yu B, Chen Y-M, Wang W, Song Z-G, et al. A new coronavirus associated with human respiratory disease in China. Nature. 2020;**579**(7798):265-269

[32] Bru D, Martin-Laurent F, Philippot L. Quantification of the detrimental effect of a single primer-template mismatch by real-time PCR using the 16S rRNA gene as an example. Applied and Environmental Microbiology. 2008;**74**(5):1660-1663

[33] Koyama T, Platt D, Parida L. Variant analysis of SARS-CoV-2 genomes. Bulletin of the World Health Organization. 2020;**98**(7):495

[34] Wang R, Hozumi Y, Yin C, Wei G-W. Mutations on COVID-19 diagnostic targets. Genomics. 2020;**112**(6):5204-5213

[35] Kaden R. Early phylogenetic diversification of SARS-CoV-2: Determination of variants and the effect on epidemiology, immunology, and diagnostics. Journal of Clinical Medicine. 2020;**9**(6):1615

[36] Lu R, Zhao X, Li J, Niu P, Yang B, Wu H, et al. Genomic characterization and epidemiology of 2019 novel coronavirus: Implications for virus origins and receptor binding. The Lancet. 2020;**395**(10224):565-574

[37] Udugama B, Kadhiresan P, Kozlowski HN, Malekjahani A, Osborne M, Li VY, et al. Diagnosing COVID-19: The disease and tools for detection. ACS Nano. 2020;**14**(4):3822-3835

[38] Hadfield J, Megill C, Bell SM, Huddleston J, Potter B, Callender C, et al. Nextstrain: Real-time tracking of pathogen evolution. Bioinformatics (Oxford, England). 2018;**34**(23): 4121-4123

[39] Tang JW, Tambyah PA, Hui DS. The emergence of a new SARS-CoV-2 variant in the UK. The Journal of Infection. 2021;**82**(4):e27-ee8

[40] Wang M, Fu A, Hu B, Tong Y, Liu R, Liu Z, et al. Nanopore targeted sequencing for the accurate and comprehensive detection of SARS-CoV-2 and other respiratory viruses. Small (Weinheim an der Bergstrasse, Germany). 2020;**16**(32):e2002169

[41] Meredith LW, Hamilton WL, Warne B, Houldcroft CJ, Hosmillo M, Jahun AS, et al. Rapid implementation of SARS-CoV-2 sequencing to investigate cases of health-care associated COVID-19: A prospective genomic surveillance study. The Lancet Infectious Diseases. 2020;**20**(11):1263-1272

[42] Moore SC, Penrice-Randal R, Alruwaili M, Randle N, Armstrong S, Hartley C, et al. Amplicon-based detection and sequencing of SARS-CoV-2 in nasopharyngeal swabs from patients with COVID-19 and identification of deletions in the viral genome that encode proteins involved in interferon antagonism. Viruses. 14 Oct 2020;**12**(10):1164

[43] Dinnes J, Deeks JJ, Berhane S, Taylor M, Adriano A, Davenport C, et al. Rapid, point-of-care antigen and molecular-based tests for diagnosis of SARS-CoV-2 infection. Cochrane Database of Systematic Reviews. 2021;(3)

[44] Apolone G, Montomoli E, Manenti A, Boeri M, Sabia F, Hyseni I, et al. Unexpected detection of SARS-CoV-2 antibodies in the pre-pandemic period in Italy. Tumori Journal. 2021;**107**(5):446-451

[45] Qiu M, Shi Y, Guo Z, Chen Z, He R, Chen R, et al. Antibody responses to individual proteins of SARS coronavirus and their neutralization activities. Microbes and Infection. 2005;7(5-6):882-889

[46] Porte L, Legarraga P, Vollrath V, Aguilera X, Munita JM, Araos R, et al. Evaluation of a novel antigen-based rapid detection test for the diagnosis of SARS-CoV-2 in respiratory samples. International Journal of Infectious Diseases: IJID: Official Publication of the International Society for Infectious Diseases. 2020;**99**:328-333

[47] Ihling C, Tänzler D, Hagemann S, Kehlen A, Hüttelmaier S, Arlt C, et al. Mass spectrometric identification of SARS-CoV-2 proteins from gargle solution samples of COVID-19 patients. Journal of Proteome Research. 2020;**19**(11):4389-4392

[48] Tan YJ, Goh PY, Fielding BC, Shen S, Chou CF, Fu JL, et al. Profiles of antibody responses against severe acute respiratory syndrome coronavirus recombinant proteins and their potential use as diagnostic markers. Clinical and Diagnostic Laboratory Immunology. 2004;**11**(2):362-371

[49] Kyosei Y, Namba M, Yamura S, Takeuchi R, Aoki N, Nakaishi K, et al. Proposal of de novo antigen test for COVID-19: ultrasensitive detection of spike proteins of SARS-CoV-2. Diagnostics. 14 Aug 2020;**10**(8):594

[50] Grant BD, Anderson CE, Williford JR, Alonzo LF, Glukhova VA, Boyle DS, et al. SARS-CoV-2 coronavirus Nucleocapsid antigen-detecting half-strip lateral flow assay toward the development of point of care tests using commercially available reagents. Analytical Chemistry. 2020;**92**(16):11305-11309

[51] Liu D, Ju C, Han C, Shi R, Chen X, Duan D, et al. Nanozyme chemiluminescence paper test for rapid and sensitive detection of SARS-CoV-2 antigen. Biosensors & Bioelectronics. 2020;**173**:112817

[52] Li HY, Jia WN, Li XY, Zhang L, Liu C, Wu J. Advances in detection of infectious agents by aptamer-based technologies. Emerging Microbes & Infections. 2020;**9**(1):1671-1681

[53] Mak GCK, Lau SSY, Wong KKY, Chow NLS, Lau CS, Lam ETK, et al. Evaluation of rapid antigen detection kit from the WHO emergency use list for detecting SARS-CoV-2. Journal of clinical Virology: The Official Publication of the Pan American Society for Clinical Virology. 2021;**134**:104712

[54] Li HY, Yin FF, Li XY, Jia WN, Ding J, Zhang L, et al. Novel aptasensor-based assay of sonic hedgehog ligand for detection of portal vein invasion of hepatocellular carcinoma. Biosensors & Bioelectronics. 2021;**174**:112738

[55] Mak GC, Cheng PK, Lau SS, Wong KK, Lau CS, Lam ET, et al. Evaluation of rapid antigen test for detection of SARS-CoV-2 virus. Journal of Clinical Virology: The Official Publication of the Pan American Society for Clinical Virology. 2020;**129**:104500

[56] Scohy A, Anantharajah A, Bodéus M, Kabamba-Mukadi B, Verroken A, Rodriguez-Villalobos H. Low performance of rapid antigen detection test as frontline testing for COVID-19 diagnosis. Journal of clinical virology:

the official publication of the Pan American Society for Clinical Virology. 2020;**129**:104455

[57] Krause PR, Fleming TR, Longini IM, Peto R, Briand S, Heymann DL, et al. SARS-CoV-2 variants and vaccines. New England Journal of Medicine. 2021;**385**(2):179-186

[58] Muñoz-Fontela C, Dowling WE, Funnell SGP, Gsell PS, Riveros-Balta AX, Albrecht RA, et al. Animal models for COVID-19. Nature. 2020;**586**(7830):509-515

[59] Singh JA, Kochhar S, Wolff J. Placebo use and unblinding in COVID-19 vaccine trials: Recommendations of a WHO expert working group. Nature Medicine. 2021;**27**(4):569-570

[60] Krause PR, Fleming TR, Longini IM, Peto R, Beral V, Bhargava B, et al. Placebo-controlled trials of Covid-19 vaccines - why we still need them. The New England Journal of Medicine. 2021;**384**(2):e2

[61] Collins R, Bowman L, Landray M, Peto R. The magic of randomization versus the myth of real-world evidence. The New England Journal of Medicine. 2020;**382**(7):674-678

[62] Fleming TR, Krause PR, Nason M, Longini IM, Henao-Restrepo AM. COVID-19 vaccine trials: The use of active controls and non-inferiority studies. Clinical Trials (London, England). 2021;**18**(3):335-342

Chapter 10

Perspective Chapter: Novel Diagnostics Methods for SARS-CoV-2

Yong Yang and Yanyan Li

Abstract

A novel coronavirus of zoonotic origin (SARS-CoV-2) has recently been recognized in patients with acute respiratory disease. COVID-19 causative agent is structurally and genetically similar to SARS and bat SARS-like coronaviruses. The drastic increase in the number of coronavirus and its genome sequence has given us an unprecedented opportunity to perform bioinformatics and genomics analysis on this class of viruses. Clinical tests such as PCR and ELISA for rapid detection of this virus are urgently needed for early identification of infected patients. However, these techniques are expensive and not readily available for point-of-care (POC) applications. Currently, lack of any rapid, available, and reliable POC detection method gives rise to the progression of COVID-19 as a horrible global problem. To solve the negative features of clinical investigation, we provide a brief introduction of the various novel diagnostics methods including SERS, SPR, electrochemical, magnetic detection of SARS-CoV-2. All sensing and biosensing methods based on nanotechnology developed for the determination of various classes of coronaviruses are useful to recognize the newly immerged coronavirus, i.e., SARS-CoV-2. Also, the introduction of sensing and biosensing methods sheds light on the way of designing a proper screening system.

Keywords: SARS-CoV-2, diagnostics, high-sensitivity, biosensors, nanotechnology

1. Introduction

In the twenty-first century, there were three outbreaks caused by massive coronavirus infection, namely Severe Acute Respiratory Syndromes (SARS) in 2003, Middle East Respiratory Syndrome (MERS) in 2012, and Corona Virus Disease 2019 (COVID-19) in 2019. In particular, the outbreak of COVID-19 caused by Severe Acute Respiratory Syndrome Coronavirus 2 (SARS-CoV-2) has aroused great concern about this major public health emergency [1, 2]. SARS-CoV-2 is highly infectious and has a high mortality rate. As of April 8, 2022, 490 million people have been infected, 6.17 million people have died, and 231 countries and regions have reported cases of infectiousness (data source: WHO). With the recent outbreak of COVID-19 in multiple waves and countries caused by SARS-CoV-2 variants, the prevention and control tend to be normalized. At present, WHO has defined five "variant of concern" (VOC) of

SARS-CoV-2, including alpha (b.1.1.7), beta (b.1.351), gamma (P.1), delta (b.1.617.2), and omicron (b.1.1.529). With Omicron BA.2 subtype appearing particularly, the basic infectiousness coefficient (R0) of BA.2 is 9.1, which is greatly enhanced compared with the wild type (R0 close to 3.0) according to Sutter health's calculation.

SARS-CoV-2 is mainly transmitted through respiratory droplets and close contacts. It is possible to transmit through aerosol when exposed to high concentration aerosol in a relatively closed environment. Since SARS-CoV-2 can be isolated from feces and urine, it should also be careful that it may cause contact transmission or aerosol transmission to the environment [3]. In order to suppress the spread of SARS-CoV-2 as soon as possible, it is necessary to develop rapid and accurate virus detection technology. The spread of the epidemic can be effectively controlled by screening infected persons and monitoring the pollution of SARS-CoV-2 in the environment to cut off the source and route of transmission timely [4].

In view of the pandemic of COVID-19, new requirements are put forward for the detection technology of SARS-CoV-2. Among the conventional diagnostic methods, enzyme-linked immunosorbent assay (ELISA), real-time fluorescent quantitative reverse transcription polymerase chain reaction (RT-qPCR), and loop-mediated isothermal amplification (LAMP) are very important for the discovery of human coronavirus. However, these methods also have limitations. For example, RT-qPCR requires skilled personnel and certain laboratory conditions and can be time-consuming. In addition, the preparation of ELISA reagents requires specific, high-affinity antibodies or expensive recombinant antibodies. In order to solve these challenges, the community of scholars and industrial circles have developed a variety of novel diagnostics methods for SARS-CoV-2 based on the research progress of nanomaterials, nano-sensing technology, and biotechnology.

2. Novel diagnostics methods for SARS-CoV-2

Nano-biosensing technology is the integration of nanotechnology and biosensing technology. The principle of nano-biosensing technology is similar to that of biosensor technology. Taking the substance to be tested as the identification element, the biological reaction is transformed into identifiable physical or chemical signals through sensitive elements (receptors) and transformation elements (transducers). On the one hand, using the unique optical, electrical, magnetic, and surface activity of nanomaterials is conducive to the construction of high-specificity and high-sensitivity biosensors. On the other hand, the size and shape of nanomaterials are easier to adjust, which is more conducive to the load and modification of targets.

2.1 SERS-based biosensors

Raman spectra could characterize the vibration of molecular chemical bonds. However, the Raman signals are weaker because of low Raman scattering cross section [5]. Therefore, surface-enhanced Raman spectroscopy (SERS) was introduced to solve the disadvantage of weak signal inherent in Raman spectroscopy technology. SERS refers to the phenomenon that Raman signals are enhanced on the surface of some rough nanomaterials. The enhancement mechanism of SERS mainly includes electromagnetic enhancement and chemical enhancement, which are caused by localized surface plasmon resonance (LSPR) of SERS-active substrate and photo-induced charge transfer (PICT) between SERS-active substrate and probe molecules, respectively [6, 7]. SERS-based sensors have high sensitivity, and the detection ability of some SERS-based sensors can even reach the level of single molecule. SERS-based sensing technology mainly depends on the performance of nano SERS-active substrate, so the properties of nanomaterials, such as high surface energy, agglomeration and dispersion, surface plasmon resonance, and the preparation technology of nanomaterials will have influence on the activity of SERS substrate [8, 9]. In medical detection, SERS-based sensing technology has been widely applied to cancer detection, virus detection, biological imaging, and other medical fields [10–12]. Limited by the inherent non-specificity of SERS substrate itself, SERS-based biosensors need to be modified by biomolecules such as proteins, antibodies, and aptamers on the surface of the SERS-active substrate to specifically capture targets to be detected [13, 14]. Because of its fast, low-cost, high sensitivity, and accuracy, SERS-based biosensors have been employed for the rapid detection of SARS-CoV-2 and the diagnosis of virus infectiousness.

SERS technology can be divided into two categories: labeled SERS technology and label-free SERS technology. Labeled SERS technology refers to label reporter molecules with high Raman scattering cross section on the SERS-active substrate. Through the reasonable design of SERS tags and SERS detection system, the Raman signals of the reported molecules are proportional to the concentration of the targeted substance, so as to obtain the concentration information of the targets. The labeled SERS technology is applicable to the molecular vibration of the target molecules, which does not have Raman activity or has weak Raman activity. Therefore, the molecules to be tested can be detected indirectly by labeling the reporter molecules with strong Raman activity. However, because the Raman signals of the molecules to be tested are not directly collected, the molecular structure cannot be analyzed. So the advantage of Raman as fingerprint spectrum is lost. Moreover, the design of SERS tags and detection system in labeled SERS technology is complex, and the stability of substrate performance is difficult to ensure.

Label-free SERS technology is to directly collect the Raman spectra of targets. It can analyze the molecular structure of the substance to be measured by analyzing the corresponding Raman vibration spectra. Especially for the identification of different viruses and variants, we can not only distinguish different viruses from the perspective of spectral vibration, but also further analyze and verify the mutation characteristics of virus nucleic acid and protein. However, for the label-free SERS detection of biological macromolecules, the weak spectral signal intensity and the poor spectral reproducibility caused by different adsorption directions of biomolecules are the major challenges [15–17].

2.1.1 Labeled SERS technology

Label-free SERS technology can not only quickly screen and diagnose SARS-CoV-2 carriers, but also further analyze SARS-CoV-2 according to the characteristic spectra of the molecules to be tested (nucleic acid, antigen, antibody, or pathogen), including the differentiation of virus subtypes, the classification of virus variants, and the identification of virus infectiousness. In SARS-CoV-2 detection, the poor reproducibility of SERS spectra is giant challenge, which is mainly due to the different adsorption sites of biomacromolecules on the surface of SERS-active substrate.

Shanghai Institute of Ceramics, Chinese Academy of Sciences has carried out systematic research in the field of accurate capture and detection of SARS-CoV-2 by label-free SERS technology and achieved a series of pioneering research results (**Figure 1a**) [18, 19]. The SERS-based biosensor designed by the team has ACE2 functionalized gold nano "forest" structure, which can selectively capture sars-cov-2, and its detection sensitivity has reached the level of single virus. The SERS-based biosensor designed by the team has ACE2 functionalized Au "virus traps" nanostructure, which can selectively capture SARS-CoV-2, and its detection sensitivity has reached the level of single virus. Due to the special "virus traps" nanostructure and high affinity of ACE2 for SARS-CoV-2 S protein, the ability of the SERS-based biosensor to enrich virus in water has been improved 106 times. Due to the multi-effect SERS enhancement mechanism produced by the specially designed Au nanostructure, the Raman signals of the SERS biosensor are enhanced by 109 times. With the help of machine learning, the identification methods of Raman signals of SARS-CoV-2 are established. The LOD of SARS-CoV-2 is 80 copies/mL, which takes only 5 min. This is of great significance for the point-of-care test (POCT) of SARS-CoV-2. A two-step SERS detection method based on ultrahigh sensitive SnS2 microsphere substrate was creatively proposed, and the SERS signals identification standard of SARS-CoV-2 S protein and RNA was established (**Figure 1b**). This identification standard is used to identify the "life or dead" and infectiousness of SARS-CoV-2 in the environment. It solves the problem of infectious diagnosis of SARS-CoV-2 in the environment that cannot be solved by RT-qPCR technology at present, which is of great significance to avoid misjudgment of the epidemic situation under the current COVID-19 pandemic [20].

Although label-free SERS technology can enhance the Raman signal intensity of the target analyte, the Raman scattering cross section of biomacromolecules is small. Even in the case of enhancement, some vibrational Raman signals of biomacromolecules are still weaker than those of dye molecules. Due to the influence of impurities in different Physiological environment and the different adsorption sites of biomacromolecules on the surface of SERS-active substrate, the Raman band assignments of SARS-CoV-2 have not been systematic. Therefore, the biomarkers of SARS-CoV-2 detected by label-free SERS technology are S protein and intact virus.

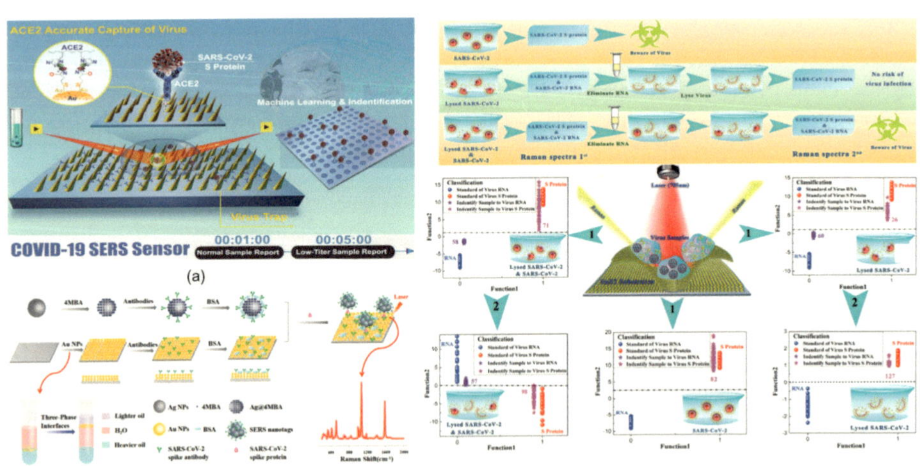

Figure 1.
a: Schematic diagram of COVID-19 SERS sensor operation procedure. b: Application of SnS2 microspheres for diagnosing the infectiousness of SARS-CoV-2 based on two-step diagnosis method. c: Schematic illustration of the SERS-based immunoassay.

2.1.2 Label-free SERS technology

Labeled SERS technology can not directly obtain the spectral information of targeted molecules, but this method has good quantitative properties, that is, the Raman intensity of SERS tags has a strong linear relationship with the concentration of the molecules to be measured [21]. Because of its high sensitivity and rapid response, the labeled SERS detection platform has been widely applied to the rapid detection of SARS-CoV-2.

Xiaomin Liu's team of Jilin University [22] used a novel method of oil/water/oil three-phase liquid-liquid interfaces self-assembly to prepare a double-layer Au nanoparticles films (**Figure 1c**). After the surface of Au nanoparticles films is modified with SARS-CoV-2 antibody, it can be used as an SERS-immune substrate to detect SARS-CoV-2 antigen. The team also designed a labeled SERS-immune detection platform, which is a "sandwich" structure composed of SERS-immune substrate, reported molecules, and Ag nanoparticles modified with antibody (SERS tags). This SERS-based immune platform will not be disturbed by impurities in physiological environment. The LOD of SARS-CoV-2 S protein in untreated saliva can reach 6.07 fg/mL, and the detection platform has excellent specificity and reproducibility. The labeled SERS technology mainly relies on the Raman signals of the reported molecules in the SERS tags to indirectly detect SARS-CoV-2, so the selection of the reported molecules and the construction of the SERS-active substrate are very important. Noble metals with strong electromagnetic enhancement such as Au/Ag nanoparticles/nanostructure are usually used as the SERS-active substrate, and reported molecules containing -SH/-NH2 functional groups such as 4-MBA, 4-ATP, and R6G are selected to form Ag/Au-S/N bonds with strong binding force through strong electrostatic interaction.

2.1.3 Application of nanotechnology in SERS-based biosensors

At present, most of the SERS-active substrates involved in the detection of SARS-CoV-2 are noble metal substrates, whether labeled or label-free SERS technology. The preparation methods of SERS-active substrate can be roughly divided into two categories: chemical method and physical method. Chemical methods include wet chemical synthesis, liquid-liquid self-assembly, hydrothermal method, etc.; physical methods include ion sputtering, magnetron sputtering, etc. [13, 18, 20, 23–26] Compared with the chemical method, the substrate prepared by the physical method has a more regular array structure, which can build a more uniform "hot spot" structure according to the detection requirements, so as to achieve higher detection sensitivity. In addition, compared with nanomaterials prepared by chemical method, substrates with nanostructures prepared by physical method are easier to be produced on a large scale. Chemical synthesis of SERS substrate has simple steps and low requirements for equipment. In order to inhibit the agglomeration of nanomaterials with high surface energy, various surfactants will be used in the process of preparing SERS-active substrate by chemical method, such as sodium citrate, PEI, PEG, and so on. Surfactants will introduce Raman bands of background, and SERS-active substrates prepared by some physical methods can effectively avoid these bands.

2.2 SPR-based biosensors

Surface plasmon resonance-based (SPR)-based biosensors realize the detection of target substances through the change of refractive index caused by the interaction between plasma resonance wave and target molecules on the metal surface. It has the advantages of real-time, label-free, high cost-effective, noninvasive nature, good reutilization, and excellent reproducibility [27, 28]. However, the sample volume and power consumption required for SPR-based biosensing detection are still large, and the sensitivity and resolution of SPR-based biosensors or devices still need to be further improved. These shortcomings hinder the application of SPR-based biosensors in biomedical detection [29]. In order to settle these problems, nanomaterials, microfluidic devices, compact and power-free pumps have been tried to be integrated into SPR-based biosensor system.

2.2.1 SPR-based biosensors for SARS-CoV-2 detection

Researchers from Huazhong University of Science and Technology, Shanghai Public Health Clinical Center affiliated to Fudan University, Liangzhun (Shanghai) Industrial Co. Ltd. [30] have successfully developed a high-sensitivity optical detection system based on a spike protein specific nano-plasmonic resonance sensor, which can quickly and specifically measure the concentration of SARS-CoV-2 virus particles without sample preparation and make it possible to quickly and noninvasively detect the asymptomatic patients of SARS-CoV-2 in the early stage of infection (**Figure 2**). The team has developed an optical nano plasma resonance chip, which has special optical properties caused by the collective oscillation of electron gases in metal metamaterial nanostructures surrounded by dielectric materials. With the help of this SPR-based biosensors, the quantitative analysis of the binding process between protein of SARS-CoV-2 surface and antibody can be completed only with conventional ordinary equipment such as optical microscope or Microplate Reader. The experimental results show that the lowest LOD of the system is 370 vp/ml, which can satisfy the requirements of rapid detection of SARS-CoV-2 in saliva. Taka-aki Yano et al. [31] constructed the "sandwich" structure composed of Au substrate, N protein of SARS-CoV-2, and antibody modified Au nanoparticles, and used SPR technology to detect novel coronavirus with fmol/L detection sensitivity of N protein. The team attributed the excellent sensitivity of the SPR-based biosensors to the coupling of surface plasmon resonance between Au nanoparticles and Au substrate and the use of large particle size Au nanoparticles (about 150 nm). Through experiments and electromagnetic field simulation, they believe that ~150 nm Au nanoparticles are more conducive to the detection of biomacromolecules than Au nanoparticles with tens of nanometers.

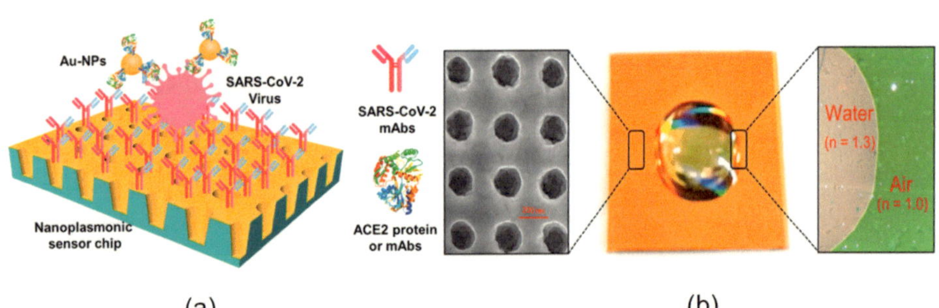

Figure 2.
a: Schematic diagram of the nanoplasmonic resonance sensor for. determination of SARS-CoV-2 pseudovirus concentration. b: Photograph (Middle) of one piece of Au nanocup array chip with a drop of water on top.

2.2.2 Application of nanotechnology for SPR-based biosensors

The sensing performance of SPR-based biosensor is directly related to the surface plasmon resonance produced by nanomaterials/nanostructures. As a result, the preparation of SPR-based biosensor materials also involves the preparation of a variety of traditional or novel preparation method of nanomaterials and micro/nanofabrication. SPR technology is mainly divided into two categories: transmitted surface plasmon resonance (commonly referred to SPR) and local surface plasmon resonance (LSPR). The kernel of substrate based on transmitted SPR technology is the design of Micro/Nano Architectures. The main preparation methods include lithography, electron beam lithography method, focused ion beam lithography method, and nanosphere self-assembly. The nanomaterials based on LSPR are related to the material quality, geometry, size, and the distance between nanoparticles [32]. The main methods for preparing LSPR-based substrate are wet chemical method, electrochemical method, and hydrothermal method. Among them, wet chemical method is the most commonly used preparation method. In order to overcome the limitation of low sensitivity of SPR-based biosensors, researchers designed composite SPR-based biosensors combined the transmitted SPR technology and LSPR technology to enable them to couple and excite each other, which greatly improved the sensing performance of the SPR-based biosensors.

2.3 Electrochemical biosensors

Electrochemical biosensors are a quantitative or semiquantitative sensing technology with high sensitivity and specificity, which works by potentiometric, amperometric, conductometric, polarographic, capacitive, or piezoelectric ways [33]. The effective physical transduce in electrochemical biosensors depends on the working electrode, and the sensitive layer is the interface between the electrode and the analyzed environment [34]. The sensing element of electrochemical biosensor must be a conductor, and the target molecules can be specifically identified and adsorbed after some modification on the conductor surface. Electrochemical biosensors have the characteristics of short detection time, simple device, low cost, and high portability, which has the potential to become a point-of-care detection tool [35, 36].

It is extremely important to select appropriate materials when designing electrochemical biosensors. When an electrochemical reaction occurs, the material must be inert at the current potential. At present, the solid electrodes employed commonly are mainly metals, such as gold, silver, nickel, copper, and so on. Metal electrodes with metal nanoparticles or nanostructure have high specific surface area and are easy to modify and label, which can improve the sensitivity, specificity, and accuracy of electrochemical biosensors. For electrochemical biosensors, suitable surface modification can shorten the detection time. Electrochemical biosensors are mainly divided into four types, including voltammetric/amperometric biosensors, impedance biosensors, potential biosensors, and field effect transistor (FET)-based biosensors.

2.3.1 Voltammetric/amperometric biosensors

Voltammetric/amperometric biosensors have the advantage of high sensitivity, which makes them the most commonly used electrochemical biosensors [37]. So far, voltammetric/amperometric biosensors have developed a variety of methods, comprising cyclic voltammetry, linear sweep voltammetry, square wave voltammetry, and differential pulse voltammetry [38]. Both voltammetric and amperometric biosensors detect the target molecules through the current generated by electrolysis caused by electrochemical oxidation and reduction on the working electrode. When the potential is applied to the indicator electrode versus the reference electrode, the signals are determined by the mass transfer rate of reactant molecules from the solution to the electrode interface. The potential applied by the working electrode increases progressively at a constant rate in voltammetric biosensors, while the potential is applied at a constant rate in potential biosensors.

Voltammetric biosensor is one of the most commonly used electrochemical biosensors, which is widely employed for the rapid detection of SARS-CoV-2. Fabiani et al. [39] facilitate the detection of S protein and N protein of SARS-CoV-2 by electrochemical biosensors based on magnetic beads and carbon-black-based screen printed electrodes (**Figure 3a**). The electrochemical biosensor can detect the target substance in untreated saliva through the change of voltammetry curve within 30 min with LOD of S protein and N protein being 19 and 8 ng/mL, respectively. Compared with the detection results of RT-qPCR, the detection results of the electrochemical biosensor showed no difference, and the detection time is faster.

2.3.2 Impedimetric biosensors

Impedimetric biosensors are another commonly used biosensors with high sensitivity and low amplitude, which realize the analysis of targets by electrochemical impedance spectroscopy (EIS) [40]. Electrochemical impedance is the ratio of the increased voltage change to the resulting current change, and the electrochemical impedance spectroscopy can determine the resistive and capacitive components of circuit through a frequency-changed small-amplitude sinusoidal AC excitation signal. When the frequency is quite high, the redox species will be blocked by the target analyte when migrating to the electrode surface and produce a rate limiting, resulting in a frequency-dependent phase lag between the AC voltage and current. Electrochemical impedance spectroscopy can be based on Faradaic and non-Faradaic modes. EIS of Faradaic mode involves charge transfer between electrodes and the adding of redox couples, while EIS of non-Faradaic mode does not need to add additional reagents.

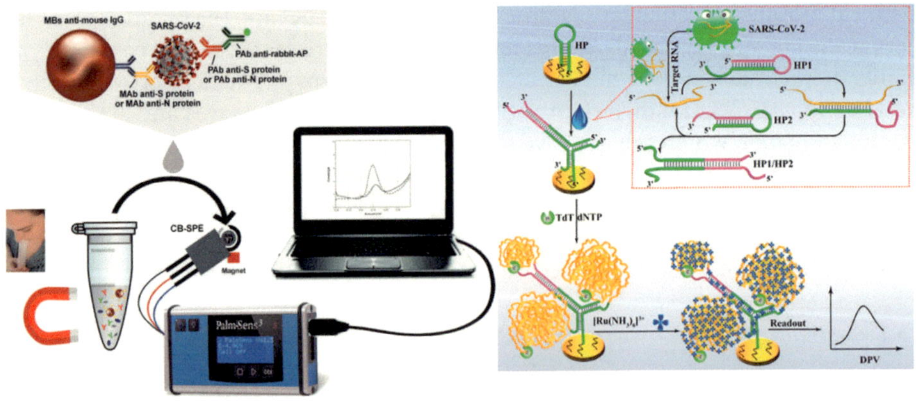

(a) (b)

Figure 3.
a: The magnetic-beads-based electrochemical assay for SARS-CoV-2 detection in untreated saliva. b: Principle of the proposed electrochemical biosensor for sensitive analysis of SARS-CoV-2 RNA.

The change of capacitive behavior is generated by charge separation at the electrode-electrolyte interface in EIS of non-Faradaic mode.

Impedimetric biosensors have also made outstanding contributions to the detection of SARS-CoV-2 antigens, antibodies, and nucleic acids. Peng et al. [41] proposed a high-sensitivity electrochemical biosensor based on impedance and voltammetry to detect the RNA of SARS-CoV-2 with the LOD of 26 fmol/L for RNA (**Figure 3b**). Target RNA will trigger the catalytic hairpin assembly circuit and cause DNA polymerization mediated by terminal deoxynucleotidyl transferase, resulting in the production of a massive of single-stranded DNA. These negatively charged single-stranded DNAs will combine with a large number of positively charged electrochemically active molecules due to electrostatic adsorption, which would amplify the electrochemical signal. The research team based on the proposed electrochemical sensor to detect clinical samples of SARS-CoV-2, which showed a high degree of stability.

2.3.3 Potentiometric biosensors

The potentiometric biosensors utilize two reference electrodes (mainly ion-selective electrode (ISEs)) to measure the charge accumulation on an electrode [42, 43]. For biological detection, potentiometric biosensors usually use enzymes to catalyze chemical reactions and generate ions near the sensing ISE. Potentiometric biosensor has the advantages of small size, fast response, easy to use, low cost, strong anti-interference ability, independent of sample volume, and has the potential to become an SARS-CoV-2 point-of-care detection tool.

After SARS-CoV-2 invades the human body, it will not only cause various antibodies in the blood, but also have a certain impact on some metabolism and enzymatic reactions. Studies have reported that the level of cholinesterase will decrease in the acute stage of severe SARS-CoV-2 infection. Pershina et al. [44] constructed a carbon-fiber-based potentiometric biosensor using polyelectrolyte multilayers to detect the ion concentration in the human biofluid of patients with SARS-CoV-2. Polyethyleneimine/polystyrene sulfonate complex has hygroscopicity and can retain ion clusters of inorganic salts, which allows the adhesion of hydrophobic ion selective membrane and produces Nernst response in miniature sensor system. This biosensor based on ion selective electrode can detect the changes of Na^{+} or K^{+} concentration in urine or blood of COVID-19 patients, and then evaluate the course of the disease. The potential biosensor has not been applied to detect the antigen, antibody, and pathogen of SARS-CoV-2 temporarily. However, this method can assess the infection status of patients by detecting the ion balance or enzymatic reaction in patients, then analyze the disease course of patients, treatment methods, and recommend the dosage of drugs.

2.3.4 FET-based biosensors

The biosensor based on field effect transistor (FET) also belongs to a kind of electrochemical biosensor, which is employed to detect the conductivity change in the electric field caused by the accumulation of charged target substances on the biosensor surface [45, 46]. FET-based biosensors have the advantages of label-free, miniaturization, easy-to-batch production, strong universality, and low cost, which are an ideal candidate for the point-of-care test of SARS-CoV-2.

Li et al. [47] constructed a graphene-based field effect transistor modified by Au nanoparticles and then modified the complementary phosphorodiamidate morpholino oligos (PMO) probe on the surface of Au nanoparticles (**Figure 4**). The FET-based biosensor can perform SARS-CoV-2 RdRp high-sensitivity test within 2 min and process low background signal caused by PMO without charge, and the LOD in throat swab is 2.29 fmol/L. In addition, the biosensor is also employed to test 30 real clinical samples, and the detection results are highly consistent with RT-qPCR. The research team further used the constructed biosensor to successfully distinguish SARS-CoV-2 RdRp and SARS-CoV RdRp. Dacheng Wei's team of Fudan University [48] constructed a electromechanical system assembling the nucleic acid fragment of SARS-CoV-2 and the graphene-based field effect transistor, which can detect the SARS-CoV-2 within 4 min.

Electrochemical biosensors have the characteristics of fast response, simple operation, low cost, and miniaturization of detection equipment, but there are still some challenges in commercialization. First of all, most of the electrochemical biosensors for detecting SARS-CoV-2 are in the laboratory stage, and some of the electrochemical biosensors have poor stability when in the external environment. Secondly, how to ensure that the structure of target molecules such as S protein or N protein will not be polluted and damaged on the unclean electrochemical detection platform, as well as the reliability of the detection results. In addition, the clinical samples are complex. The biological environment of virus/protein/nucleic acid is complicated, and the components of preservation solution will be different. Whether the sensitivity of electrochemical sensor will be affected and whether the stability of the results can be guaranteed is a problem. Of course, how to ensure that the detection personnel are not infected by the targeted virus is also a key problem for all kinds of novel biosensors.

2.3.5 Application of nanotechnology in electrochemical biosensors

In electrochemical biosensors, nanomaterials are mainly applied for modifying the sensitive interface of the biosensors or immobilizing biomolecules. Because of its large specific surface area and high surface energy, nanomaterials can become an

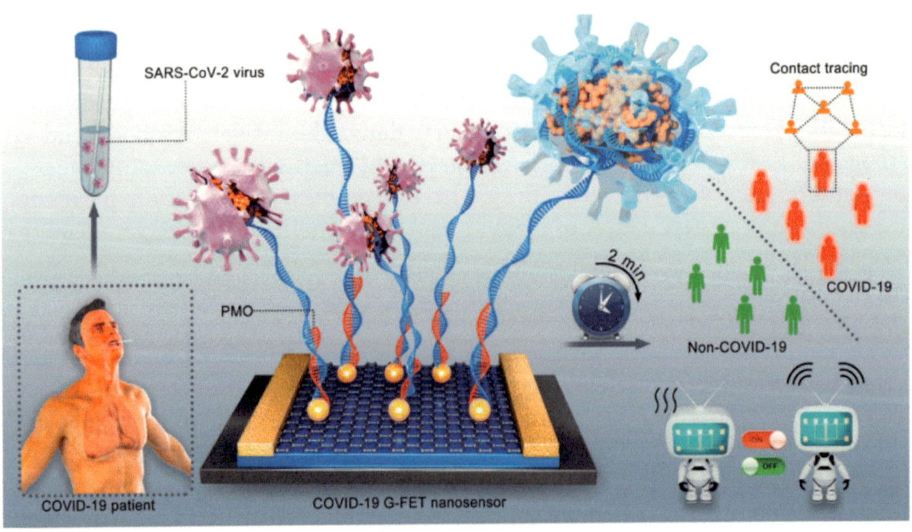

Figure 4.
Schematic diagram of rapid direct identification of SARS-CoV-2 using the PMO-functionalized G-FET nano-sensors.

active electron acceptor or electron donor. The electrode modified by nanomaterials can significantly improve the specific surface area of the electrode, improve the conductivity of the electrode, load more biomolecules, improve the sensitivity and stability of the biosensors, and speed up the response of the biosensor [49].

Nanomaterials commonly used in electrochemical biosensors include noble metal nanomaterials, carbon nanotubes, graphene, magnetic oxide nanoparticles, and so on. Noble metal nanoparticles represented by gold nanoparticles not only have large specific surface area and high surface energy, but also have high catalytic efficiency, strong adsorption, and excellent biocompatibility, which can effectively load and label target biomolecules. In addition, gold nanoparticles have excellent electrochemical activity and can effectively improve the electron transmission efficiency. Au nanoparticles can also form strong covalent binding through Au-S bond and Au-N bond, which is conducive to the coordination of biomolecules containing -SH and -NH2. Carbon-based materials such as carbon nanotubes and graphene have large specific surface area and strong electron conduction ability. The modification of this kind of carbon-based nanomaterials can greatly improve the electrochemical activity of the electrode, improve the detection sensitivity, increase the current signal, and improve the response time of the electrochemical biosensors [50]. Magnetic nanoparticles can be modified on the surface of the electrode to improve the specific surface area of the electrode, which can also be applied for immobilizing biomolecules to improve the selectivity and specificity of electrochemical detection and avoid the interference of other impurities in the biological environment to the target molecules.

2.4 Magnetic biosensors

Magnetic biosensors have attracted extensive attention of researchers in the past two decades. The biosensors can be divided into surface-based and volume-based magnetic biosensors, which are widely used in the detection of viruses, pathogens, and cancer biomarkers [51–53]. In magnetic biosensors, magnetic nanoparticles modified by suitable antibodies or DNA/RNA probes are usually used as magnetic nanotags, which can skillfully convert the concentration of analytes into magnetic signals [54]. Compared with optical, plasma, and electrochemical biosensors, magnetic biosensors have lower background noise. Because the biological environment of most biomolecules is non-magnetic, the magnetic biosensors will not be disturbed by the biological environment, so as to produce more accurate and reliable detection results [55]. Magnetic biosensors can be roughly divided into three categories: magnetoresistive (MR) biosensors, magnetic particle spectroscopy (MPS) platforms, and nuclear magnetic resonance (NMR) platforms.

2.4.1 Magnetoresistive biosensor

Magnetoresistive biosensor is a surface-based sensing technology, which is very sensitive to the stray field from generated by magnetic nanoparticles close to the sensor surface, so as to convert the binding of magnetic nanoparticles with analytes into readable electrical signals [56, 57]. Magnetic nanotags in magnetoresistive biosensors need to produce high magnetic moment without losing paramagnetic properties.

At present, there are few studies on magnetoresistive biosensors for the detection of SARS-CoV-2, and we infer main reason is that magnetic nanoparticles would inevitably reduce the magnetic moment when their size decreases. Jinhong Guo's team at the University of Electronic Science and technology of China [58] constructed an LFIA detection platform based on superparamagnetic nanoparticles and giant magnetoresistive sensing system to detect the immunoglobulin IgM and IgG of SARS-CoV-2 at the same time. Among them, the giant magnetoresistive sensing platform can transmit medical data to smart phones through Bluetooth, which is convenient for medical personnel to obtain patient information. Superparamagnetic nanoparticles with an average size of 68 nm were synthesized by a simple and rapid coprecipitation method with excellent dispersion and magnetic properties. This sensing technique has the advantages of low cost, rapidity, easy operation, and high sensitivity, which can simultaneously detect two antibodies of SARS-CoV-2 within 10 min with the LOD of 10 ng/mL for IgM and the LOD of 5 ng/mL for IgG.

2.4.2 Nuclear magnetic resonance (NMR) platform

The nuclear magnetic resonance (NMR) platform uses magnetic nanoparticles as contrast enhancer, which causes the nonuniformity of local magnetic field and disturbs the precession frequency variations of surrounding water protons [59]. Therefore, the development of high-sensitivity NMR platform essentially depends on the application of appropriate magnetic nanoparticles with high transverse relaxation.

Siwei Yang's team of Shanghai Institute of Microsystems and Information Technology, Chinese Academy of Sciences [60] reported a rapid and highly sensitive detection of SARS-CoV-2 pathogens based on ultralow-field NMR relaxometry (**Figure 5a**). This method utilizes magnetic graphene quantum dots modified by SARS-CoV-2 antibody as a probe to construct a magnetic relaxation switch to specifically detect novel coronavirus. It is worth noting that closed-tube one-step strategy is safer for experimenters without samples preparation. This one-step detection method has the characteristics of excellent sensitivity and rapid detection with 248 particles/mL within 2 min.

NMR spectroscopy, like infrared spectroscopy and Raman spectroscopy, can analyze the structure of the molecules to be measured. Different from infrared spectroscopy and Raman spectroscopy, which can directly reflect the molecular structure information, NMR spectroscopy obtains the skeleton structure of the molecules to be tested by analyzing the ^{1}H, ^{13}C, and ^{15}N NMR spectra. Nuclear magnetic resonance spectroscopy is also widely applied to the screening of antibodies of SARS-CoV-2 and the characterization of protein and nucleic acid structures. Magnetic nanoparticles can be used as a signal amplification tags in this technology to improve the sensitivity of detection. Schoenle et al. [61] reported the sequence-specific backbone assignment of the SARS-CoV-2 RBD and proved that biomolecular NMR spectroscopy chemical shift perturbation (CSP) mapping can quickly and successfully identify the molecular epitopes of RBD-specific antibodies. CSP mapping combined with other detection technology of biomolecules could help us accurately recognize the interaction between RBD and antibody, which is of great significance for antibody screening and further vaccine development.

2.4.3 Magnetic particle spectroscopy platform

Magnetic particle spectroscopy platform is a volume-based detection technology, which directly detects the dynamic magnetic responses of magnetic nanoparticles [62, 63]. Therefore, for this kind of biosensor, the properties of excitation magnetic field, saturation magnetization, and anisotropy should be considered. Rosch et al. [64] reported a novel SARS-CoV-2 nucleic acid detection platform based on

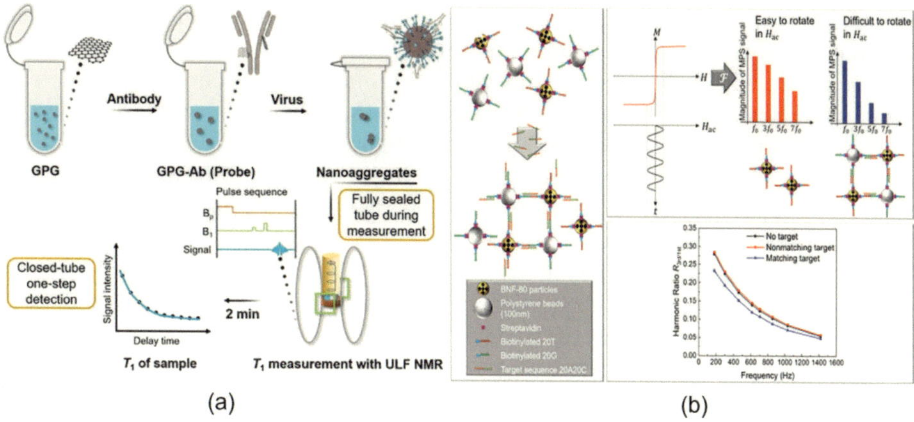

Figure 5.
a: The detection process of SARS-CoV-2 of the magnetic relaxation switches assay with ULF NMR. b: The schematic diagram of the detection of SARS-CoV-2 RNA based on magnetic particle spectroscopy biosensors.

magnetic response changes of magnetic nanoparticles (**Figure 5b**). The specific modified magnetic nanoparticles and target molecules mediated assembling will lead to the increase of hydrodynamic radius, which can be measured by the magnetic particles spectrum in alternating magnetic field. This sensing technology has high sensitivity for the detection of SARS-CoV-2 RNA, with LOD of 0.28 nmol/L, and the biological environment such as saliva will not affect the performance of the detection platform.

Compared with optical biosensors, magnetic biosensors have simpler sample processing steps in the detection process, and magnetic tags are safer than electrochemical biosensors. Because of its high sensitivity, accuracy, and specificity, magnetic sensing technology is expected to be employed for on-site detection tools to restrain the spread of SARS-CoV-2.

2.4.4 Application of nanotechnology in magnetic biosensors

The unique magnetic relaxation properties and good biocompatibility of magnetic nanomaterials give many biosensors high sensitivity and selectivity. In the process of designing magnetic biosensors, which rely on magnetic nanoparticles tags, the size of magnetic nanotags is required to match that of analytes [65]. However, with the decrease of the size of magnetic nanoparticles, these magnetic nanotags often have low magnetic moment and uneven particle size distribution. In addition, the serious surface defects on the surface of nanoparticles and the unavoidable magnetocaloric effect will cause the fluctuation of magnetic signal in the detection of low-concentration analytes. Therefore, the development of magnetic biosensors should focus on how to prepare magnetic nanoparticles with uniform size and good dispersion and the point-of-care detection of magnetic biosensors.

3. Conclusions

Up to now, SARS-CoV-2 has continued to diffuse and spread all over the world, and the epidemic of COVID-19 is facing the dilemma of globalization and time sustainability. Especially in view of the continuous variants of SARS-CoV-2 with increasing transmission speed, concealment, and the proportion of immune escape, even new variants still pose a serious and death threat to people with low immunity and the elderly. Therefore, it is necessary to further improve the conventional detection methods and break through the limitations of the original detection methods and develop new methods as a supplement or substitute for future monitoring and detection tools. Especially in some developing countries with a shortage of medical resources, it is particularly important to develop rapid, simple, high-throughput, and intelligent detection methods.

The nanotechnology attached to the novel nano-biosensing technology has developed relatively mature, but the application of biomacromolecules detection still needs to be further improved, such as the biological toxicity of nanomaterials, the modification of biomolecules on the surface of nanomaterials, the large-scale manufacturing of nanomaterials, and so on. For the novel diagnostics methods, the following aspects need to be considered:

1. High-sensitivity detection. At present, the accuracy of various PCR diagnostic kits at home and abroad is acceptable, and the limitation of detection can reach 200 ~ 500 copies/ml. However, false negatives may still occur in the detection of COVID-19 patients with low viral load. In view of the screening and future monitoring needs of the normalized management of SARS-CoV-2, it is still very necessary to develop a highly sensitive detection method that is less affected by the sampling method and sample quality in order to detect the infected person as soon as possible.

2. High-throughput detection. The simultaneous detection of a large number of samples can alleviate the detection pressure caused by the large-scale outbreak of the epidemic.

3. Multi-pathogen detection. Strengthen the ability to identify and detect a variety of pathogens, viruses, and variants. The differential diagnosis of multiple pathogens under normal management can save manual labor, material resources, and time.

4. Detection of environmental virus and identification of virus infectiousness. For the cured cases, virus detection in the environment, air, and freight develops intelligent detection technology that can distinguish the death and life of the virus, which can accurately identify the virus and avoid unnecessary false alarm and huge social cost consumption. At this stage, a new rapid and highly sensitive pathogen detection method that can distinguish the activity of SARS-CoV-2 is developed to fill the gap of current detection methods.

5. On-site detection. For different application scene such as hospitals, customs, communities, and even families, develop portable, economical, and miniaturized instruments to realize on-site rapid detection, which will greatly help to improve the timeliness of monitoring.

6. Automation and integrated detection of multiple technologies. Single detection technology always has its disadvantages. The novel diagnostic methods integrate sample pretreatment, nucleic acid extraction, amplification, and detection to truly realize "sample in-result out." By integrating the new diagnostic technology

with the existing nucleic acid, antibody, and pathogen detection methods and complementing their advantages, the combined use of them is expected to achieve the accurate and rapid detection of SARS-CoV-2. This method not only provides a powerful means for the current outbreak of COVID-19 and the detection of unknown pathogens in the future, but also has important practical significance for the future application in the fields of respiratory disease differential diagnosis, environmental monitoring, food safety assessment, etc.

7. Intelligent detection. Standardize the high-throughput screening results, instrument interpretation results, and analysis results for large population to avoid the lag and subjectivity of manual interpretation. The interpretation results are not only comparable, but also can be output in time for on-site or remote research and judgment.

Conflict of interest

The authors declare no conflict of interest.

Author details

Yong Yang[1*] and Yanyan Li[2,3,4]

1 Shanghai Institute of Ceramics, Chinese Academy of Sciences, Shanghai, China

2 State Key Laboratory of High-Performance Ceramics and Superfine Microstructures, Shanghai Institute of Ceramics, Chinese Academy of Sciences, Shanghai, People's Republic of China

3 Graduate School of the Chinese Academy of Sciences, Beijing, People's Republic of China

4 Center of Materials Science and Optoelectronics Engineering, University of Chinese Academy of Sciences, Beijing, China

*Address all correspondence to: yangyong@mail.sic.ac.cn

References

[1] Yuce M, Filiztekin E, Ozkaya KG. COVID-19 diagnosis—A review of current methods. Biosensors and Bioelectronics. 2021;**172**:112752. DOI: 10.1016/j.bios.2020.112752

[2] Ji TX, Liu ZW, Wang GQ, et al. Detection of COVID-19: A review of the current literature and future perspectives. Biosensors and Bioelectronics. 2020;**166**:112455. DOI: 10.1016/j.bios.2020.112455

[3] Xue X, Ball JK, Alexander C, et al. All surfaces are not equal in contact transmission of SARS-CoV-2. Matter. 2020;**3**:1433-1441. DOI: 10.1016/j.matt.2020.10.006

[4] Cui FY, Zhou HS. Diagnostic methods and potential portable biosensors for coronavirus disease 2019. Biosensors and Bioelectronics. 2020;**165**:112349. DOI: 10.1016/j.bios.2020.112349

[5] Baro B, Rodo P, Ouchi D, et al. Performance characteristics of five antigen-detecting rapid diagnostic test (Ag-RDT) for SARS-CoV-2 asymptomatic infection: A head-to-head benchmark comparison. Journal of Infection. 2021;**82**:269-275. DOI: 10.1016/j.jinf.2021.04.009

[6] CLM M, Paraskevaidi M, Cui L, et al. Standardization of complex biologically derived spectrochemical datasets. Nature Protocols. 2019;**14**:1546-1577. DOI: 10.1038/s41596-019-0150-x

[7] Yang LL, Yang Y, Ma YF, et al. Fabrication of semiconductor ZnO nanostructures for versatile SERS application. Nanomaterials (Basel). 2017;7:398. DOI: 10.3390/nano7110398

[8] Shan YF, Yang Y, Cao YQ, et al. Synthesis of wheatear-like ZnO nanoarrays decorated with Ag nanoparticles and its improved SERS performance through hydrogenation. Nanotechnology. 2016;**27**:145502. DOI: 10.1088/0957-4484/27/14/145502

[9] Yang Y, Nogami M, Shi JL, et al. Self-assembled semiconductor capped metal composite nanoparticles embedded in BaTiO3 thin films for nonlinear optical applications electronic. Journal of Materials Chemistry. 2003;**13**:3026-3032. DOI: 10.1039/b306590a

[10] Yang LL, Peng YS, Yang Y, et al. Green and sensitive flexible semiconductor SERS substrates: Hydrogenated black TiO2 nanowires. ACS Applied Nano Materials. 2018;**1**:4516-4527. DOI: 10.1021/acsanm.8b00796

[11] Kim H, Kang H, Kim HN, et al. Development of 6E3 antibody-mediated SERS immunoassay for drug-resistant influenza virus. Biosensors and Bioelectronics. 2021;**187**:113324. DOI: 10.1016/j.bios.2021.113324

[12] Wang JF, Wu XZ, Wang CW, et al. Facile synthesis of Au-coated magnetic nanoparticles and their application in bacteria detection via a SERS method. ACS Applied Materials Interfaces. 2016;**8**:19958-19967. DOI: 10.1021/acsami.6b07528

[13] Pramanik A, Gao Y, Patibandla S, et al. The rapid diagnosis and effective inhibition of coronavirus using spike antibody attached gold nanoparticles. Nanoscale Advances. 2021;**3**:1588-1596. DOI: 10.1039/d0na01007c

[14] Lin CL, Liang SS, Peng YS, et al. Visualized SERS imaging of single molecule by Ag/Black phosphorus

nanosheets. Nano-Micro Letters. 2022;**14**:75. DOI: 10.1007/s40820-022-00803-x

[15] Wu YX, Dang HJ, Park SG, et al. SERS-PCR assays of SARS-CoV-2 target genes using Au nanoparticles-internalized Au nanodimple substrates. Biosensors and Bioelectronics. 2022;**197**:113736. DOI: 10.1016/j.bios.2021.113736

[16] Sanchez JE, Jaramillo SA, Settles E, et al. Detection of SARS-CoV-2 and its S and N proteins using surface enhanced Raman spectroscopy. RSC Advances. 2021;**11**:25788-25794. DOI: 10.1039/d1ra03481b

[17] Li YY, Lin CL, Peng YS, et al. High-sensitivity and point-of-care detection of SARS-CoV-2 from throat and nasal swabs by magnetic SERS biosensor. Sensors and Actuators B Chemical. 2022;**365**:131974, 9 pages. DOI: 10.1016/j.snb.2022.131974

[18] Yang Y, Tanemura M, Huang ZR, et al. Aligned gold nanoneedle arrays for surface-enhanced Raman scattering. Nanotechnology. 2010;**21**:325701. DOI: 10.1088/0957-4484/21/32/325701

[19] Yang Y, Peng YS, Lin CL, et al. Human ACE2-functionalized gold "virus-trap" nanostructures for accurate capture of SARS-CoV-2 and single-virus SERS detection. Nano-Micro Letters. 2021;**13**:109. DOI: 10.1007/s40820-021-00620-8

[20] Peng YS, Lin CL, Li YY, et al. Identifying infectiousness of SARS-CoV-2 by ultra-sensitive SnS2 SERS biosensors with capillary effect. Matter. 2022;**5**:694-709. DOI: 10.1016/j.matt.2021.11.028

[21] Li JR, Wuethrich A, Edwardraja S, et al. Amplification-free SARS-CoV-2 detection using nanoyeast-scFv and ultrasensitive plasmonic nanobox-integrated nanomixing microassay. Analytical Chemistry. 2021;**93**:10251-10260. DOI: 10.1021/acs.analchem.1c01657

[22] Zhang M, Li XD, Pan JL, et al. Ultrasensitive detection of SARS-CoV-2 spike protein in untreated saliva using SERS-based biosensor. Biosensors and Bioelectronics. 2021;**190**:113421. DOI: 10.1016/j.bios.2021.113421

[23] Zhang DY, Zhang XL, Ma R, et al. Ultra-fast and onsite interrogation of severe acute respiratory syndrome coronavirus 2 (SARS-CoV-2) in waters via surface enhanced Raman scattering (SERS). Water Research. 2021;**200**:117243. DOI: 10.1016/j.watres.2021.117243

[24] Marques AC, Pinheiro T, Morais M, et al. Bottom-up microwave-assisted seed-mediated synthesis of gold nanoparticles onto nanocellulose to boost stability and high performance for SERS applications. Applied Surface Science. 2021;**561**:150060. DOI: 10.1016/j.apsusc.2021.150060

[25] Sitjar J, Xu HZ, Liu CY, et al. Synergistic surface-enhanced Raman scattering effect to distinguish live SARS-CoV-2 S pseudovirus. Analytica Chimica Acta. 2022;**1193**:339406. DOI: 10.1016/j.aca.2021.339406

[26] Chen H, Park SK, Joung Y, et al. SERS-based dual-mode DNA aptasensors for rapid classification of SARS-CoV-2 and influenza A/H1N1 infection. Sensors and Actuators: B. Chemical. 2022;**355**:131324. DOI: 10.1016/j.snb.2021.131324

[27] Chen C, Wang JS. Optical biosensors: An exhaustive and comprehensive review. Analyst. 2020;**145**:1605-1628. DOI: 10.1039/c9an01998g

[28] Firdous S, Anwar S, Rafya R. Development of surface plasmon resonance (SPR) biosensors for use in the diagnostics of malignant and infectious diseases. Laser Physics Letters. 2018;**15**:065602. DOI: 10.1088/1612-202X/aab43f

[29] Lynn NS, Dandy DS. Passive microfluidic pumping using coupled capillary/evaporation effects. Lab on a Chip. 2009;**9**:3422-3429. DOI: 10.1039/b912213c

[30] Huang LP, Ding LF, Zhou J, et al. One-step rapid quantification of SARS-CoV-2 virus particles via low-cost nanoplasmonic sensors in generic microplate reader and point-of-care device. Biosensors and Bioelectronics. 2021;**171**:112685. DOI: 10.1016/j.bios.2020.112685

[31] Yano TA, Kajisa T, Ono M, et al. Ultrasensitive detection of SARS-CoV-2 nucleocapsid protein using large gold nanoparticle-enhanced surface plasmon resonance. Scientific Reports. 2022;**12**:1060. DOI: 10.1038/s41598-022-05036-x

[32] Kajiura M, Nakanishi T, Iida H, et al. Biosensing by optical waveguide spectroscopy based on localized surface plasmon resonance of gold nanoparticles used as a probe or as a label. Journal of Colloid and Interface Science. 2009;**335**:140-145. DOI: 10.1016/j.jcis.2009.03.016

[33] Torrente-Rodriguez RM, Lukas H, Tu J, et al. SARS-CoV-2 rapidPlex: A graphene-based multiplexed telemedicine platform for rapid and low-cost COVID-19 diagnosis and monitoring. Matter. 2020;**3**:1981-1998. DOI: 10.1016/j.matt.2020.09.027

[34] Akshath US, Shubha LR, Bhatt P, et al. Quantum dots as optical labels for ultrasensitive detection of polyphenols. Biosensors and Bioelectronics. 2014;**57**:317-323. DOI: 10.1016/j.bios.2014.01.038

[35] Nishitani S, Sakata T. Enhancement of signal-to-noise ratio for serotonin detection with well-designed nanofilter-coated potentiometric electrochemical biosensor. ACS Applied Materials Interfaces. 2020;**12**:14761-14769. DOI: 10.1021/acsami.9b19309

[36] Dai Y, Liu CC. Recent advances on electrochemical biosensing strategies toward universal point-of-care systems. Angewandte Chemie (International Edition in English). 2019;**58**:12355-12368. DOI: 10.1002/anie.201901879

[37] Bollella P, Gorton L. Enzyme based amperometric biosensors. Current Opinion in Electrochemistry. 2018;**10**:157-173. DOI: 10.1016/j.coelec.2018.06.003

[38] Chen A, Chatterjee S. Nanomaterials based electrochemical sensors for biomedical applications. Chemical Society Reviews. 2013;**42**:5425-5438. DOI: 10.1039/c3cs35518g

[39] Fabiani L, Saroglia M, Galata G, et al. Magnetic beads combined with carbon black-based screen-printed electrodes for COVID-19: A reliable and miniaturized electrochemical immunosensor for SARS-CoV-2 detection in saliva. Biosensors and Bioelectronics. 2021;**171**:112686. DOI: 10.1016/j.bios.2020.112686

[40] MDT T, WR d A, LF d L, et al. Low-cost biosensor for rapid detection of SARS-CoV-2 at the point of care. Matter. 2021;**4**:2403-2416. DOI: 10.1016/j.matt.2021.05.003

[41] Peng Y, Pan YH, Sun ZW, et al. An electrochemical biosensor for

sensitive analysis of the SARS-CoV-2 RNA. Biosensors and Bioelectronics. 2021;**186**:113309. DOI: 10.1016/j.bios.2021.113309

[42] Kimmel DW, Leblanc G, Meschievitz ME, et al. Electrochemical sensors and biosensors. Analytical Chemistry. 2012;**84**:685-707. DOI: 10.1021/ac202878q

[43] Luo XL, Davis JJ. Electrical biosensors and the label free detection of protein disease biomarkers. Chemical Society Reviews. 2013;**42**:5944-5962. DOI: 10.1039/c3cs60077g

[44] Pershina LV, Grabeklis AR, Isankina LN, et al. Determination of sodium and potassium ions in patients with SARS-Cov-2 disease by ion-selective electrodes based on polyelectrolyte complexes as a pseudo-liquid contact phase. RSC Advances. 2021;**11**:36215-36221. DOI: 10.1039/d1ra04582b

[45] Gutierrez-Sanz O, Andoy NM, Filipiak MS, et al. Direct, label-free, and rapid transistor-based immunodetection in whole serum. ACS Sensors. 2017;**2**:1278-1286. DOI: 10.1021/acssensors.7b00187

[46] Kang H, Wang XJ, Guo MQ, et al. Ultrasensitive detection of SARS-CoV-2 antibody by graphene field-effect transistors. Nano Letters. 2021;**21**:7897-7904. DOI: 10.1021/acs.nanolett.1c00837

[47] Li JH, Wu D, Yu Y, et al. Rapid and unamplified identification of COVID-19 with morpholino-modified graphene field-effect transistor nanosensor. Biosensors and Bioelectronics. 2021;**183**:113206. DOI: 10.1016/j.bios.2021.113206

[48] Wang LQ, Wang XJ, Wu YG, et al. Rapid and ultrasensitive electromechanical detection of ions, biomolecules and SARS-CoV-2 RNA in unamplified samples. Nature Biomedical Engineering. 2022;**6**:276-285. DOI: 10.1038/s41551-021-00833-7

[49] You CC, Chompoosor A, Rotello VM. The biomacromolecule-nanoparticle interface. Nano Today. 2007;**2**:34-43. DOI: 10.1016/s1748-0132(07)70085-3

[50] Banks CE, Crossley A, Salter C, et al. Carbon nanotubes contain metal impurities which are responsible for the “electrocatalysis” seen at some nanotube-modified electrodes. Angewandte Chemie International Edition in English. 2006;**45**:2533-2537. DOI: 10.1002/anie.200600033

[51] Aytur T, Foley J, Anwar M, et al. A novel magnetic bead bioassay platform using a microchip-based sensor for infectious disease diagnosis. Journal of Immunological Methods. 2006;**314**:21-29. DOI: 10.1016/j.jim.2006.05.006

[52] Hash S, Martinez-Viedma MP, Fung F, et al. Nuclear magnetic resonance biosensor for rapid detection of vibrio parahaemolyticus. Biomedical Journal. 2019;**42**:187-192. DOI: 10.1016/j.bj.2019.01.009

[53] Su DQ, Wu K, Krishna VD, et al. Detection of influenza a virus in swine nasal swab samples with a wash-free magnetic bioassay and a handheld giant magnetoresistance sensing system. Frontiers in Microbiology. 2019;**10**:1077. DOI: 10.3389/fmicb.2019.01077

[54] Pastucha M, Farka Z, Lacina K, et al. Magnetic nanoparticles for smart electrochemical immunoassays: A review on recent developments. Mikrochimica Acta. 2019;**186**:312. DOI: 10.1007/s00604-019-3410-0

[55] Schotter J, Kamp PB, Becker A, et al. Comparison of a prototype

magnetoresistive biosensor to standard fluorescent DNA detection. Biosensors and Bioelectronics. 2004;**19**:1149-1156. DOI: 10.1016/j.bios.2003.11.007

[56] Baibich MN, Broto JM, Fert A, et al. Giant magnetoresistance of (001)Fe/(001)Cr magnetic superlattices. Physical Review Letters. 1988;**61**:2472-2475. DOI: 10.1103/PhysRevLett.61.2472

[57] Binasch G, Grunberg P, Saurenbach F, et al. Enhanced magnetoresistance in layered magnetic structures with antiferromagnetic interlayer exchange. Physical Review B: Condensed Matter. 1989;**39**:4828-4830. DOI: 10.1103/physrevb.39.4828

[58] Bayin Q, Huang L, Ren CH, et al. Anti-SARS-CoV-2 IgG and IgM detection with a GMR based LFIA system. Talanta. 2021;**227**:122207. DOI: 10.1016/j.talanta.2021.122207

[59] Zalesskiy SS, Danieli E, Blumich B, et al. Miniaturization of NMR systems: Desktop spectrometers, microcoil spectroscopy, and "NMR on a chip" for chemistry, biochemistry, and industry. Chemical Reviews. 2014;**114**:5641-5694. DOI: 10.1021/cr400063g

[60] Li YQ, Ma PX, Tao Q, et al. Magnetic graphene quantum dots facilitate closed-tube one-step detection of SARS-CoV-2 with ultra-low field NMR relaxometry. Sensors and Actuators: B. Chemical. 2021;**337**:129786. DOI: 10.1016/j.snb.2021.129786

[61] Schoenle MV, Li Y, Yuan M, et al. NMR based SARS-CoV-2 antibody screening. Journal of the American Chemical Society. 2021;**143**:7930-7934. DOI: 10.1021/jacs.1c03945

[62] Zhang X, Reeves DB, Perreard IM, et al. Molecular sensing with magnetic nanoparticles using magnetic spectroscopy of nanoparticle Brownian motion. Biosensors and Bioelectronics. 2013;**50**:441-446. DOI: 10.1016/j.bios.2013.06.049

[63] Znoyko SL, Orlov AV, Bragina VA, et al. Nanomagnetic lateral flow assay for high-precision quantification of diagnostically relevant concentrations of serum TSH. Talanta. 2020;**216**:120961. DOI: 10.1016/j.talanta.2020.120961

[64] Rösch EL, Zhong J, Lak A, et al. Point-of-need detection of pathogen-specific nucleic acid targets using magnetic particle spectroscopy. Biosensors and Bioelectronics. 2021;**192**:113536. DOI: 10.1016/j.bios.2021.113536

[65] Wu K, Saha R, Su DQ, et al. Magnetic-nanosensor-based virus and pathogen detection strategies before and during COVID-19. ACS Applied Nano Materials. 2020;**3**:9560-9580. DOI: 10.1021/acsanm.0c02048

Chapter 11

Perspective Chapter: Microfluidic Technologies for On-Site Detection and Quantification of Infectious Diseases – The Experience with SARS-CoV-2/COVID-19

Andres Escobar and Chang-qing Xu

Abstract

Over the last 2 years, the economic and infrastructural damage incurred by the severe acute respiratory syndrome coronavirus 2 (SARS-CoV-2) has exposed several limitations in the world's preparedness for a pandemic-level virus. Conventional diagnostic techniques that were key in minimizing the potential transmission of SARS-CoV-2 were limited in their overall effectiveness as on-site diagnostic devices due to systematic inefficiencies. The most prevalent of said inefficiencies include their large turnaround times, operational costs, the need for laboratory equipment, and skilled personnel to conduct the test. This left many people in the early stages of the pandemic without the means to test themselves readily and reliably while minimizing further transmission. This unmet demand created a vacuum in the healthcare system, as well as in industry, that drove innovation in several types of diagnostic platforms, including microfluidic and non-microfluidic devices. In this chapter, we will explore how integrated microfluidic technologies have facilitated the improvements of previously existing diagnostic platforms for fast and accurate on-site detection of infectious diseases.

Keywords: microfluidics, SARS-CoV-2, covid-19, diagnostics, healthcare, on-site, infectious diseases

1. Introduction

Severe acute respiratory syndrome coronavirus 2 (SARS-CoV-2) is a type of highly infectious pathogen that is unique compared to many other viruses seen in recent history [1]. The virulent nature of SARS-CoV-2 has allowed it to set the stage for the current global pandemic that continues to plague our society, known as coronavirus disease 2019 (COVID-19) [1]. Over the last 2 years, COVID-19 has drastically altered the way in which humans have lived and is expected to continue with no foreseeable end. As a result of the pandemic, people, businesses, and governments alike have been forced to adapt to continuously changing situations. The changes in people's daily routines, workplace habits, and social interactions over the past 2 years, only account for a fraction of the seemingly permanent COVID-19-induced changes [2]. Otherwise known as the COVID-19 experience, these adaptations and changes to our society are not limited to the experiences of average citizens. SARS-CoV-2 has also fundamentally altered how institutions such as the healthcare industry and governments respond to potentially pandemic-level infectious diseases, both in terms of diagnostic capabilities and social practices [2].

Unlike many other viruses in the same coronavirus family, SARS-CoV-2 was found to be sufficiently infectious and complex that it was not readily or accurately diagnosed in the early stages of the pandemic. SARS-CoV-2 almost always initially presents itself as a mild case of the common cold or seasonal flu virus [1]. These near-asymptomatic early-stage primary infections, coupled with the limitations in early diagnostic testing, have led to some of the highest rates of lethality and long-lasting symptoms seen in the last century [3]. As of March 2022, it has been reported that COVID-19 has been officially linked to over 6,000,000 deaths worldwide. At one time, it was the second-leading cause of global deaths in both children and adults [3]. SARS-CoV-2's unique characteristic of presenting seemingly mild or asymptomatic cases continues to be one of the most difficult aspects of managing the spread and treatment of infected patients. In one study, it has been reported that roughly 50% of all new SARS-CoV-2 infections were estimated to have originated from asymptomatic individuals [4], which included both individuals who transmitted prior to the development of symptoms (42%) and individuals who never developed symptoms (8%) [4]. Studies such as these reinforced the unnerving truth that transmission between primary infections and secondary infections was just as likely to originate from a seemingly asymptomatic individual as a symptomatic individual. In the early stages of the pandemic, this inability to discern between infected and uninfected COVID-19 patients forced researchers and healthcare professionals around the world to collaborate and assess the potential for the initial epidemic of COVID-19 to evolve into a pandemic. To do so, researchers and healthcare professionals evaluated the risk of reaching a pandemic status through epidemiological studies, with various empirical techniques [5]. One of the best-established techniques for assessing risk is the reproduction number (R_0).

As seen in **Figure** 1, R_0 represents a well-established epidemiological concept that measures the potential for an infectious disease to spread by determining the average number of secondary infections that one primary case will generate [5]. Assuming nobody is either immune or vaccinated, an R_0 value less than zero would represent the infections eventually stopping on their own, whereas an R_0 greater than zero would estimate exponential growth in the number of cases in the given population. With R_0 values averaging over 2.0 in most parts of the world, COVID-19 was expected to reach pandemic levels by the start of the second year [6]. Prior to December 2020 (when vaccines became mass-produced and widely distributed), SARS-CoV-2 was a global virus that would endure for many years to come. Without an accurate means of diagnosing individuals for SARS-CoV-2, there were no reliable means for quickly managing potential outbreaks and secondary infections. The high risk of lethality and seemingly permanent post-infection symptoms thus prompted urgent and necessary advancements in vaccine technology, but more importantly in diagnostic technology [1–4].

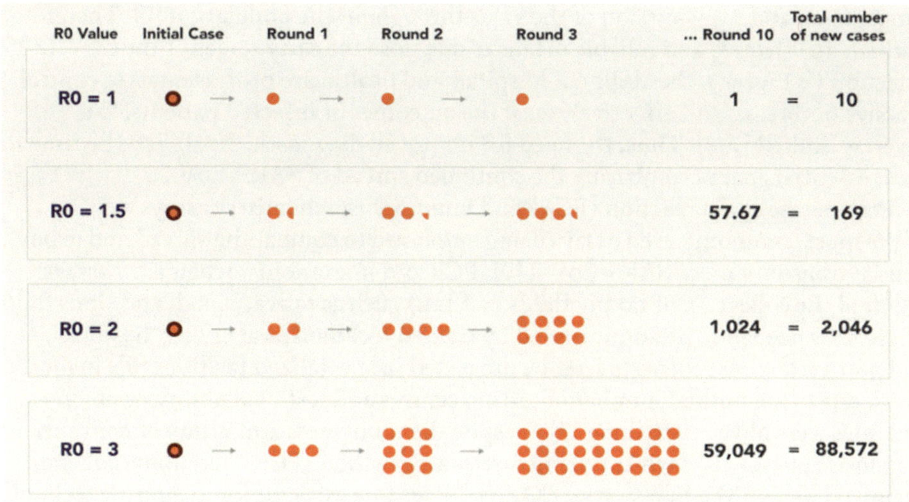

Figure 1.
A schematic for visualizing the practical significance of R_0 values. Adapted from Ref. [5].

2. The COVID-19 "Experience"

SARS-CoV-2 has become the most persistent and lethal virus seen in the last century. After more than 2 years, to date, the COVID-19 pandemic has drastically changed the lives of people across the globe. Although the pandemic is an ongoing issue, there are two major time periods which each contain several important milestones in the evolution and management of life during the COVID-19 pandemic. The first year preceded the mass administration and distribution of vaccines and diagnostic testing [2]. While the second year saw more focus on the amelioration of the post-mass-vaccination testing capabilities and societal norms of countries worldwide [6]. By highlighting some of the milestones within the 2 years, the progression of the COVID-19 "experience" can be traced.

2.1 Year one

In the pre-vaccination stage of the COVID-19 pandemic, between December 2019 and 2020, most people's "experience" with COVID-19 included a constant fear of unknowingly being infected with SARS-CoV-2 [1–4]. At the time, a significant amount of immune-compromised and seemingly healthy individuals infected with SARS-CoV-2 were readily being admitted to the hospital with a range of symptoms as mild as incessant coughs to more severe symptoms such as shortness of breath and even death [4]. As vaccines had not yet been developed, most people had not yet developed innate or induced immunological defences to this novel virus and feared the uncertainty in symptoms severity [4, 6, 7]. This concern was further magnified after reports of hospitalized COVID-19 patients presenting little to no symptoms, symptoms often indistinguishable from the symptoms of the more common seasonal flu, during the early stages of infection. The ambiguity of symptom development coupled with the high transmissibility of SARS-CoV-2 resulted in an increased likelihood of unreported transmission, and an even greater difficulty in tracking the propagation and transmission of the virus throughout the population [7]. Therefore, without an effective and reliable means to diagnose the early stages of the COVID-19 infection (< 1 week), the ability of hospitals and healthcare professionals to control massive outbreaks and effectively treat the outcomes of infected patients, was severely limited [7, 8]. Thus, the need for improved diagnostic capabilities became the most essential goal in combating the continued spread of SARS-CoV-2.

Polymerase chain reaction (PCR) and immunohistochemistry assays were two of the most commonly used assays being employed to combat the spread and exponential transmission of SARS-CoV-2 [9]. PCR and immunohistochemistry assays required the collection of bodily fluids (> 1 mL) such as saliva, blood, and sinus fluid. These tests needed to be administered by trained technicians at clinics, hospitals, and pop-up testing centres to later be processed in specialized facilities [6]. In most cases, due to the limited number of testing centres and test-availability, wait-times and lines were always very long [7]. Despite the robustness and utility of conventional diagnostic platforms, such as polymerase chain reaction (PCR) and immunohistochemistry assays, the first year of COVID-19 became difficult for diagnostic technologies to match the increasing global demand [9, 10]. The need for improved diagnostic capabilities became increasingly apparent, forcing the requirements for conventional diagnostic platforms to evolve as well. PCR tests sported a limit of detection (LOD) and specificity that was yet unmatched by alternative testing technology like immunohistochemistry assays [2, 9]. In the early to middle stages of the first year, this practice of diagnosing patients experiencing flu-like symptoms, who are potentially infected with SARS-CoV-2, with PCR tests became the gold standard. For a time, it allowed healthcare professionals to better manage and track primary infections, from mild to severe symptomatic infections, by providing a superficial means to control potential outbreaks through contact tracing [2, 9, 10]. In addition, it allowed for better-directed resources and healthcare efforts for those positively infected with SARS-CoV-2. This, however, would prove to eventually become less and less viable as a diagnostic method, due to the test speed at which transmissions between primary and secondary infections were occurring.

Although PCR tests are normally able to process tests within 1 week of submission, the delay in onset of symptoms and high transmissibility of SARS-CoV-2, severely hindered its effectiveness to facilitate tracing and resource management in the healthcare system [11]. To further hinder the efforts of PCR testing, testing backlogs at processing facilities resulted in a delay of over two weeks to receive testing results. This coupled with the understanding that SARS-CoV-2 was often transmitted before the onset of symptoms (< 1 week) meant that people were now not able to confirm their state of infectiousness until their infectious period had already passed. The sheer speed and virality of SARS-CoV-2 left PCR tests incapable of forewarning primary infections of their risk of transmission. PCR tests, shown in **Figure 2**, remained the gold standard for the diagnosis of SARS-CoV-2. However, exploring other detection methods may address some tests' inherent limitations.

The newly observed limitations of PCR testing, highlighted by the exponential growth of SARS-CoV-2 cases across the globe, demonstrated that future prospective diagnostic tests required less turnaround time and greater accessibility to the public [12]. Near the end of the first year, in response to the growing need for even faster SARS-CoV-2 diagnostic technology, funding and research into "rapid" immunohistochemistry tests began to grow exponentially [2, 13]. At the time, rapid tests based on immunohistochemistry were difficult to mass-produce with enough rigor to reliably diagnose patients for SARS-CoV-2, while also being logistically difficult to meet its

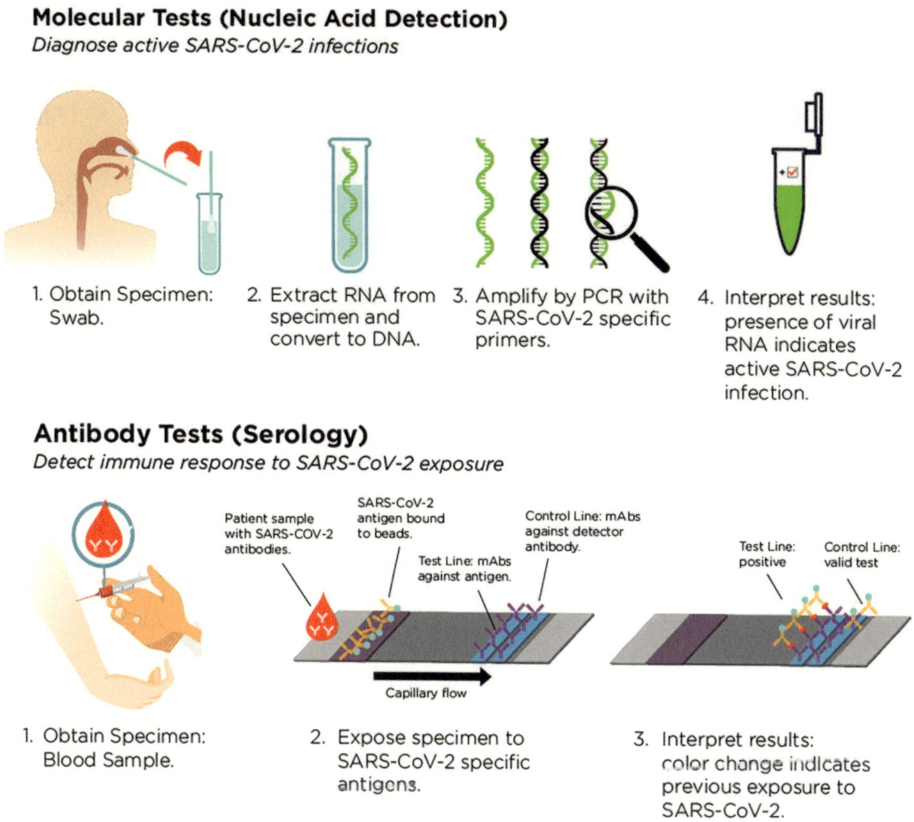

Figure 2.
A visualization of the testing procedures involved in PCR and immunohistochemistry assays. Adapted from Ref. [12].

demand [9, 13, 14]. At minimum, future rapid tests would now need to be more accessible such that people might be able to test in any environment without specialized equipment while producing results within the first week of suspected infection to help prevent primary infections from spreading. Moreover, the production and distribution of these potential tests would require great logistical improvements, which would not be possible without a great deal of continued funding. These obstacles meant PCR tests, for a little while longer, would remain the gold-standard for SARS-CoV-2 diagnostics over other detection methods, including immunohistochemical assays. This growing list of requirements jumpstarted the need for the technological advancements that would lead to the mass-production of rapid, accurate, low-cost, on-site tests seen in the second year of the COVID-19 pandemic [2, 8]. The improvements that earlier quantitative and qualitative rapid tests required to meet the needs of society could have been addressed more readily, in the short-term, with immunohistochemical detection methods, but were not the most viable long-term solution [12, 13].

2.2 Year two

By early 2021, the fear of unknowingly acquiring and transmitting SARS-CoV-2 prompted governments, healthcare professionals and businesses to enter a state of stasis; with the hopes, it would mitigate the transmission and persistence of SARS-CoV-2 [2, 14]. Under the advisement of healthcare professionals, people were now forced to restrict their social interactions and to experience heightened levels of caution between one another for necessary tasks. This time of stasis created a loop of financial and emotional hardships between consumers and businesses in ways the world had never experienced before. The speed at which SARS-CoV-2 was transmitted between individuals was not the only concern researchers were trying to address by improving our qualitative and quantitative diagnostic capabilities. Variants of the SARS-CoV-2 virus were slowly emerging and becoming an increasing cause for concern during the spring of 2021 [15]. The emergence of the SARS-CoV-2 variants had now provoked a resurging fear across the globe.

With the introduction of vaccines in early 2021, the potential prevention and reduction of SARS-CoV-2 infections quickly turned much of the first year's fear, uncertainty, and general unease into hope [2, 11, 15]. The hopeful end to COVID-19, at this time, was further supported by a large increase in the production and accessibility of rapid (< 30 min) diagnostic tests that helped to control the spread of SARS-CoV-2 variants. Despite the emergence of the virus variants, people were hoping to return to some sense of normalcy. To facilitate this transition, some governments and healthcare professionals began relaxing health policies as vaccinations were being regularly administered to a large portion of the population. This hope would, however, prove to be short-lived as novel discoveries demonstrated the virus's ability to replicate and mutate into several increasingly more infectious variants [15]. Almost exclusively across the second year of the pandemic, five COVID-19 variants of note were recorded by the World Health Organization (WHO) [15]. These variants of note included Alpha and Beta (discovered in December 2020), Gamma (January 2021), Delta (April 2021), and Omicron (November 2021) [15]. Each variant of note is structurally similar to that of the original strain, often referred to as the "index virus," in that they all contain a lipid shell that houses viral genetic material and spike proteins on the surface of the lipid shell, which facilitates the anchoring and fusion of viral cells to healthy cells [2]. However, each subsequently discovered variant of SARS-CoV-2 demonstrates slight differences in the structure of the spike proteins that occupy the outer lipid shell [2]. Normally, our bodies are built to naturally defend against repeated infections from viruses by producing antibodies that specifically target the surface proteins of a previously introduced virus, as well as antibodies with slight modifications to try and prevent infections from similarly structured viruses [7, 9]. Unfortunately, the slight variations in spike proteins of subsequent SARS-CoV-2 variants proved to be significant enough that the body could not recognize or defend against them, resulting in increased infectiousness that bypasses both the induced and innate immune response against infections. This meant that despite the induced protection from the SARS-CoV-2 vaccines, these new variants could once again infect a person without presenting symptoms in the early stages of infection. Mass-production of diagnostic rapid tests was now, more than ever, in direct need of improvements to aid in combating the spread of SARS-CoV-2 and its variants. The previously established quantitative and qualitative tests, such as PCR and **ELISA, offered their own strengths and limitations, but neither could meet the needs of the healthcare system to help control the spread of SARS-CoV-2 independently. Therefore, alternative diagnostic technologies were being explored. Microfluidic systems continued to show great promise in addressing the shortcomings of the diagnostic testing platforms currently available, as well as the logistical limitations in mass-producing these tests [16].

3. The evolution of diagnostic technology throughout the COVID-19 pandemic

By December of 2019, SARS-CoV-2 became a newly established virus, which meant that researchers and scientists did not yet have a thorough understanding of how SARS-CoV-2 transmission occurred or exactly how infectious and deadly it would become [12, 16]. This meant that many of the established conventional diagnostic technologies were not yet optimized for the accuracy, sample processing speed, and capacity for mass production that was required to help control mass outbreaks like the COVID-19 pandemic. As a result, many of the deaths and infections unknowingly caused by COVID-19 in the first year could not have been averted. The obstacles to outbreak management and tracing caused by a strain on the healthcare systems around the world almost certainly led to the underestimation of both the transmission rate, severity, and the capacity of COVID-19 as a pandemic-level threat. In effect, the world was not prepared for the rampant shortages of hospital beds, cleaning supplies, and masks which were essential for mitigating people's exposure risk to the virus [16]. Eventually, SARS-CoV-2 diagnostic tests would be able to accurately diagnose patients in a reasonable amount of time. However, it took roughly 1 year and a half to achieve a sufficient level of reliable testing capabilities utilizing improvements on previously established diagnostic systems [16].

3.1 The cost of technological advancement

Given the rampant fear brought on by the uncertainty of the first year of the pandemic, it was given that a collective effort across worldwide industry, healthcare professionals, and governments would be necessary to tackle the logistical and technological shortcomings of developing rapid diagnostic tests. In response, many resource-abundant countries promised to commit billions of dollars worth of funding to promote the development and manufacturing of rapid tests [17]. Due to the large influx of funding, the attraction for developing increasingly robust rapid tests prompted many small and large-scale companies to try and compete to mass-produce effective tests faster than each other. By the summer of 2021, there was increased access to rapid, 30-minute tests, which allowed people to slowly gain clarity on how to go more carefully about their daily lives while reducing the spread of COVID-19 [17]. These rapid tests empowered people to monitor their own social behaviours and individual health to a greater degree than what was previously possible, providing them with the knowledge to minimize their risk for exposure and transmission. This short-term competition between companies had lent itself to exponential advancements in the development and production of rapid tests which resulted in some countries eventually being able to give out limited numbers of rapid tests for free. Within countries that were fortunate enough to have ready access to a combination of vaccines and rapid tests, the number of COVID-19 cases saw a gradual reduction, over an extended period of time [2, 10]. Conversely, the risk for continued viral transmission was not effectively addressed in resource-limited countries. Other less-equipped countries were unable to produce, receive or distribute as many rapid tests as their more fortunate counterparts, to their own citizens. The disparity between countries for access to rapid tests was observed to have, in part, a direct correlation with population size and density, as well as the economic state of a country's wellbeing [7, 10]. Thus, the short-term reliance on rapid diagnostic tests that were too costly to produce or distribute in resource-limited countries highlighted the possibility of conventional diagnostic techniques not being ideal in globally addressing the importance of fair access to accurate and rapid testing.

3.2 Progression of PCR and immunohistochemical diagnostics

Accurately tracking the state of active infectiousness in a person with SARS-CoV-2 is an essential tool in managing and combating potential outbreaks by providing people with primary infections some insight into a timeline for when and how long they should be self-isolating to reduce the risk of propagating secondary infections [17]. The progression of an individual's infection, otherwise known as active infectiousness, can ideally be monitored by quantifying the viral load of a person, the number of viral copies in a unit volume of bodily fluid. Measuring the viral load can in turn provide healthcare professionals and researchers with useful data pertaining to the time required for the onset of symptoms and the state of a person's active infectiousness.

Quantifying the concentration of individual units of double-stranded template genetic material (DNA) in a unit volume of sample is possible through PCR. By cycling through the three major steps of PCR (denaturation, annealing, and elongation), one individual copy of DNA can be multiplied exponentially [8]. However, assessing the "active infectiousness" of a person involves quantifying individual units of viral genetic material, which are instead, units of single-stranded mRNA [8, 17]. To use single-stranded mRNA as the substrate for the replication of genetic material, we first require a molecular complex known as a reverse-transcriptase (RT) to create a complementary strand of DNA (cDNA) to the template single-stranded mRNA [8, 9]. By introducing the RT to the template mRNA, a double-stranded DNA template that can be further amplified in a downstream PCR reaction, is created. This technique combines these two processes to create RT-PCR (rtPCR) which will inevitably allow for the amplification of genetic material from mRNA. To later quantify mRNA samples previously amplified through rtPCR, the use of a fluorescent reporter molecule must be used [8]. This reporter molecule could be in the form of a dye or a molecular complex, such as a probe. These reporter molecules will then bind to double-stranded DNA, if it is a dye or a specific target sequence if it is a genetic probe [8]. By measuring the increase in fluorescence of the sample, a quantitative PCR (qPCR) analysis can be achieved. The fewer number of cycles it takes for the sample to fluoresce beyond a certain threshold, the greater the concentration of genetic material, and vice versa. This process allows for the detection of targeted sequences in very low concentrations as well as quantification of viral loads through the addition of fluorescence-based reporter probes. PCR assays have shown their use in reliably diagnosing infectious diseases, with a reasonable amount of accuracy, but require higher costs and turnaround times than other methods such as immunohistochemistry assays.

Immunohistochemical assays, such as in **Figure 3**, offer qualitative detection methods that do not rely on a genetic component but instead on the intrinsic binding properties of antibodies and aptamers to biomarkers of interest [17, 18]. Qualitative, immunohistochemical assay, rapid 30-minute tests were designed to target some of the most common antibodies present in people infected with SARS-CoV-2, namely IgG, IgM, and IgA, but lacked the ability to track the progression of an individual's infection [2, 18]. Due to the potential specificity of antibodies and aptamers to biomarkers of interest, false positives in immunohistochemical assays are not common, however, false negatives are not so uncommon in rapid diagnostic systems [19]. Due to the strictly qualitative nature of the test, the concentration of target molecules

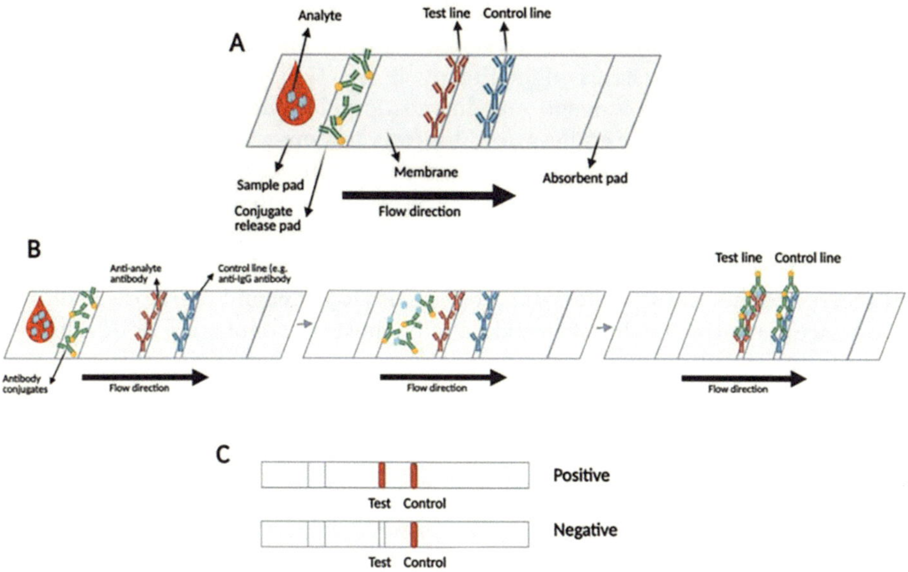

Figure 3.
A visualization of the qualitative nature of a rapid immunohistochemistry diagnostic test. Adapted from Ref. [11].

must reach a certain threshold before resulting in an observable positive result and can result in false negatives [19]. As a trade-off, these assays can instead gain a greater amount of modularity, selectivity, and specificity compared to other assays by researching and testing combinations of detector and target molecules to optimize the detection technique. One important example of an immunohistochemical assay with proven applications in medical diagnostics is the enzyme-linked immunosorbent assay (ELISA). ELISA assays bind antigens onto an absorbent surface that would facilitate the even distribution of a test buffer and sample mixture across the entire surface through capillary action [17, 19]. When a target antibody moves across some of the bound antigens on the surface, they will bind and be fixed onto the surface in a particular orientation [17]. Afterward, the secondary detection antibody, designed to be complimentary to the antibody at the other end of the target antibody, then subsequently becomes fixed onto the surface allowing for conformational changes in the detection antibody. This conformational change then allows for a reporter gene to be activated and create a colour change that can be qualitatively assessed by the naked eye [17]. However, unlike PCR tests, this technology is not capable of achieving quantitative diagnostic capabilities.

Despite the numerous technological advances in diagnostic technology, many conventional detection techniques such as immunohistochemistry and PCR have yet to comprehensively address the requirements for a mass-producible, rapid, on-site diagnostic test that is capable of both quantitative and qualitative results [19]. Many of these diagnostic tests are too costly to manufacture in resource-limited parts of the world, increasing their intrinsic cost and restricting their access from the general-public. In addition, the on-site requirements of many of these available tests are too great either structurally or logistically to be reliably used and shipped across the globe. For example, several types of cost-effective tests cannot withstand extreme changes in weather conditions through transit and could be compromised in terms of their accuracy. Many currently available rapid tests (< 30 min) have insufficient detection limits to provide an accurate diagnosis across the early stage (0–7 days) of infection, where primary cases might already be infectious to surrounding people [2, 19]. The limitations of conventional diagnostic techniques are continuously magnified by the seemingly endless need for tests as more and more variants, with greater infectiousness than their predecessor, begin to make our healthcare practices less effective over time. Moreover, the benefits of such technological and health-related advancements were limited to wealthier countries, which celebrated earlier access to both vaccines and rapid tests, long before other less fortunate countries had access to either of these life-saving resources [16]. It would therefore be of great importance to continue to innovate existing diagnostic technologies, or develop new ones, to try and address the socioeconomic disparity between countries in the pursuit of preventing further mass outbreaks.

Throughout the COVID-19 pandemic, the main goals of conventional rapid-test manufacturers and researchers were to increase the reproducibility and reliability of the unit tests, while reducing overall costs in production and logistics [11, 16]. Improving the technology of more readily available diagnostic tests, such as rapid PCR and immunohistochemistry tests, would prove to be an extremely useful tool in reducing the transmission of COVID-19 around the world. However, it would still be necessary to explore alternate diagnostic technologies which were also expected to advance our diagnostic capabilities, such as microfluidic devices. Microfluidic devices offer not only some promising prospects to address many of the limitations of previous conventional devices through their modularity and reproducibility, but also offer the ability to enhance previously established diagnostic techniques.

4. Microfluidic devices as diagnostic platforms for SARS-CoV-2/COVID-19

Microfluidic devices utilize fluid systems on the micro-scale that behave differently than that of fluids at volumes seen in day-to-day life. The main difference between micro and macro-scale fluid dynamics is seen in the readiness of micro-scale fluids to achieve a state of flow known as laminar flow [2]. Laminar flow describes a state of fluid flow where the fluid moves in continuous parallel layers, without any disruption between the layers of fluid [20]. In practice, this means that even at lower velocities, the fluid is not subjected to unwanted lateral mixing and the particles within the fluid itself are moving in straight, parallel, lines with one another. This directly contrasts with the type of flow ordinarily seen in macro-scale volumes, turbulent flow, which would instead experience rapid and chaotic variations in pressure and flow velocity across any given period. In turbulent fluids, particles are unevenly distributed and are subjected to random changes, which are undesirable traits when attempting to measure or work with systems that require a great deal of accuracy [20]. In the context of microfluidics, by taking advantage of the readily achievable laminar flow states, researchers and scientists can perform extremely useful and precise experiments that would normally be impossible with larger volumes [20, 21]. Interestingly, microfluidic technology was originally invented in the 1950s by Siemens-Elema, not as a diagnostic technique but as a subset of printing technology used to efficiently transport ink [21].

It was not until the turn of the millennium that this microfluidic technology really began seeing more practical medical applications [21]. As seen in **Figure 4**, the

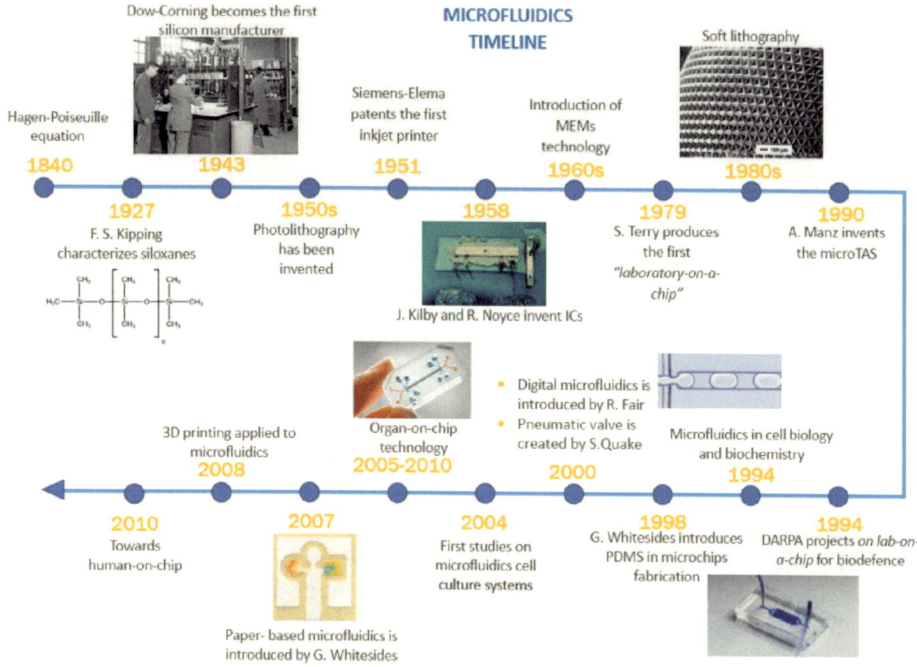

Figure 4.
A timeline of the historical milestones achieved with microfluidics [21].

number of microfluidic applications has seen a steady increase since the early 2000s, largely in part to the extremely fast development of computing power and computational hardware, which allowed for many combinations of microfluidic technology, integrated with digital processing [19–21]. Therefore, the number of potential future microfluidic applications appears limitless.

4.1 Microfluidic classification and scientific relevance

Over the years, microfluidics has grown in a way that several classifications of microfluidic technology exist to aid in organizing the myriad of its applications. The biggest classification of microfluidics distinguishes microfluidic systems between continuous-flow and droplet-based systems, sometimes called segmented flow.

As seen in **Figure 5**, Continuous-flow microfluidic systems utilize the characteristics of laminar flow to facilitate experimental processes that often require controlled mixing of micro-scale reagent and sample volumes [20]. Moreover, these continuous-flow systems can serve as ideal platforms for other slow-processing experiments such as microfluidic-based PCR quantification and even real-time sample separation techniques. Conversely, droplet microfluidics allows for more instances of chaotic mixing to occur in a highly controlled environment, essentially facilitating numerous independent mixing phenomena to occur [20].

The differences in how these techniques can be achieved or improved upon with microfluidics depend on the micro-channel design of the system. In continuous-flow microfluidics, the four main categories of channel design include serpentine, spiral, oscillating-flow, and straight microchannels [22]. Each design channel design serves its own unique purpose when being used in microfluidics. For instance, serpentine

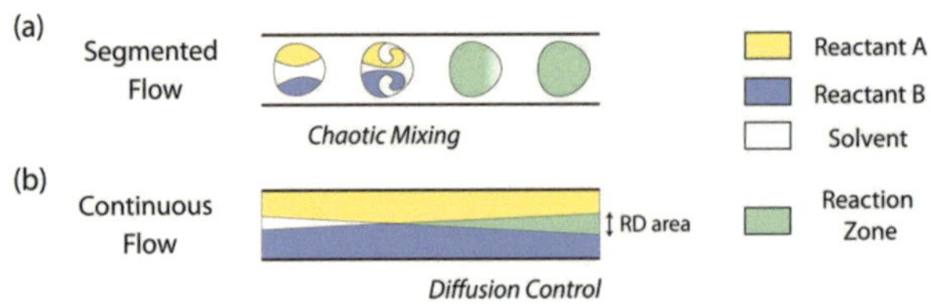

Figure 5.
A visualization of (a) droplet, and (b) continuous-flow microfluidics fluid dynamic mixing [20].

microchannels can be used to extend the time in which a fluid is exposed to external factors, such as UV light for crosslinking or heat to promote a particular reaction, across a more unified and even distribution of the fluid [18, 22]. Oscillatory continuous-flow microfluidics has been used to increase the effectiveness of liquid-liquid separations as well as aid in sample concentration techniques to improve detection outcomes in downstream processes [22]. These continuous-flow adaptations allow microfluidic systems to intrinsically offer more freedom for the experimental design than conventional techniques and can use a smaller working volume to make better use of smaller and costlier reagents. In general, continuous-flow microfluidic systems have seen an increase in popularity over the years due to their modularity, but do not compare in popularity to droplet microfluidic systems.

Droplet microfluidic systems forego the continuous laminar flow physics that is innate in continuous-flow systems, but instead make use of the micro-scale laminar flow physics to facilitate the production of individual droplet microenvironments [23]. These droplet microenvironments, shown in **Figure 6**, are discrete microlitre volumes that are formed through the controlled flow of a sheath (transporter) fluid across one or more sample fluids at a common junction [23]. Thus, repeatedly partitioning the sample fluids in a controlled manner and encapsulating the mixture of sample fluids into droplets. What makes droplet microfluidics so important and unique, even compared to continuous-flow microfluidics, is that it can allow for both high throughput experimentation and an increase in resolving power [2, 24]. Droplet microfluidic systems have been demonstrated to effectively process, in high throughput, experimental analysis in resolutions as high as single-cell resolutions; something many other platforms cannot achieve on their own [23, 24]. The various forms of droplet microfluidic systems can be classified into three main categories: high and ultrahigh throughput droplet microfluidics (htDM/uhtDM), digital droplet microfluidics (dDM), and controlled droplet microfluidics (cDM) [23]. In htDM and uhtDM, the main purpose of the system is to generate as many stable and uniform droplet microenvironments as possible to facilitate increased resolution and turnaround time. The production of thousands of comparable droplet microenvironments in a controlled manner promotes increased reaction efficiency as well as both qualitative and quantitative analysis through integration with digital technology. This integration between htDM and uhtDM with digital technology does not necessarily overlap with the dDM classification but does experience some similarities in that they can both utilize automation to enhance their analyses [24]. dDM systems aim to achieve complete automation through their integration with droplet microfluidics. However, it does not often utilize high throughput processing [23, 24]. Instead, purely dDM systems often generate multiple types of droplets in one system and have these different droplets interact with one another, in a highly controlled manner [23]. By utilizing components of both htDM/uhtDM systems and dDM systems,

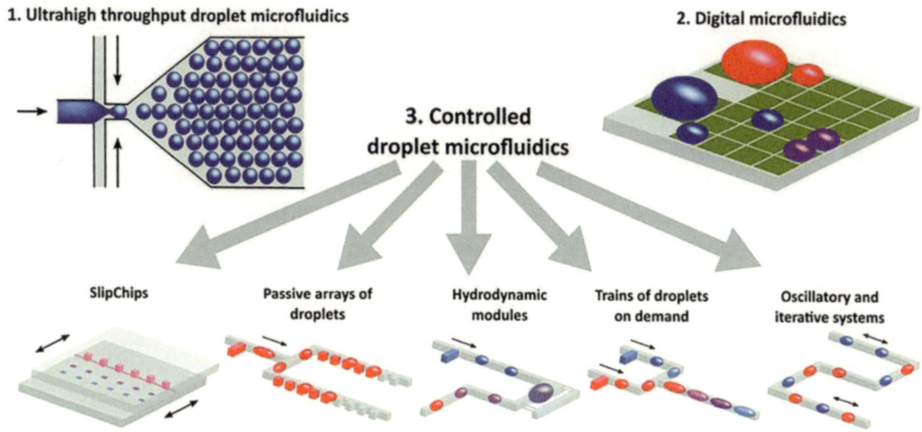

Figure 6.
A graphic highlighting the various droplet microfluidic classifications [23].

researchers can achieve systems that are classified as controlled droplet microfluidic systems. These controlled droplet microfluidic systems gain some of the advantages of the other two systems and offer even greater modularity than either of those systems independently. As a result, the use of digital integration along with controlled droplet microfluidic systems microfluidics permits microfluidic platforms to be one of the most promising cost-reducing diagnostic platforms in both current and future diagnostic research.

4.2 Advantages of microfluidic integration in diagnostic tools

The increased efficiency of sample-reagent interactions is a particularly attractive characteristic of microfluidic devices which drives research towards improved diagnostic applications of microfluidic technology [25]. Normally, diagnostic technologies utilizing sample-reagent interactions between molecules of relatively weak binding affinities are regarded as non-optimal, in macro-scale volumes, due to the inefficiencies and potential overconsumption of resources [25]. Resources such as reagents, samples, and equipment can often be extremely resource-intensive and expensive, which can result in fewer tests per unit volume of sample and may discourage researchers from moving forward with a particular combination of cost-effective and practical diagnostic material. Ideal detection molecules for diagnostic purposes should offer an acceptable balance between cost, binding efficiency, and selectivity to the target molecule of interest. Finding this balance of characteristics in a detection molecule often requires lengthy amounts of research and testing, which would further incur operational costs. However, these limitations associated with non-microfluidic technologies can be improved upon with the use of microfluidic technology. Therefore, microfluidic integration can overcome many of the limitations associated with non-microfluidic systems and gain some advantages unique to microfluidics.

4.2.1 Cost-reduction

Conventional diagnostic techniques often require costly materials as well as logistical and operational costs, all of which create barriers limiting the access of these techniques to resource-limited settings [26]. Furthermore, due to the COVID-19 pandemic, unmet demand for conventional diagnostic tests had significantly increased the prices of individual tests, leaving several countries and low-income individuals with fewer options for obtaining these potentially lifesaving items [19, 26]. In 2021, it was found that a single COVID-19 rapid antigen test could have costed consumers upwards of $20 USD, per test [2, 19, 25]. These essential diagnostic tools are often subject to the whim of the companies that produce and distribute the tests, which can only further limit access to lower-income individuals [16, 17]. By integrating microfluidic technology with previously existing platforms, microfluidics has the potential to reduce the overall costs of mass-producing rapid and accurate diagnostic tests for the detection and quantification of SARS-CoV-2.

4.2.1.1 Fabrication

To better optimize the costs for mass-producing diagnostic tests, microfluidic integration may help to reduce costs by permitting more variety in the materials used to fabricate tests. As seen in **Table 1**, commonly used materials in producing several microfluidic integrated systems including silicon, glass, polymers, and paper; each material, offers its own respective advantages and disadvantages [2, 26].

Silicon and glass were two of the most used materials in the fabrication of microfluidic devices due to their abundance [2]. These two materials offered great modularity in the type of potential applications the microfluidic systems would supplement. However, both suffered from high material costs [2, 26]. As technology advanced and other synthesized materials became more affordable, these two abundant microfluidic materials became less and less viable for the mass-production of diagnostic tests [16, 26]. As a result, materials such as polymers and paper became more attractive microfluidic substrates. Coupled with their simplified fabrication and processing methods, both paper-based and polymer microfluidic devices share stronger potential as on-site SARS-CoV-2 diagnostic tests, as compared to glass or silicon-based systems [16, 18, 19].

In addition to the reduction of microfluidic substrate costs, microfluidics reduces the inherent costs associated with reagent use since only microlitre volumes are used in the system. Each individual microfluidic test would, ideally, only require microlitre volumes of any reagents and samples to be effectively analyzed. Lower fluid volumes required for the successful operation of each test reduce the cost of fabrication per test and might allow for a better redistribution of financial resources.

4.2.1.2 Operations

A microfluid integrated diagnostic device has the potential to greatly reduce operational costs associated with processing samples. By reducing the number of experienced operators required to pilot the device or removing the need for expensive equipment to process samples, a large portion of the cost (per test) incurred by the consumer can be greatly reduced. This operational cost reduction can be achieved by developing a system with self-contained microfluidic tests that are qualitatively and quantitatively analyzed by a small portable test analyzer, with a single operator.

By developing a portable microfluidic analyzer that can independently process multiple diagnostic tests, in sequence or in parallel, only one unit operator would be required to perform on-site diagnoses. Depending on the design and software of the analyzer, the operator might not always require a great deal of experience to collect, process, and record samples. In the case where diagnostic sample processing

	Glass	Silicon	Polymer	Paper
Fabrication Techniques	• Photolithography • Etching	• Bulk or surface micromachining • Nano-imprint lithography • Electron beam irradiation	• Soft lithography • Injection moulding • 3D printing	• Wax and inkjet printing • Photolithography
Advantages	• Transparent • Inert and stable • Solvent compatible • Hydrophilic	• Mechanically strong • Thermostable • Chemical resistance	• Transparent • Easy fabrication • Low cost	• Flexible and lightweight • Low cost • Biocompatible • Recyclable
Limitations	• Brittle • Not flexible • High cost	• High cost • Biocompatibility	• Hydrophobic • Short shelf life	• Humidity and temperature sensitive • Difficult to design and integrate into single chip

Adapted from Ref. [2] with permission.

Table 1.
A summary of several different microfluidic substrate types and their respective characteristics.

includes whole-sample mediums, such as whole blood, saliva, and mucosal liquids, a potential biohazardous risk to the collector could exist [24, 25]. These potentially biohazardous samples can be collected by trained personnel swabbing the patient's sinuses or mouth, as well as through the drawing of blood [25]. These collection techniques are used to require trained operators to wear personal protective equipment (PPE) to minimize potential transmission and required processing off-site. In the early stages of the pandemic, it was common for diagnostic tests being administered by a healthcare professional wearing PPE to take more than a week to produce results. Many of these early tests still required millilitre-volume samples that lead to lowered detection-sensitivity issues [17]. Conversely, in the later stages of the pandemic, more and more diagnostic tests were being self-administered, and taking less time, as diagnostic technology continued to advance. However, these self-administered tests were often restricted to qualitative detection methods that could not yet provide a measure of an individual's "active infectiousness". In theory, microfluidic technology is expected to allow for a single portable microfluidic analyzer to both qualitatively and quantitatively diagnose large numbers of samples, with only one operator.

An equally important feature of microfluidic systems is its ability to facilitate on-site and on-device pre-treatment of samples. Some form of molecular separation or enhanced sample concentration was usually required to accurately process samples for diagnostic purposes [2]. In addition, this pre-treatment usually required some equipment that was both non-portable and difficult to operate. However, microfluidic technology has allowed for some of these pre-treatment techniques to be automated and contained within the test itself, for improved on-site capabilities [11]. The separation of unwanted molecules, from the sample, and the enhanced concentration of the target analyte could now be performed on-device and increase accuracy and sensitivity. One way in which microfluidics can facilitate this is by introducing a mixture of channel designs and reagents into the microfluidic device to initiate this pre-treatment of samples, directly inside the microfluidic device. The self-containing design principle intrinsic to most on-site microfluidic systems readily facilitates this feat and can be integrated into a myriad of diagnostic techniques such as qPCR [16]. Furthermore, by integrating these on-device pre-treatment steps into each individual test, the microfluidic analyzer would be able to capture and process data in real-time. Thereby, reducing some operational costs while improving the assay's sensitivity and limit of detection (LOD) significantly. By enhancing the modularity of diagnostic tests through microfluidic integration and a portable microfluidic analyzer, not only can the number of operators and trained personnel be reduced but can also provide quantitative analysis.

4.2.1.3 Logistics

Diagnostic platforms integrated with microfluidic systems may offer advantages over other non-microfluidic platforms such as portability, size, structural integrity, and reproducibility that can reduce logistical costs associated with the mass-production and distribution of tests. One of the most important measures of on-site diagnostic validity is the ability to efficiently reproduce, store and distribute tests without affecting quality or accuracy of the device [19].

Paper-based and polymer-based microfluidic designs offer a greater amount of reproducibility and modularity compared to non-microfluidic tests [2]. The moulds used to imprint upon the paper and polymer substrates in microfluidic devices can be readily fabricated through methods such as lithography and etching [2]. These fabrication methods allow for microfluidic devices to remain relatively small and highly reproducible. Despite the moulds requiring expensive equipment to fabricate, only a few moulds need to be made to continuously produce a large number of microchannels for the intended devices. Thus, testing devices can be manufactured at high capacity. By separating the testing platform and the analyzer, one can significantly reduce costs associated with quality control and large-scale production.

Storage of the diagnostic tests depends on both the reagent lifespan used in the tests as well as the rigor of the test itself. Reagents used in diagnostic analysis often have expiration dates that are meant to limit quality control issues in the reagents themselves, which may lead to inaccurate testing results [22]. In general, most diagnostic reagents have a recommended shelf-life of 1 year, which would provide ample time for a microfluidic-based device to be stored and distributed with little worry. The additional rigor added to diagnostic devices through microfluidic integration refers to the thermostability and structural integrity of the devices themselves. If a test must be stored and transported in a temperature-controlled environment, the logistical costs for transporting those tests would significantly increase. Similarly, if the tests are not structurally sound, the need for more delicate transportation would also add to the costs of storing and transporting the tests. Thus, microfluidics offers a useful advantage in both scenarios as the self-containing principle behind ideal microfluidic diagnostic devices, can be applied. Therefore, through microfluidic integration, these important logistical metrics may be readily met, promoting continued mass-production of diagnostic tests.

4.2.2 Decreased turnaround time

Prior to the advent of the technological revolution of the 2000s, microfluidic technologies were extremely limited in their automation capacity due to many of the automation-driven adaptations being hindered by the cost of computational processing, the size of the equipment required to process the experiments, and the time required for the experiment to complete [21]. The increased accessibility for computational processing and digital analysis over the last two decades has allowed microfluidics to achieve significant improvements in diagnostic technology, such as increased automation and high throughput analysis. Turnaround times in both microfluidic and non-microfluidic diagnostic tests have significantly improved over the last 2 years, from times greater than 1 week to less than 30 minutes [25]. Microfluidic automation and high throughput processing improved transmission prevention, and potentially improved treatment outcomes might be possible by more accurately diagnosing SARS-CoV-2 at an earlier stage.

4.2.2.1 Automation

Microfluidic integration of digital automation can allow for several simultaneous processes to occur, which can exponentially decrease the time it takes to analyze a certain number of samples. Greater computational processing power and more robust software and hardware have provided microfluidic technologies with the means to explore previously unfathomable feats in diagnostic testing [23, 24]. Inconsistencies such as human error in sample analysis or device fabrication can more easily be avoided, further reducing costs to the producer. This in turn will create a greater incentive for microfluidic research, further driving down prices and effectively creating a feedback loop. Equipment can be coded to operate machinery, treat samples, and even provide qualitative and quantitative insight that would have been difficult for operators to observe. Through automation, the reliance on manual operation, experienced operators, and expensive equipment for diagnostic techniques is severely mitigated and can be adapted to process samples at speeds impossible for humans to do, otherwise known as high throughput processing.

4.2.2.2 High throughput processing

The benefits of high throughput processing achieved through microfluidic integration can be easily observed in microfluidic-based techniques such as droplet microfluidics. In droplet microfluidics, hundreds if not thousands of individual droplet microenvironments can be formed to initiate microscopic bioreactions in series, which can be later processed or analyzed in parallel [23, 27]. The processing speed in which high throughput analyses works, coupled with the micro-scale volumes used in microfluidics, presents a unique advantage that is not easily achieved in other detection methods [24]. Therefore, by integrating high throughput analysis through microfluidics, exponentially shorter turnaround times can be achieved.

4.2.3 Accuracy and LOD

The effectiveness of conventional non-microfluidic diagnostic techniques can often be hindered by their limit of detection (LOD) and their accuracy [19]. Microfluidic devices can, in some cases, overcome these limitations. Accuracy is defined by the ability of the test to correctly discern between a state in which a target condition is met and when that target condition is not met [2, 19]. By establishing benchmarks for accuracy in non-microfluidic diagnostic techniques, we can compare it to the accuracy seen in similar microfluidic techniques. In many situations, since microfluidic integration does not necessarily change the detection method primarily used, the accuracy might not significantly improve. In most immunohistochemical assays, the accuracy of a diagnostic test varies significantly with differences in viral loads [17, 18]. As the concentration of virus particles increases, so does the accuracy of most immunohistochemical tests, not necessarily in a linear manner. Conversely, through microfluidic implementation, a pre-treatment step can be applied to concentrate and separate the target molecules from other unwanted material into standardized volumes [22]. In doing so, the variance in accuracy from samples with low viral loads can be mitigated. The modularity of microfluidic systems may offer a means to improve the LOD, as well as improved accuracy.

Target molecules at low concentrations found in macro-scale volumes of sample fluid are not always readily detected by non-microfluidic devices [23–25]. This limitation of non-microfluidic devices becomes more important when dealing with molecules that are not easily replicated by conventional means, such as protein biomarkers found on the surface of a SARS-CoV-2 cell. As a result, single-cell-resolution droplet microfluidic systems can be designed to generate thousands of microlitre droplet microenvironments to capture biomarkers, in extremely low concentrations, normally too difficult to detect through conventional means [27].

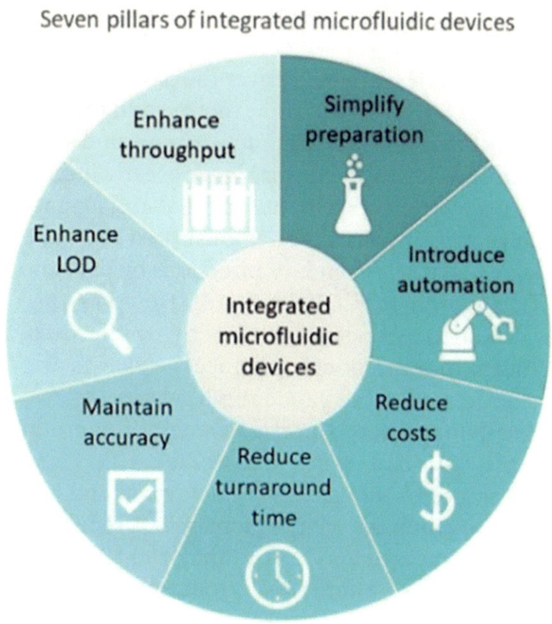

Figure 7.
The 7 pillars for assessing effective on-site diagnostic devices. Adapted from Ref. [2] with permission.

5. Standards for ideal on-site diagnostic microfluidic devices

Microfluidic devices that would like to be tested and sold as on-site diagnostic devices, must first adhere to a standardized set of criteria set out by the WHO. The WHO published a list of criteria that states that on-site diagnostic devices must be "affordable, sensitive, user-friendly, rapid and robust, equipment-free and deliverable to end-users" [2]. These criteria are the 6 basic standards that prospective on-site diagnostic devices should strive to achieve, otherwise known as ASSURED. The ASSURED criteria allow researchers and healthcare professionals to assess the effectiveness of prospective on-site diagnostic devices [2]. The six criteria can be further divided into two main categories for evaluation, the technical and the practical criteria. The technical criteria include: "sensitivity", "rapid and robust", as well as "equipment-free". While the practical criteria include: "affordable", "user-friendly" and "deliverable to end users". While some criteria are not necessarily related to one another, they are nevertheless all equally important in designing an idealized on-site microfluidic device. However, the ASSURED criteria are not easy to be simultaneously and effectively implemented. Therefore, to improve the overall potential of a microfluidic device as an effective on-site diagnostic tool, several other more measurable criteria must also be addressed; as seen in **Figure 7**.

Effective diagnostic microfluidic devices that manage to address the ASSURED criteria, as best as possible, may still struggle to measure how they are addressing these criteria [2]. **Figure 7** summarizes a list of seven more measurable criteria that simplify and quantify the characteristics that best represent an ideal on-site microfluidic device used for diagnostic purposes. These "seven pillars" of integrated microfluidic device design will aid in providing developers with quantifiable metrics to better evaluate their device's efficacy and on-site diagnostic potential.

6. Current state of microfluidic systems in SARS-CoV-2 diagnostics

Advancements in diagnostic technology over the past 2 years have allowed for infectious diseases, such as SARS-CoV-2, to be more readily and accurately diagnosed [2, 9, 11]. Improvements made to costs, accuracy, turnaround times, and processing speeds in non-microfluidic diagnostic tests have greatly improved the ability of healthcare workers and governments to better prevent and manage mass outbreaks [12]. For example, rapid antigen tests have demonstrated their effectiveness in reducing the number of potential secondary infections by providing people with a qualitative means of diagnosing for COVID-19 [14]. However, this does not mean that these tests and their detection technology cannot still be improved upon. Microfluidic technology offers a means to continuously advance the world's diagnostic capabilities and preparation for the next potential pandemic-level virus.

The past decade has demonstrated the effectiveness of microfluidics in the on-site diagnosis of various infectious pathogens, such as Zika, HIV-1 and more recently SARS-CoV-2 [2]. The errant lack of tests, medical devices, and human resources seen throughout the pandemic, prompted a large increase in the demand for technology capable of being remotely operated and readily analyzed [18, 20]. Advancements in information technology and computational processing created a revolution of new approaches by which microfluidic devices can accurately diagnose COVID-19

material	microfluidic device	detection target	duration	sample type	selection
gold@Fe3O4 nanocomposite	electrochemical sensor	nucleic acid		artificial and clinical RNA samples	against SARS-CoV-2, MERS-CoV, HCoV-OC43
gold nanoislands	plasmonics and photothermal effect	nucleic acid		synthesized samples	against SARS-CoV-2
gold nanoparticles	paper-based electrochemical sensor	nucleic acid	<5 min	COVID-19 positive patients	against MERS-CoV and SARS-CoV-2 viral RNA
graphene sheet	field-effect transistor	spike (S) protein	real-time electrical response	clinical sample for COVID-19patients	
gold nanoparticles	surface plasmon resonance and colorimetric assay	nucleic acid	10 min	isolated RNA	against MERS-CoV viral RNA

Figure 8.
Various microfluidic diagnostic devices for SARS-CoV-2 [25].

	Immunoassay (rapid antigen test)	RT-PCR	Nanoparticle	Microflow Cytometry
Reagent consumption	10 μg (in tube)	20 μL (in tube)	Negligible	50 μL (in tube)
Target of detection	IgG, IgA, IgM	N gene, E gene	Gold-spiked	IgM, IgG
Limit of detection	0.4 ng/L	1–10 copy/μL	0.08 mg/L	0.06–0.10 mg/L
Total assay time	30 minutes	2 hours	2–5 hours	30 minutes
Sample volume	20 μL	120 μL	1 μL	10 μL
Assay control	Automated	Manual	Manual	Automated
Cost per test	~ 6 (USD)	~ 4 (USD)	~ 10 (USD)	~ 5 (USD)
Quantitative	No	Yes	Yes	Yes
Mobile	Yes	Yes	No	No

Adapted from Ref. [2] with permission.

Table 2.
Comparison of rapid test to microfluidic diagnostic tests.

patients, on-site [21, 24]. **Figure 8** highlights several of the most current, digitally integrated, microfluidic platforms capable of diagnosing SARS-CoV-2.

In many of the diagnostic platforms highlighted in **Figure 8**, smartphones are used as an imaging processor to read fluorescent signals through machine learning and artificial intelligence [25]. With the ever-increasing global access to the internet, smartphone-enabled microfluidic diagnostic devices can produce results that can be uploaded to a data-cloud to be immediately stored. Moreover, these smartphone-enabled devices can reduce the turnaround time for qualitatively diagnosing SARS-CoV-2 to, on average, less than 15 minutes.

Despite the processing speed advantages which smartphone-enabled systems offer, there is still unmet need for faster and more robust microfluidic devices capable of quantitative analysis [26]. As seen in **Table 2**, several types of existing quantitative microfluidic diagnostic tools are slowly becoming more comparable even the most current rapid diagnostic tests for SARS-CoV-2. It is only a matter of time before quantitative microfluidic-based tests will be able to either perform comparably, or better, than the rapid antigen tests.

7. Conclusions

This chapter deals with the experience of COVID-19 over the last 2 years and highlights the significance of microfluidics to the history and advancement of SARS-CoV-2 diagnostic technology. In these years, conventional rapid PCR and ELISA COVID-19 technology has advanced greatly. However, limitations in their modularity, sensitivity, turnaround time and cost greatly reduce their future viability as on-site diagnostic tools. The current state of microfluidic, information and smartphone technology allow microfluidic-based diagnostics to address many limitations associated with conventional on-site/rapid tests. The advantages of microfluidic integration into medical diagnostics are discussed throughout this chapter. The expectation is that microfluidics will advance our future diagnostic abilities to help better prepare for, and manage, the next possible pandemic-level threat.

Acknowledgements

The authors would like to acknowledge Alexander Diab-Liu and Kamaya Bosland for their help in proofreading this work.

Conflict of interest

The authors declare no conflict of interest.

Notes/thanks/other declarations

Thank you to Dr. Xu and IntechOpen for the opportunity to work on this chapter.

Author details

Andres Escobar[1*] and Chang-qing Xu[2]

1 Faculty of Engineering, School of Biomedical Engineering, McMaster University, Hamilton, Ontario, Canada

2 Faculty of Engineering, McMaster University, Department of Engineering Physics and School of Biomedical Engineering, Hamilton, Ontario, Canada

*Address all correspondence to: escoba3@mcmaster.ca

References

[1] Kocadagli O, Kose AM, Gokmen Inan N, Ozer E, Kocadagli Y, Bostanci E. Important factors affecting the transmission rate of COVID-19 in G20 and EU. Sigma Journal of Engineering and Natural Sciences. 2022;**40**:208-218. DOI: 10.14744/sigma.2022.00017

[2] Escobar A, Chiu P, Qu J, Zhang Y, Xu CQ. Integrated microfluidic-based platforms for on-site detection and quantification of infectious pathogens: Towards on-site medical translation of SARS-CoV-2 diagnostic platforms. Micromachines. 2021;**12**:1-25. DOI: 10.3390/mi12091079

[3] World Health Organization. WHO Coronavirus (COVID-19) Dashboard. [Internet]. 2022. Available from: https://covid19.who.int//

[4] Johansson MA, Quandelacy TM, Kada S, et al. SARS-CoV-2 transmission from people without COVID-19 symptoms. JAMA Network. 2021;**4**(1):1-8. DOI: 10.1001/jamanetworkopen.2020.35057

[5] DiSalvo S. A Primer for R_0 for Infectious Diseases. [Internet]. 2020. Available from: https://www.mastersindatascience.org/resources/r0-infectious-diseases/ [Accessed: May 5, 2022]

[6] Locatelli I, Trachsel B, Rousson V. Estimating the basic reproduction number for COVID-19 in Western Europe. PLoS One. 2021;**16**(3):e0248731. DOI: 10.1371/journal.pone.0248731

[7] Duffy RB, Zio E. Prediction of COVID-19 infection, transmission, and recovery rates: A new analysis in global societal comparisons. Safety Science. 2020;**129**:1-15. DOI: 10.1016/j.ssci.2020.104854

[8] Botes M, de Kwaadsteniet M, Cloete TE. Application of quantitative PCR for the detection of microorganisms in water. Analytical and Bioanalytical Chemistry. 2013;**405**:91-108. DOI: 10.1007/s00216-012-6399-3

[9] Chittoor-Vinod V. Molecular biology of PCR testing for COVID-19 diagnostics. In: Biotechnology to Combat COVID-19. London: IntechOpen; 2021. pp. 1-14. DOI: 10.5772/intechopen.96199

[10] Romero-Severson EO, Hengartner N, Meadors G, Ke R. Change in global transmission rates of COVID-19 through may 6 2020. PLoS One. 2020;**15**(8):1-12. DOI: 10.1371/journal.pone.0236776

[11] Shaffaf T, Ghafar-Zadeh E. COVID-19 diagnostic strategies part II: Protein-based technologies. Bioengineering. 2021;**4**(1):1-8. DOI: 10.3390/bioengineering8050054

[12] Hagen A. COVID-19 Testing FAQs. [Internet]. 2020. Available from: https://asm.org/Articles/2020/April/COVID-19-Testing-FAQs [Accessed: May 5, 2022]

[13] Alhalabi O, Iyer S, Subbiah V. Testing for COVID-19 in patients with cancer. EClinicalMedicine. 2021;**4**(1):1-8. DOI: 10.1001/jamanetworkopen.2020.35057

[14] U.S. Food & Drug Safety Administration. FDA Approves First COVID-19 Vaccine. [Internet]. 2021. Available from: https://www.fda.gov/news-events/press-announcements/fda-approves-first-covid-19-vaccine [Accessed: May 5, 2022]

[15] World Health Organization. Tracking SARS-CoV-2 Variants. [Internet]. 2022. Available from: https://www.who.int/en/activities/tracking-SARS-CoV-2-variants [Accessed: May 5, 2022]

[16] Sachdeva S, Davis RW, Saha AK. Microlfuidic point of care testing: Commercial landscape and future directions. Frontiers in Bioengineering and Biotechnology. 2021;**8**:1-14. DOI: 10.3389/fbioe.2020.602659

[17] Microfluidic Detection of Human Diseases. From liquid biopsy to COVID-19 diagnosis. Journal of Biomechanics. 2021;**117**:1-9. DOI: 10.1016/j.jbiomech.2021.110235

[18] Tayyab M, Sami AS, Raji H, Mushnoori S, Javanmard M. Potential microfluidic devices for COVID-19 antibody detection at point-of-care (POC): A review. IEEE Sensors Journal. 2021;**21**:4007-4017. DOI: 10.1109/JSEN.2020.3034892

[19] Ainsworth M, Andersson M, Auckland K, Baillie JK, Barnes E, Beer S, et al. Performance characteristics of five immunoassays for SARS-CoV-2: A head-to-head benchmark comparison. The Lancet Infectious Diseases. 2020;**20**:1390-1400. DOI: 10.1016/S1473-3099(20)30634-4

[20] Gonidec M, Puigmarti-Luis J. Continuous- versus segmented-flow microfluidic synthesis in materials science. Crystals. 2019;**9**(12):1-1. DOI: 10.3390/cryst9010012

[21] Dellaquila A. Five Short Stories on The History of Microfluidics. [Internet]. 2017. Available from: https://www.elveflow.com/microfluidic-reviews/general-microfluidics/history-of-microfluidics/ [Accessed: May 5, 2022]

[22] Kopparthy VL, Crews ND. A versatile oscillating-flow microfluidic PCR system utilizing a thermal gradient for nucleic acid analysis. Biotechnology and Bioengineering. 2020;**117**(5):1525-1535. DOI: 10.1002/bit.27278

[23] Kaminski TS, Garstecki P. Controlled droplet microfluidic Systems for Multistep Chemical and Biological Assays. Chemical Society Reviews. 2017;**46**:6210-6226. DOI: 10.1039/C5CS00717H

[24] Li Z, Bai Y, You M, Hu J, Yao C, Cao L, et al. Fully integrated microfluidic devices for qualitative, quantitative, and digital nucleic acids testing at point of care. Biosensors & Bioelectronics. 2021;**177**:112952. DOI: 10.1016/j.bios.2020.112952

[25] Kumar A, Parihar A, Panda U, Parihar DP. Microfluidics-based point-of-care testing (POCT) devices in dealing with waves of COVID-19 pandemic: The emerging solution. ACS: Applied BioMaterials. 2022:1-23. DOI: 10.1021/acsabm.1c01320

[26] Scott S, Ali Z. Fabrication methods for microfluidic devices: An overview. Micromachines. 2021;**12**:319. DOI: 10.3390/mi12030319

[27] Funari R, Chu K, Shen AQ. Detection of antibodies against SARS-CoV-2 spike protein by gold nanospikes in an optomicrofluidic chip. Biosensors & Bioelectronics. 2020;**169**:112578. DOI: 10.1016/j.bios.2020.112578

Chapter 12

Perspective Chapter: Recent Progressions on the Colorimetric Diagnosis of SARS-CoV-2 by Loop-Mediated Isothermal Amplification (LAMP) Assay

Galyah Alhamid and Huseyin Tombuloglu

Abstract

A simple, fast, and accurate diagnosis of SARS-CoV-2 is of great importance for the patient's isolation, treatment, and the control of the COVID-19 pandemic. Although RT-qPCR is accepted as the gold standard, studies to improve fast, simple, and more reliable diagnostic methods are continuing. Colorimetric reverse transcription loop-mediated isothermal amplification (RT-LAMP) is a method that allows visual detection of SARS-CoV-2 without needing expensive fluorescence readers. However, the performance of the assay depends on some factors, such as selection of a target gene (*i.e.*, *N*, *RdRp*, *S*, *E*, *M*), primer design, the dye used for visual observation—neutral red, calcein, cresol red, or phenol red—and the reaction conditions such as the buffer pH, reaction temperature, and enzyme concentration. In the last 2 years, plenty of research has been conducted to obtain the best performance. In this chapter, the recent progressions on colorimetric RT-LAMP assay for the diagnosis of SARS-CoV-2 are comprehensively elucidated.

Keywords: SARS-CoV-2, RT-LAMP, COVID-19, colorimetric, diagnosis

1. Introduction

For over 2 years from its emergence, the coronavirus disease 2019 (COVID-19) pandemic, caused by the severe acute respiratory syndrome coronavirus 2 (SARS-CoV-2) has infected over 500 million cases and 6.2 million deaths worldwide as of May 2022 [1]. This highly contagious disease spreads through the respiratory tract via sneezing, coughing, and talking and causes a range of symptoms from mild, like coughing, to severe, like pneumonia. Most patients are asymptomatic and do not require hospitalization; however, high-risk groups—elders over 65 years old, patients with obesity, impaired immune system, and chronic diseases—may develop serious complications that lead to septic shock, multi-organ failure, and eventually, death. However, asymptomatic patients are 75% more likely to spread the disease to others compared to symptomatic cases, which hinders the control of this pandemic [2–5]. It overtook both SARS and MERS outbreaks in terms of infectivity and spread [6]. This crisis still poses a threat to public health and socioeconomics globally ever since its appearance in late 2019. SARS-CoV-2 is from a family of viruses that undergo frequent mutations that alter its characteristics like infectiousness and the rate of transmission.

To control the spread of the pandemic, expanded and rapid point of care (POC) testing is of utmost importance. The reverse transcription-quantitative polymerase chain reaction (RT-qPCR) molecular testing is the gold standard according to world health organization (WHO). This bulky and expensive instrument requires special facilities and must be operated by experts, which makes expanded testing challenging in resource-poor regions. Alternative testing methods are needed for simple and fast POC testing to resolve the demand for reagents and diagnostic equipment in such regions. Therefore, fast, affordable, and practical alternative diagnostic tests to detect the novel SARS-CoV-2 are being investigated, one of which meets these criteria is the loop-mediated isothermal amplification (LAMP). LAMP is a molecular test that provides simple detection methods including the colorimetric LAMP, which relies on a color change in the presence of viral nucleic acids and can be detected via the naked eye. Addition of reverse transcriptase (RT-LAMP) enables the detection of RNA pathogens in a one tube reaction. This single-step technique does not require sophisticated equipment, as the reaction takes place isothermally. This chapter summarizes the most recent developments on the colorimetric RT-LAMP assay for the diagnosis of COVID-19.

2. Principle of RT-LAMP

Founded by Notomi [7], RT-LAMP is a molecular diagnostic technique that detects and amplifies nucleic acids (DNA or RNA) using 4–6 primers that identify six regions in a gene, these include forward and backward inner primers and forward and backward outer primers designated as FIP, BIP, F3, and B3, respectively, in addition to forward and backward loop primers (LF and LB) to increase the amplification rate. Unlike RT-qPCR, RT-LAMP is a single-step isothermal reaction that takes place in a heat block or water bath heated to 60–70°C (depending on the enzyme used), thus eliminating the need of a thermal cycler, and the results can be obtained as early as 15 minutes [8]. This technique caught the attention of scientists during COVID-19 pandemic because it provides a cheaper POC testing alternative while maintaining sensitivity and specificity.

RT-LAMP reaction takes place in a single tube containing reverse transcriptase, DNA polymerase, and 4–6 primers. It starts by converting the viral RNA to cDNA via reverse transcriptase enzyme. Then, FIP anneals to its complementary region, initiating DNA synthesis via DNA polymerase with strand displacement activity. Subsequently, F3 anneals outside FIP to its complementary region and starts polymerization and displaces the strand synthesized by FIP. This released strand has a complementary region at 5` end and thus forms a stem-loop structure, which becomes a template strand for BIP. At the other end, BIP binds to its complementary region and similarly starts polymerization, forming a new strand that is displaced by B3. The released BIP strand has complementary sequences at both ends that form a dumbbell structure, which serves as a starting point of LAMP amplification cycle at loop regions by inner and loop primers. This repeated annealing and displacing cycle rapidly releases

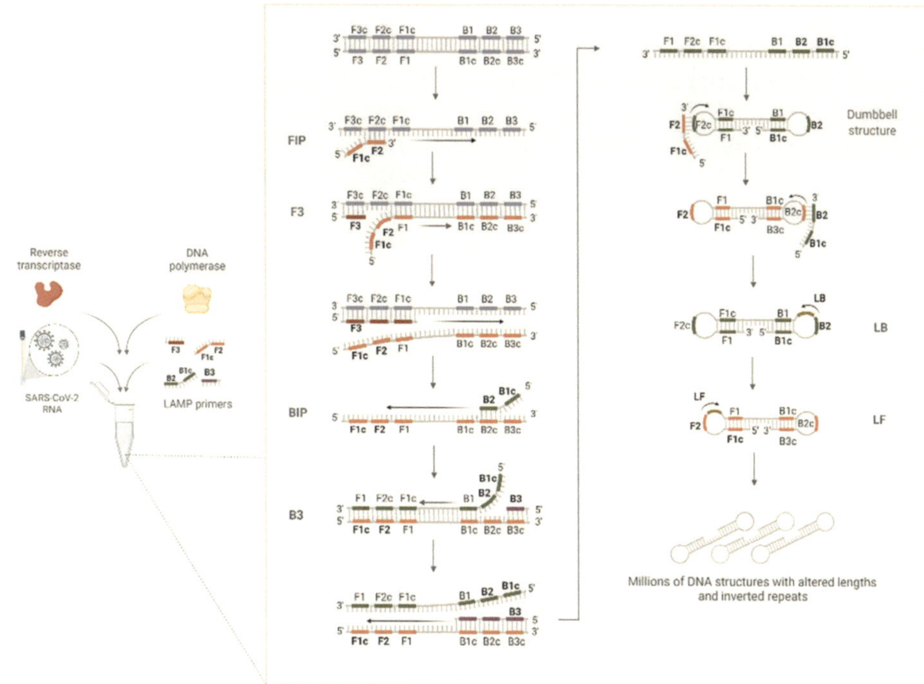

Figure 1.
Main components and primers binding mechanism of loop-mediated isothermal amplification (LAMP) reaction. For the detection of SARS-CoV-2, the reaction tube must be composed of reverse transcriptase, DNA polymerase, primers, and SARS-CoV-2 RNA template, in addition to the reaction building blocks and cofactors like dNTPs and $MgSO_4$. The amplification starts by binding the forward inner primer (FIP) to its complementary target sequence that results in synthesizing a new strand via DNA polymerase. FIP is then displaced by the outer forward primer F3 annealing and similarly starts polymerization. The released FIP becomes the template strand in which both backward inner and outer primers (BIP and B3) bind and start polymerization and strand displacement as well. Both FIP and BIP form dumbbell structure that become the starting point of loop primers amplification cycle, resulting in millions of DNA target sequences with different lengths and inverted repeats.

millions of the targeted DNA structures with different lengths and inverted repeats (**Figure 1**) [7].

Many studies proved the high specificity of RT-LAMP against SARS-CoV-2 [9–13]. RT-LAMP products can be detected by different methods including the colorimetry, fluorometry, turbidity, and gel electrophoresis, with the colorimetry being the most attractive for its accessibility since it does not require additional instruments for the results' interpretation. Researchers are developing colorimetric RT-LAMP kits to be commercially used for COVID-19 *in vitro* diagnosis (IVD) in hospitals, airports, or in-home self-testing. These kits provide a fast and simple diagnosis that can be visualized by a robust color change between positive and negative specimens. For instance, FastProof™ 30 min-TTR SARS-CoV-2 RT-LAMP is a kit that obtained an FDA approval. This kit targets the *N* gene and gives the results within 30 minutes <https://zenosticbio.com/fastproof-30-min-ttr-sars-cov-2-rt-lamp-kit/>. Several studies validated the performance of this kit. For example, Promlek et al. collected 315 clinical specimens from a hospital during the fourth wave of COVID-19 in Thailand. The assay had a 100% positivity rate in specimens with Ct < 31 in RT-qPCR. However, the accuracy decreased for samples that had higher Ct values. They revealed that the kit was able to detect the infection with high accuracy, particularly in symptomatic patients [14]. Also, the Color SARS-CoV-2 RT-LAMP Diagnostic Assay has been authorized for emergency use by FDA. The FDA recommends using an internal control in these assays to assure a successful reaction [15]. A five-month multicenter prospective observational study evaluated the diagnostic accuracy of the colorimetric RT-LAMP in resource-limited areas in parts of Africa. The study included 1657 symptomatic and asymptomatic individuals and the results were compared with the gold standard RT-qPCR. They obtained 87% overall sensitivity that reaches up to 98% in high viral load samples (Ct < 30) [16]. These results suggest that the colorimetric RT-LAMP is reliable and applicable for POC testing, especially in poor resources areas for offering a cheaper alternative to the gold standard, with a comparable accuracy.

3. Colorimetric RT-LAMP in the detection of SARS-CoV-2

The colorimetric RT-LAMP is one of the simplest detection methods offered in this technique because it can be qualitatively visualized by the naked eye. The color change in the solution post-reaction is due to the accumulation of pyrophosphate ions (PPi) produced during amplification, which causes a pH drop. On average, the pH value drops from 8 to 6 before and after the colorimetric RT-LAMP reaction, respectively [9]. The pH-sensitive dyes that are capable changing color around the reaction pH include phenol red, neutral red, and cresol red. These dyes can be added to the reaction as an amplification indicator. Also, some DNA intercalating dyes such as propidium iodide (PI), SYBR green, SYTO-9, etc., can show a distinguished change in positive samples both colorimetrically and under UV visualization. Additionally, the color change can be quantified using the spectrophotometer via measuring the absorbance at 434 nm and 560 nm wavelengths.

3.1 pH-sensitive dyes

The selection of the pH-sensitive dye is crucial for the best visual detection. The color transition zone of the dye should cover the initial and final reaction pH. In general, when using a minimal reaction buffer (26 μM Tris), the pH should be adjusted to 8.8 with 1 M KOH [17]. After 1 h incubation at 65°C, the estimated pH drops around 6.0–6.5, which is a > 2 pH unit drop due to acidification. The dye stock solution can be prepared in large quantities (50–100 mM) with distilled water and should be diluted to 2.5 mM (25×). However, the dye concentration to be used in the reaction mixture is changeable according to the dye type. In general, a final concentration of 100 μM provides more striking visual detection for most of the dyes. However, cresol red demonstrates more obvious color difference when used at lower concentration (50–100 μM) [18]. Before the reaction, the pH of the reaction solution should be adjusted above the indicating threshold [17]. Therefore, only the dyes that react to the pH of the reaction mixture can be used in the LAMP reaction; these dyes are phenol red, neutral red, bromothymol blue, m-cresol purple, and cresol red. Other than these dyes, a higher pH requiring dye (>pH 9.5) such as naphtholphthalein and thymol blue can be used in visual detection. However, the reaction pH should be adjusted to a higher pH value than usual. In this case, the reaction takes longer time due to the suboptimal pH conditions for polymerase and reverse transcriptase enzymes. The most suitable pH-sensitive dyes with corresponding color changes at low and high pH, and transition pH range for colorimetric RT-LAMP are indicated in **Table 1**.

Dye	Final conc.	Color change	Low pH color	High pH color	pH range
Phenol Red	100 μM	Red to Yellow	Yellow	Red	6.8–8.2
Cresol Red	50 μM	Red to Yellow	Yellow	Reddish-purple	7.2–8.8
Neutral Red	100 μM	Yellow to Red	Red	Yellow	6.8–8.0
m-Cresol Purple	100 μM	Purple to Yellow	Yellow	Purple	5.2–6.8
Bromothymol Blue	100 μM	Blue to Yellow	Yellow	Blue	6.0–7.6

Table 1.
pH-sensitive dyes for the colorimetric RT-LAMP reactions.

Recently, Amaral et al. [19] suggested a new assay to ease the distinguishing of color by naked eye. A complexometric indicator, namely murexide (MX), obviously forms pink color in positive samples, while remaining yellow in negative ones. The working principle of the dye based on the complexation of MX (2 μL of 5 mM) with Zinc ions (Zn^{+2}) (1 μL of 50 mM of $ZnCl_2$) that are added to the post-reaction (30 min). In the presence of Zn^{+2}, MX possesses yellow color (negative); whereas it turns to pink (positive) in the absence of Zn^{+2}. Pyrophosphates (PPi), as the byproduct of LAMP, strongly interacts with Zn^{+2} ions and prevents MX-Zn^{+2} interaction. This competition leads to a color formation in LAMP-positive samples as pink.

3.2 Intercalating dyes

In addition to pH-sensitive dyes, intercalating dyes such as propidium iodide (PI), ethidium bromide, SYBR green, SYTO-9, Eva green, and GeneFinder can be used to distinguish positive or negative test results. These dyes are added to the reaction mix at the end of the reaction and visualized either by the naked eye or under UV transilluminator. For example, for the visual inspection, PI at a concentration of 1 mg/mL can be mixed to the end point RT-LAMP product. Although the use of these dyes facilitates the interpreting of results, they can lead to results misinterpretation owing to the abundant primer concentration of the reaction mixture. In negative or non-template control (NTC) samples, binding of the dye to the primers and non-specific amplicons leads bright transillumination under UV, which makes distinguishing between positives and negatives difficult. Also, the addition of dye at the end of the reaction necessitates opening the reaction tube, which maximizes the carry-over contamination risk. To minimize it, some studies have suggested adding the dye to the tube cap prior to the reaction, this way it can be called a cap-tube assay.

Yu et al. [20] used GeneFinder™ (D039 from Bridgen) to improve the fluorescent signal and sensitivity of the RT-LAMP. The SARS-CoV-2 positive samples are observed as green under blue light, while it was pink in the negative samples. Addition of 2 μL of SYBR Green I (1:10 dilution in TAE buffer) or 0.5 μL of 50× SYBR green into the positive reaction tubes (25 μL) changed the solution color from orange to yellow [21]. In addition, the positive tubes can be observed under UV and/or by loading the product in agarose gel. A ladder-type banding pattern is the typical positive RT-LAMP result.

In addition, dye combinations can improve the visual observation. For instance, adding PI dye to the end-point reaction of neutral red-stained LAMP improves the color difference (data not shown). Moreover, the addition of PI enables the detection of the reaction under UV, which helps to verify colorimetric results in the case of intermediate results. Pre-addition of colorimetric fluorescence indicator (CFI), a color mixture composed of 0.7% (v/v) 10,000× Gelgreen (Biotium, Freemont, 108 CA) in 12 mM Hydroxynapthol blue (Sigma-Aldrich, Oakville, ON) re-suspended in dH_2O, changes the reaction color from orange to yellow in positive samples. The color change can be detected by the naked eye after excitation of gel green in the reaction with a blue LED light. The sensitivity of the assay was 50 copies/reaction, and the reaction time was 30 min by targeting the *S* gene [22].

Another study by Zhang et al. [23] reported that the addition of guanidium chloride improves the sensitivity for colorimetric and fluorometric SARS-CoV-2 detection about five to ten folds. Moreover, addition of 40–50 mM of guanidine chloride solution (pH $\sim$ 8 adjusted with KOH) speed up the LAMP reaction time about two-fold, corresponding to $\sim$40% improvement. Additionally, no nonspecific amplification was detected after the incubation period, which enables better colorimetric and fluorometric LAMP discrimination. The mechanism of action of guanidine hydrochloride in the RT-LAMP reaction has not yet been clarified. According to Zhang et al., [23] guanidine hydrochloride improves the base pairing between primers and target sequences. The addition of guanidine also significantly shortens reaction times for helicase-dependent amplification. The increase is probably not the result of modulation of enzyme activity, as additional enzyme such as reverse transcriptase or Bst 2.0 DNA polymerase had no such effect.

4. Selection of target genes

SARS-CoV-2 genome is comprised of a positive and single-stranded $\sim$30 kb in length RNA. The subgenomic RNA (sgRNA) encodes conserved structural proteins (spike protein [S], envelope protein [E], membrane protein [M], and nucleocapsid protein [N]), and several accessory proteins. In addition, non-structural protein coding genes such as *nsp12*, which harbors *RNA-dependent RNA polymerase* (*RdRp*) gene responsible for replication, reside in the viral genome. *ORF1ab* as the largest gene, encodes for two polyproteins PP1ab and PP1a, can also be a target. Dong et al. [24] reported that an *N* gene-based RT-LAMP assay is more sensitive in detecting SARS-CoV-2 than those based on other genes. Among the target genes, *N* gene possesses the most abundant expression of subgenomic mRNA during infection [19, 25]. Therefore, it can be the most suitable target for LAMP reaction, especially in the low viral loaded specimens. In parallel, it was reported that RT-PCR assay detected single gene *N*, but not *orf1ab* gene upon 9–10 days from the onset of the disease. After 2 weeks, both genes resulted in positive amplification, pointing out the sensitivity of *N* gene over *orf1ab* [26, 27]. It should be also noted that because of the high-frequency mutation rate of the SARS-CoV-2 genome, the sequence of the target genes is evolving. A recent study estimated that the nucleotide mutation rate of the SARS-CoV-2 genome is 6.677×10^{-4} substitution/site/year [28]. For instance, the *S* gene of the Omicron variant harbors double number of mutations compared to that of the Delta variant, which caused 29 amino acid substitutions and one insertion mutations [29]. Due to this dynamic nature of the genome as well as the viral recombination, the genome is very prone to mutations, which can lead to loss of assay's sensitivity [30]. This requires at least monthly checking and updating of existing primer sequences.

In addition to selecting a single mRNA target, some studies have reported improved RT-LAMP sensitivity upon using two gene targets simultaneously. According to Zhang and Tanner [31], combining two primer sets that target the same or different genes in the same LAMP reaction led to a higher sensitivity (~12.5 SARS-CoV-2 RNA copies/reaction) compared to the reactions used one primer set. In addition, some dual primer sets exhibited higher sensitivity at lower temperatures (60°C). However, utilizing the LAMP reaction with triple primer sets instead of dual ones showed no advantage over dual sets.

5. Advantages and drawbacks of the colorimetric RT-LAMP

The colorimetric RT-LAMP technique is gaining popularity in diagnosing a variety of pathogenic diseases, one of which is the most recent COVID-19 pandemic. Due to the large number of infections per day, the global demand for reagents, facilities, and healthcare workers increases, and thus RT-qPCR falls short under these circumstances. The simplicity and accessibility of the colorimetric RT-LAMP enables testing a large number of people in a shorter time without the need of complicated instruments like a thermal cycler. Also, since this test does not require advanced laboratory setting and experienced personnel to be operated, it can be used in rural areas with low resources or POC settings like airports and emergency departments. In addition, the use of four to six primers improves the amplification selectivity for the target sequence, and thus this technique is highly specific for SARS-CoV-2 and not for other viruses, including respiratory and other coronaviruses. Regardless, the results from RT-LAMP must be validated with RT-qPCR when developing new assays to assure high sensitivity [11].

One of the most common limitations in this technique is the formation of unwanted primer secondary structures that lead to misamplification in negative samples, which leads to false positive diagnosis. Therefore, primers must be well designed to avoid forming these structures. Some open-source LAMP primer design platforms have been developed such as Primer Explorer V5 by Eiken (https://primerexplorer.jp/e/), LAMP Primer Design Tool by NEB (https://lamp.neb.com/). However, the classical empirical testing of primers often yields suboptimal results. To acquire the best sensitivity and specificity, several LAMP primer sets should be designed [31]. For instance, Yang et al. [32] tested 35 sets, and Joung et al. [33] designed 29 primer sets that target different genes. Recently, 18 primer sets, mostly from previous publications, were screened to find the most sensitive primer set. Based on the sensitivity, they were classified as sensitive (eight sets), medium (seven sets), and poor (three sets) [31]. In general, only a few sets that possess a satisfactory result are further suggested as a robust method. The others result in lower sensitivity or false-positive results in NTC. To tackle this issue, some algorithms have been developed to find out the robust primer set. Recently, Huang et al. [34] developed an algorithm and suggested to shorten the FIP and BIP primers, which are the longest ones that have a poor annealing efficacy than other primers. The shortening of these primers led to a significant time-to-threshold (TT) improvement in comparison to that of non-truncated ones. According to the suggested protocol, the optimal stem length was in between 12 and 17 bp with a melting temperature (Tm) of >45°C. By means of this strategy, the sensitivity of the RT-LAMP assay has been improved to detect 1.5 copies/μL of SARS-CoV-2 particles in saliva [34].

Together with the abovementioned limitations, the sensitivity of the colorimetric RT-LAMP decreases when testing samples with low viral loads. Some studies reported indeterminate color change—between positive and negative—in lower viral copies samples [9, 10]. The sensitivity also depends on the days from which symptoms of the disease appeared. It was reported that 5 days was the optimum time in which this technique gives the most accurate results, whereas sensitivity reduces if more than 7 days since the onset of the symptoms have passed [10]. To overcome these limitations, studies suggested using internal controls to evaluate primers' performance and confirm the success of reaction. In addition, it was found that skipping RNA extraction step, especially in saliva specimens, affects the pH of the solution, leading to false diagnosis. Therefore, RNA extraction step is crucial to assure the accuracy of the colorimetric RT-LAMP results [12].

6. Conclusions and future prospect

Since its emergence, RT-qPCR was the only approved gold standard molecular diagnostic technique that detects SARS-CoV-2. However, once studies started to utilize the colorimetric RT-LAMP for a faster and cheaper alternative, they proved the success of this technology in diagnosing COVID-19. Hence, some developed RT-LAMP SARS-CoV-2 detection kits received the approval by the FDA like the AQ-TOP™ COVID-19 Rapid Detection Kit, the Color SARS-CoV-2 RT-LAMP Diagnostic Assay, FastProof™ 30 min-TTR SARS-CoV-2 RT-LAMP, or the Lucira COVID-19 All-In-One Test Kit Labeling for emergency use authorization (EUA). Thanks to its simplicity and accessibility for end-users, this technology can be easily adapted for custom-use. For instance, Davidson and colleagues developed a paper-based colorimetric assay that contains lyophilized reagents for room temperature storage and distribution [18]. Also, some colorimetric RT-LAMP reagents, especially enzymes, can be made in-house to reduce the cost of the assay. To improve the efficiency of the detection, RT-LAMP can be combined with other technologies like CRISPR [35], nanotechnology [36], and many more. Therefore, the colorimetric RT-LAMP method must be further investigated not only for the detection of SARS-CoV-2, but also for broader applications such as human, plant, or animal-hosted viral pathogens.

Acknowledgements

BioRender < https://biorender.com/> is used to generate **Figure 1**.

Conflict of interest

The authors declare no conflict of interest.

Author details

Galyah Alhamid[1,2] and Huseyin Tombuloglu[1*]

1 Department of Genetics Research, Institute for Research and Medical Consultations (IRMC), Imam Abdulrahman bin Faisal University, Dammam, Saudi Arabia

2 Biotechnology Master Program, Imam Abdulrahman bin Faisal University, Dammam, Saudi Arabia

*Address all correspondence to: htoglu@iau.edu.sa

References

[1] COVID Live - Coronavirus Statistics. Worldometer; [cited 2022 May 7]. Available from: https://www.worldometers.info/coronavirus/

[2] Ferguson N, Laydon D, Nedjati Gilani G, Imai N, Ainslie K, Baguelin M, et al. Report 9: Impact of Non-pharmaceutical Interventions (NPIs) to Reduce COVID19 Mortality and Healthcare Demand. London: Imperial College; 2020 [cited 2021 Oct 28]. Available from: http://spiral.imperial.ac.uk/handle/10044/1/77482

[3] Khan S, Tombuloglu H, Hassanein SE, Rehman S, Bozkurt A, Cevik E, et al. Coronavirus diseases 2019: Current biological situation and potential therapeutic perspective. European Journal of Pharmacology. 2020;**886**: 173447

[4] Wang MY, Zhao R, Gao LJ, Gao XF, Wang DP, Cao JM. SARS-CoV-2: Structure, biology, and structure-based therapeutics development. Frontiers in Cellular and Infection Microbiology. 2020;**10**:587269

[5] Zhou P, Yang XL, Wang XG, Hu B, Zhang L, Zhang W, et al. A pneumonia outbreak associated with a new coronavirus of probable bat origin. Nature. 2020;**579**(7798):270-273

[6] Hu B, Guo H, Zhou P, Shi ZL. Characteristics of SARS-CoV-2 and COVID-19. Nature Reviews. Microbiology. 2021;**19**(3):141-154

[7] Notomi T. Loop-mediated isothermal amplification of DNA. Nucleic Acids Research. 2000;**28**(12):63e-663e

[8] Notomi T, Mori Y, Tomita N, Kanda H. Loop-mediated isothermal amplification (LAMP): Principle, features, and future prospects. Journal of Microbiology. 2015;**53**(1):1-5

[9] Aoki MN, de Oliveira CB, Góes LGB, Minoprio P, Durigon EL, Morello LG, et al. Colorimetric RT-LAMP SARS-CoV-2 diagnostic sensitivity relies on color interpretation and viral load. Scientific Reports. 2021;**11**(1):9026

[10] de Oliveira CB, Sanchuki HBS, Zanette DL, Nardin JM, Morales HMP, Fornazari B, et al. Essential properties and pitfalls of colorimetric reverse transcription loop-mediated isothermal amplification as a point-of-care test for SARS-CoV-2 diagnosis. Molecular Medicine. 2021;**27**(1):30

[11] Dao Thi VL, Herbst K, Boerner K, Meurer M, Kremer LP, Kirrmaier D, et al. A colorimetric RT-LAMP assay and LAMP-sequencing for detecting SARS-CoV-2 RNA in clinical samples. Science Translational Medicine. 2020;**12**(556): eabc7075

[12] Bokelmann L, Nickel O, Maricic T, Pääbo S, Meyer M, Borte S, et al. Point-of-care bulk testing for SARS-CoV-2 by combining hybridization capture with improved colorimetric LAMP. Nature Communications. 2021;**12**(1):1467

[13] Lu R, Wu X, Wan Z, Li Y, Jin X, Zhang C. A novel reverse transcription loop-mediated isothermal amplification method for rapid detection of SARS-CoV-2. International Journal of Molecular Sciences. 2020;**21**(8):2826

[14] Promlek T, Thanunchai M, Phumisantiphong U, Hansirisathit T, Phuttanu C, Dongphooyao S, et al. Performance of colorimetric reverse transcription loop-mediated isothermal amplification as a diagnostic tool for

SARS-CoV-2 infection during the fourth wave of COVID-19 in Thailand. International Journal of Infectious Diseases. 2022;**116**:133-137

[15] Food and Drug Administration (FDA). Color SARS-CoV-2 RT-LAMP Diagnostic Assay - EUA Summary. Vol. 252021. https://www.fda.gov/media/138249/download

[16] Baba MM, Bitew M, Fokam J, Lelo EA, Ahidjo A, Asmamaw K, et al. Diagnostic performance of a colorimetric RT -LAMP for the identification of SARS-CoV-2: A multicenter prospective clinical evaluation in sub-Saharan Africa. EClinicalMedicine. 2021;**40**:101101

[17] Tanner NA, Zhang Y, Evans TC. Visual detection of isothermal nucleic acid amplification using pH-sensitive dyes. BioTechniques. 2015;**58**(2):59-68

[18] Davidson JL, Wang J, Maruthamuthu MK, Dextre A, Pascual-Garrigos A, Mohan S, et al. A paper-based colorimetric molecular test for SARS-CoV-2 in saliva. Biosensors and Bioelectronics: X. 2021;**9**:100076

[19] Amaral C, Antunes W, Moe E, Duarte AG, Lima LMP, Santos C, et al. A molecular test based on RT-LAMP for rapid, sensitive and inexpensive colorimetric detection of SARS-CoV-2 in clinical samples. Scientific Reports. 2021;**11**(1):16430

[20] Yu L, Wu S, Hao X, Dong X, Mao L, Pelechano V, et al. Rapid detection of COVID-19 coronavirus using a reverse transcriptional loop-mediated isothermal amplification (RT-LAMP) diagnostic platform. Clinical Chemistry. 2020;**66**(7):975-977

[21] Lamb LE, Bartolone SN, Ward E, Chancellor MB. Rapid detection of novel coronavirus/severe acute respiratory syndrome coronavirus 2 (SARS-CoV-2) by reverse transcription-loop-mediated isothermal amplification. Kalendar R, editor. PLoS One. 2020;**15**(6):e0234682

[22] Mohon AN, Hundt J, van Marle G, Pabbaraju K, Berenger B, Griener T, et al. Development and Validation of Direct RT-LAMP for SARS-CoV-2. Infectious Diseases (except HIV/AIDS); 2020. [cited 2022 May 7]. Available from: http://medrxiv.org/lookup/doi/10.1101/2020.04.29.20075747

[23] Zhang Y, Ren G, Buss J, Barry AJ, Patton GC, Tanner NA. Enhancing colorimetric loop-mediated isothermal amplification speed and sensitivity with guanidine chloride. BioTechniques. 2020;**69**(3):178-185

[24] Dong Y, Wu X, Li S, Lu R, Li Y, Wan Z, et al. Comparative evaluation of 19 reverse transcription loop-mediated isothermal amplification assays for detection of SARS-CoV-2. Scientific Reports. 2021;**11**(1):2936

[25] Kim D, Lee JY, Yang JS, Kim JW, Kim VN, Chang H. The architecture of SARS-CoV-2 transcriptome. Cell. 2020;**181**(4):914-921.e10

[26] Lv DF, Ying Q m, Weng Y s, Shen C b, Chu J g, Kong J p, et al. Dynamic change process of target genes by RT-PCR testing of SARS-Cov-2 during the course of a coronavirus disease 2019 patient. Clinica Chimica Acta. 2020;**506**:172-175

[27] Tombuloglu H, Sabit H, Al-Khallaf H, Kabanja JH, Alsaeed M, Al-Saleh N, et al. Multiplex real-time RT-PCR method for the diagnosis of SARS-CoV-2 by targeting viral N, RdRP and human RP genes. Scientific Reports. 2022;**12**(1):2853

[28] Wang S, Xu X, Wei C, Li S, Zhao J, Zheng Y, et al. Molecular evolutionary

characteristics of SARS-CoV-2 emerging in the United States. Journal of Medical Virology. 2022;**94**(1):310-317

[29] Venkatakrishnan A, Anand P, Lenehan P, Suratekar R, Raghunathan B, Niesen MJM, et al. Omicron Variant of SARS-CoV-2 Harbors a Unique Insertion Mutation of Putative Viral or Human Genomic Origin. Open Science Framework; 2021. DOI: 10.31219/osf.io/f7txy

[30] Tahamtan A, Ardebili A. Real-time RT-PCR in COVID-19 detection: Issues affecting the results. Expert Review of Molecular Diagnostics. 2020;**20**(5): 453-454

[31] Zhang Y, Tanner NA. Improving RT-LAMP detection of SARS-CoV-2 RNA through primer set selection and combination. Dykeman EC, editor. PLoS One. 2022;**17**(4):e0254324

[32] Yang J, Petitjean SJL, Koehler M, Zhang Q, Dumitru AC, Chen W, et al. Molecular interaction and inhibition of SARS-CoV-2 binding to the ACE2 receptor. Nature Communications. 2020; **11**(1):4541

[33] Joung J, Ladha A, Saito M, Kim NG, Woolley AE, Segel M, et al. Detection of SARS-CoV-2 with SHERLOCK one-pot testing. The New England Journal of Medicine. 2020;**383**(15):1492-1494

[34] Huang X, Tang G, Ismail N, Wang X. Developing RT-LAMP assays for rapid diagnosis of SARS-CoV-2 in saliva. eBioMedicine. 2022 Jan;**75**:103736

[35] Selvam K, Najib M, Khalid M, Mohamad S, Palaz F, Ozsoz M, et al. RT-LAMP CRISPR-Cas12/13-based SARS-CoV-2 detection methods. Diagnostics. 2021;**11**(9):1646

[36] Moitra P, Alafeef M, Dighe K, Frieman MB, Pan D. Selective naked-eye detection of SARS-CoV-2 mediated by N gene targeted antisense oligonucleotide capped Plasmonic nanoparticles. ACS Nano. 2020;**14**(6):7617-7627

Section 3

Genomics, Bioinformatics and Immunology

Chapter 13

Perspective Chapter: Bioinformatics Study of the Evolution of SARS-CoV-2 Spike Protein

Črtomir Podlipnik, Radostina Alexandrova, Sebastian Pleško, Urban Bren and Marko Jukič

Abstract

SARS-CoV-2 belongs to the family of coronaviruses, which are characterized by spikes that sit densely on the surface of the virus. The spike protein (Spro) is responsible for the attachment of the virus to the host cell *via* the ACE2 receptor on the surface of the host cell. The strength of the interaction between the receptor-binding domain (RBD) of the highly glycosylated spike protein of the virus and the host cell ACE2 receptor represents the key determinant of the infectivity of the virus. The SARS-CoV-2 virus has mutated since the beginning of the outbreak, and the vast majority of mutations has been detected in the spike protein or its RBD. Since specific mutations significantly affect the ability of the virus to transmit and to evade immune response, studies of these mutations are critical. We investigate GISAID data to show how viral spike protein mutations evolved during the pandemic. We further present the interactions of the viral Spro RBD with the host ACE2 receptor. We have performed a large-scale mutagenesis study of the Spro RBD-ACE2 interface by performing point mutations *in silico* and identifying the ambiguous interface stabilization by the most common point mutations in the viral variants of interest (beta, gamma, delta, omicron).

Keywords: spike protein, spro, point mutations, SARS-CoV-2, receptor binding domain, ACE2

1. Introduction

The SARS-CoV-2 virus has been with us for more than 2 years now. More than half a billion people have contracted the virus in a little over 2 years, and more than 6 million people have died from the virus [1, 2]. Subsequent pandemic waves of the disease can be prevented by social distancing during local outbreaks and vaccination. In spite of current pandemic, coronaviruses have always been present and are commonly the cause of colds. The first virus from the family mentioned above, isolated in 1962,

IntechOpen

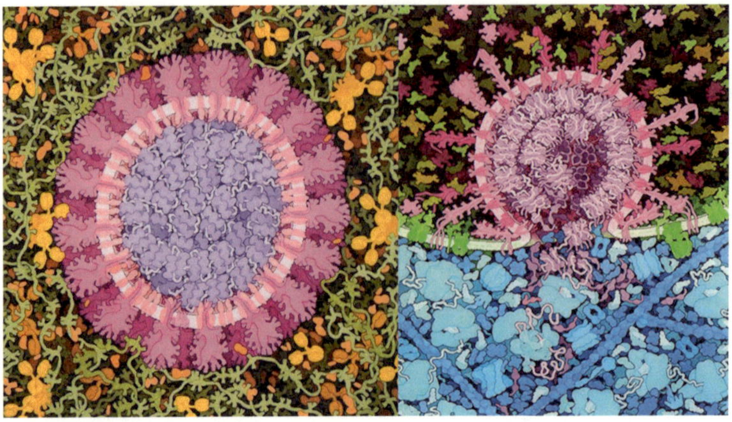

Figure 1.
The cross-section of SARS-CoV-2 with characteristic spikes at the virus's surface (left) and the fusion of the virus with the cell membrane (right). The figure is the artwork of David Goodsell (PDB-101: Educational resources supporting molecular explorations through biology and medicine [3]).

was classified as an enveloped, single-stranded (+ssRNA) RNA virus. The new virus family was named after its characteristic morphological appearance, the crown spikes (spike protein or Spro) on its surface (**Figure 1**) [4].

Until the outbreak of the SARS (Severe Acute Respiratory Syndrome; causative virus named SARS-CoV) pandemic in mainland China and Hong Kong in 2003, coronaviruses did not receive so much attention from the scientific community. Timely action at that time prevented the outbreak and evolution to the pandemic. However, in 2012, the respiratory syndrome coronavirus (MERS-CoV) led to an outbreak of the Middle East respiratory syndrome (MERS) in Saudi Arabia, mainland China, the United Arab Emirates, and the Republic of Korea [2, 5, 6]. In late 2019, SARS-CoV-2, a member of the *Coronaviridae* family, emerged in Wuhan, China. As a result, a creeping spread among the human population began, and the WHO declared a pandemic on March 11, 2020 [7, 8]. At the time of writing, COVID-19 disease (caused by SARS-CoV-2) has spread worldwide, claiming more than 6.5 million lives. As the SARS-CoV-2 virus has become a critical health concern, scientists immediately began research on this topic. COVID-19 disease is of great concern worldwide because, while the majority of cases have mild symptoms, a variable percentage (0.2 to >5%!) of patients progresses to pneumonia and multiple organ failure, which can lead to death especially without medical assistance [9, 10].

Vaccines against SARS-CoV-2 are now available, few therapeutic options have been authorized for emergency use by FDA and only one antiviral agent has been approved for COVID-19 treatment, however novel drug research is ongoing [11–16]. Since vaccines are the poster child in the fight against the COVID-19 pandemic, a high viral mutation rate may lead to changes in the structures of essential viral proteins, rendering available vaccines ineffective [17]. This concern is exacerbated by the fact that, with the exception of inactivated SARS-CoV-2 vaccines, all other vaccines (RNA vaccines, Adenovirus-based and protein-based vaccines) currently in clinical use are targeted at the same structure in the virus – the spike protein from the viral envelope. Its biological functions and surface location, make it a major target for the formation of neutralizing antibodies. However, this also determines the high frequency of mutations in this region, which can help the virus escape from the immune response [18].

The first identified mutations and respectively recognized subtypes / variants of the virus were announced in March and April 2020 [19, 20]. In late 2020, the first SARS-CoV-2 variant of concern (VOC) was reported—the B.1.1.7 variant (UK variant, designated *alpha* by WHO as of June 7, 2021; https://www.who.int/). Alpha is often designated by canonical mutations: N501Y, 69/70 deletion, P681H. This was followed by the appearance of several other variants of concern—*beta, gamma, delta and omicron*, as well as a number of variants of interest (VOI; for variant classification the reader is referred to a wonderful classification at CDC: https://www.cdc.gov/coronavirus/2019-ncov/variants/variant-classifications.html). The second in the list of VOC was B.1.351 variant (*beta;* canonical mutations: K417N, E484K, N501Y) or South African variant [21, 22]. Both variants carry an N501Y mutation in the RBD (receptor binding domain) of the Spro, which is associated with increased viral transmission [23]. In addition, the South African variant carries mutations K417N and E484K, which may be responsible for decreased binding to host antibodies [24]. P.1 (*gamma*, canonical mutations: K417T, E484K, and N501Y) variant has been reported in Brazil with the known N501Y, E484K and the novel K417T mutations [25]. *Epsilon* or B.1.427 or B.1.429 followed with canonical mutations: S13I, W152C, L452R, D614G. In early 2021, a novel SARS-CoV-2 variant B.1.617.2 (*delta*, canonical mutations: L452R, T478K, D614G, and P681R) nicknamed "the double mutant" or Indian variant was reported to cause infections in India and slowly spread throughout the world via global travel practices [26]. Acquired critical mutations in the Spro, particularly in the receptor-binding domain (RBD), are currently under heavy investigation (Delta Plus variant) as they may have higher infectivity and transmissibility or even escape the host immune response [27]. Last but not least is the observed *omicron* or B.1.1.529 variant first detected in Botswana and then in South Africa in November 2021. Omicron is described with at least 34 mutations in Spro, of which 15 are in RBD, 7 in the NTD and 3 close to the furin cleavage site.

2. The structure of the spike protein and its role

Since the first announcement of the existence of the new virus, many scientific groups around the world began an intensive search for a suitable drug. In their attempts to develop drugs to treat COVID-19, scientists are focusing on a variety of strategies, including identifying / creating agents that attack and neutralize the virus; agents that affect inflammation, prevent the formation of blood clots, etc. [28]. The structure of the Spro, as well as its biological properties and its role in the entry of SARS-CoV-2 into the cell have been the subject of extensive studies and are the key towards development of adequate preventive and curative approaches [29, 30]. The spike glycoprotein is the crucial protein that determines viral host selection and pathology and thus one of the most important targets for diagnosis and therapy. With a total length of 1273 amino acids, the Spro consists of an extracellular N-terminus, a transmembrane domain anchored in the viral membrane (TM), and a short intracellular C-terminal segment. Bound to the protein are specific polysaccharides whose function is to prevent the host immune system from recognizing the viral protein. Once the virus interacts with the host cell, the conformational changes of the Spro lead to the fusion of the virus with the host cell membrane. The protein consists of the signaling protein (1-13) and the S1 (14-685) and S2 (686-1273) subunits. In addition, the S1 domain, which is responsible for receptor binding, is divided into an N-terminal domain (NTD; 14-305) and a receptor-binding domain (RBD; 319-541).

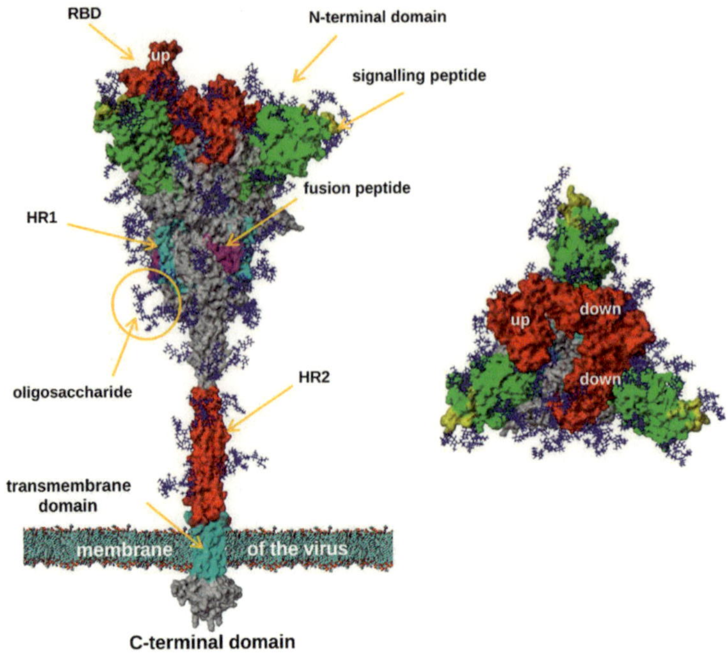

Figure 2.
The structure of the Spro with labeled domains. The model is based on the cryo-EM structure of SARS-CoV-2 spike glycoprotein trimer in prefusion conformation with a single receptor-binding domain (RBD) in "up" conformation (PDB-ID: 6vsb) [31].

The S2 subunit, whose function is fusion, consists of the fusion peptide (FP) (788-806 residues), heptapeptide repeat sequence 1 (HR1) (912-984), HR2 (1163-1213), the TM domain (1213-1237), and the cytoplasmic domain (1237-1273). A polybasic insertion (PRRAR) characteristic of joining the S1/S2 and S′ domains of SARS-CoV-2 can be cleaved by furin, and this cleavage is essential for membrane fusion. The model of the Spro with labeled domains shown in **Figure 2** and results from a detailed all-atom molecular dynamics simulation (μs trajectory timeframe) of the fully glycosylated full-length Spro in a viral membrane [32].

The Spro is densely coated with polysaccharides. Each monomer of SARS-CoV-2 Spro has 22 N-linked glycans, 18 of which were conserved between SARS-CoV and SARS-CoV-2 Spro [33]. The glycan shielding has several effects on Spro folding, its processing by host cell proteases, immune evasion, and the elicitation of a humoral immune response. Extensive glycan shielding of the Spro, which blocks the surface of the protein, can thereby hide specific epitopes from neutralization by antibodies, masking them and facilitating immune evasion [33]. In addition, it has been observed that both glycosylated and de-glycosylated S ectodomains bind with almost identical affinity to ACE-2 (1.7 nM vs. 1.5 nM); therefore, it has been suggested that glycosylation of the Spro does not alter the binding affinity of the Spro to ACE-2 [18]. However, the glycan shield of the Spro of SARS-CoV-2 is thought to be less dense and less effective compared to glycoproteins of other viruses such as HIV-1, which may be advantageous for the induction of humoral immunity and vaccine development. Therefore, there is great interest in investigating the potential immunogenicity of glycan components as vaccine candidates [34]. Furthermore, the structure bound to ACE2 shows that the *omicron* variant

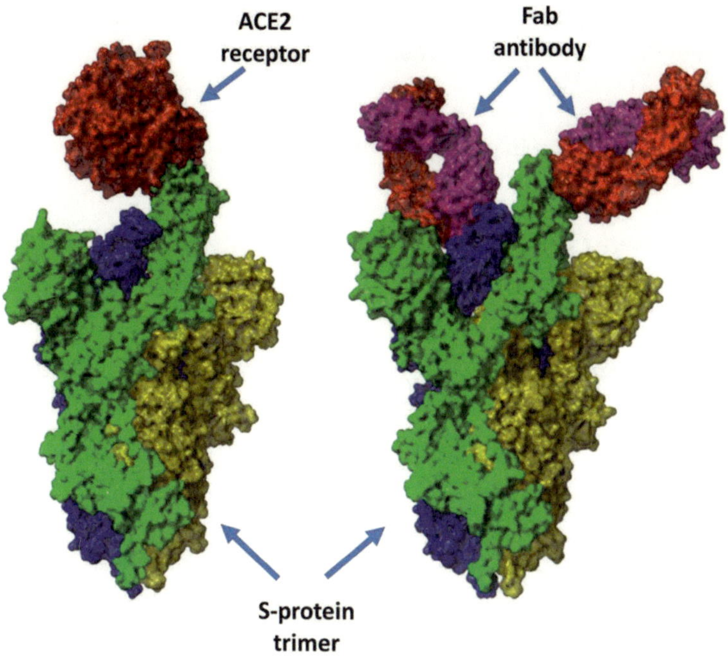

Figure 3.
The structure of SARS-CoV-2 (omicron variant) Spro trimer in complex with ACE2 receptor (PDB ID: 7wpa, left) and with Fab antibody (PDB ID: 7wpf, right) [35].

spike trimer contains an unusual RBD-RBD interaction and other interactions at the ACE2-RBD interface, both of which contribute to the higher affinity of ACE2 for the *omicron* spike trimer, which is six to nine times higher than that of the wild type, WT. The structural analysis of the *omicron* spike trimer also explains why the *omicron* escapes the most therapeutic antibodies and reduces the efficacy of vaccinations. The interaction of *omicron* spike trimer with ACE2 and Fab antibody is shown in **Figure 3** [35].

3. SARS-CoV-2 variants and mutations in the spike protein

Genetic sequencing studies have revealed numerous neutral or mildly deleterious mutations, mainly single nucleotide polymorphisms (SNPs) and insertions/deletions (indels). However, a small percentage of mutations can alter fitness and help the virus adapt. These substitutions or deletions can alter peptide polarity and affect the structure and functionality of viral proteins responsible for infectivity, transmissibility, and antigenicity [36]. Several databases and nomenclature systems have been established to classify genome sequences and track the epidemiology and genetic evolution of SARS-CoV-2. GISAID (The Global Initiative on Sharing All Influenza Data, https://www.epicov.org) contains millions of SARS-CoV-2 whole-genome sequences [37]. The GISAID nomenclature categorizes genomes into clades (based on marker mutations) that help understand large-scale diversity patterns and geographic dispersal. Pango nomenclature (https://cov-lineages.org/) is one of the most widely used nomenclatures that assigns newly identified genomes to a lineage based on the global phylogenetic tree. Based on the extensive sequencing data and observations available, the WHO has classified the SARS-CoV-2 variants that may pose an increased public health risk into the following three groups:

- *Variants of Concern (VOC)*: VOC is defined by increased transmissibility and virulence or a decrease in practiced public health and social interventions and available therapeutics.

- *Variants of Interest (VOI)*: VOI is defined by variants that have been observed to spread in the community and occur in multiple cases or clusters or have been detected in different countries.

- *Variants under Surveillance (VUM)*: VUM is defined as a variant with genetic alterations that are believed to affect viral properties, and that may pose some risk to public health and safety in the future. Increased surveillance and ongoing assessment are needed to gather evidence of these variants' phenotypic or epidemiologic impact.

According to comprehensive data provided by WHO as of May 2, 2021 (https://www.who.int/en/activities/tracking-SARS-CoV-2-variants/), the above groups are summarized in **Table 1**.

RNA viruses have the highest mutation rates, 1:10,000 to 1:1,000,000 mutations per base pair, due to the lack of proofreading ability of RNA-dependent RNA polymerases (RdRp) [38]. However, coronavirus family viruses have a proofreading

WHO label	Pango lineage	GISAID clade	Earliest documented amples	Date of designation
Alpha	B.1.1.7	GRY	UK, Sep-20	VOC: 18-Dec-20
Beta	B.1.351	GH/501Y.V2	South Africa, May-20	VOC: 18-Dec-20
Gamma	P.1	GR/501Y.V3	Brazil, Nov-20	VOC: 11-Jan-21
Delta	B.1.617.2	G/478 K.V1	India, Oct-20	VOI: 4-Apr-21; VOC: 11-May-21
Epsilon	B.1.427	GH/452R.V1	USA, Mar-20	VOI: 5-Mar-21
Zeta	P.2	GR/484 K. V2	Brazil, Apr-20	VOI: 17-Mar-21
Eta	B.1.525	G/484 K.V3	Multiple countries, Dec-20	VOI: 17-Mar-21
Theta	P.3	GR/1092 K. V1	Philippines, Jan-21	VOI: 24-Mar-21
Iota	B.1.526	GH/253G.V1	USA, Nov-20	VOI: 24-Mar-21
Kappa	B.1.617.1	G/452R.V3	India, Oct-20	VOI: 4-Aprl-21
Lambda	C.37	GR/452Q.V1	Peru, Dec-20	VOI: 14-Jun-21
Mu	B.1.621	GH	Colombia, Jan-21	VOI: 30-Aug-21
Omicron	B.1.1.529	GR/484A	Multiple countries, Nov-21	VUM: 24-Nov-21; VOC: 26-Nov-21

Table 1.
Summary of VOI, VOC, and VUM as published by the WHO.

No.	Mutation	Region	Virus variant	Impact in viral pathogenicity
1	D614G	RBD	several lineages	the most prevalent mutation, increase spike density.
2	N501Y	RBD	B.1.1.7,B.1.351,P.1	antibody escape, may effect host tropism
3	E484K/K/Q/A	RBD	B.1.351,P.1, B.1.617.1, B.1.1.529	antibody escape, increase ACE binding
4	K417N/T	RBD	B.1.351,P1	antibody escape, vaccine ineffectiveness, reinfection
5	L452R, T478K	RBD	B.1.617	increase ACE binding, antibody escape resistance to antibody drugs
6	Q677P/H	S1/S2	Several lineages	Increasing virus fusion with human cell
7	T478K, Q493K, Q498R	RBD	B.1.1.529	Increase ACE2-RBD binding
8	Δ69–70	NTD	B.1.1.7,B.1.1.529	Immune escape

Table 2.
Collected key mutations of SARS-CoV-2, which have a substantial impact on the viral pathogenicity.

mechanism due to the exoribonuclease (ExoN) domain of nsp14 [39]. Although this was expected to contribute to a low mutation rate, more than 6 million viral genomes were captured within 2 years (GISAID). Furthermore, the first fitness-enhancing mutation at the spike protein was identified only a few months after SARS-CoV-2 emerged [40]. These findings could be a consequence of the sheer magnitude of infection numbers on a global scale. In addition, Gribble et al. [41] have experimentally demonstrated that nsp14-ExoN may play a critical role in RNA recombination events during viral replication that can generate genetic variants (**Table 2**).

As we see in **Table 2**, the most essential mutations of the SARS-CoV-2 are found on the spike protein's receptor-binding domain (RBD), but that is not the whole story. Other important regions are critical to the success of different lineages, like mutations in the antibody binding regions found on/near the RBD, on the N-terminal domain (NTD) and the S2 domain. Such mutations mainly contribute to the lineages' antibody escape. Some mutations stabilize binding with stabilization of the open conformation and add/remove glycosylation sites which are also important. There is also the furin cleavage site, one of the vital mutation points that was present in the *delta* variant. The other aspect of mutations is also the influence on testing capabilities. For example the mutation S:69/70del that caused the so-called S-drop out in the PCR testing, which was caused by the mutation in the PCR primer region. This mutation was later cleverly exploited to quickly distinguish between *alpha* and non-*alpha* infections and *omicron* and non-*omicron*. There are also mutations on the N-gene that are present mainly in the omicron lineage, which cause lower sensitivity and even failure of detection using lateral flow tests (so-called quick antigen tests). Lastly, there are also mutations in other proteins that are significant for novel drug design. The phylogenetic analysis of SARS-CoV-2 is presented in **Figure 4** (The reader is referred to an excellent resource: https://covariants.org/).

The *omicron* variant mutations potentially attenuate the efficacy of therapeutic antibodies and enhance the binding of ACE2. Of even more significant concern, *omicron* infections have been reported in individuals vaccinated in South Africa and Hong Kong [44]. The recent study by Yin et al. reported the biochemical and structural

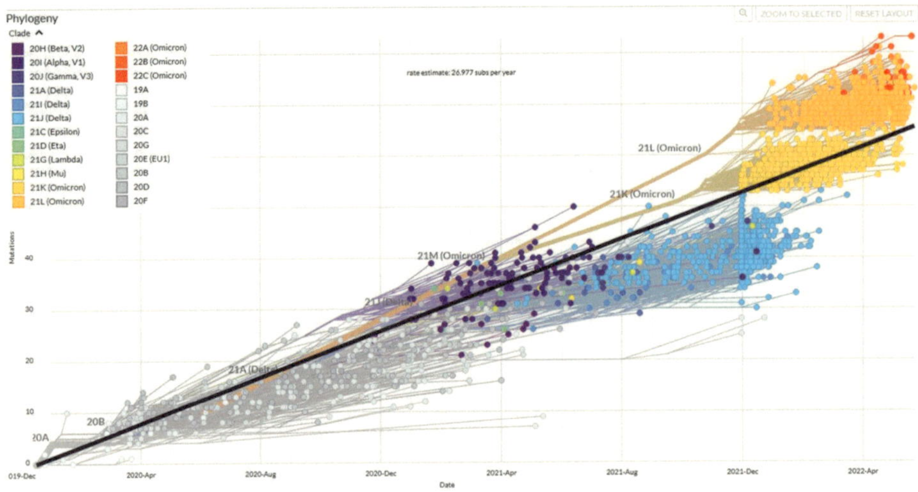

Figure 4.
On the chart we can see the molecular clock, i.e. the number of mutations in a particular sequence dependent on the time of sampling. The colors represent variants (clades). The thick line represents the average mutation rate. We can see that 21 L (BA.2) omicron, as well as 22A (BA.4), 22B (BA.5), 22C (BA.2.12.1), clearly deviate from the average. Nextstrain; 2022-05-31 [42, 43].

characterization of the spike protein trimer of SARS-CoV-2 *omicron* variant and its binding to ACE2. Data show that *omicron* variant RBD is less stable and more dynamic than WT RBD. [35] *Omicron* differs significantly from all previous versions of SARS-CoV-2. These mutations in turn have led to important consequences in the behavior of the virus, including significant epidemiological characteristics [42, 43]. Namely, mutations altered the area recognized by neutralizing antibodies and reduced the effectiveness of the immune response elicited by previous variants and vaccines. Of particular interest are the neutralizing antibodies that still recognize the virus, because knowing them will help us to improve prophylactic and therapeutic strategies and to respond adequately to future variants. There is excellent research done on antibody escape by J.D. Bloom et al. [45]. Bloom's lab plotted the antibody escape in dependence on the spike mutation site for Moderna's vaccine serum and convalescent serum. From the plots presented in **Figure 5** it's nicely seen that the mutation on 484 or 456 sites would cause an antigen to escape from any previously acquired immunity. The mutation on 484th residue, present in *beta* and *gamma* lineages as E484K and in *omicron* as E484A, confirmed Bloom's work. The mutation 456 on the other hand, is not present so far in any of the WHO's variants of interests.

Omicron variant mutations thus contributed to the successful transmission of the virus from person to person and its faster spread. Surprisingly, the virus with so many mutations continues to effectively bind to the ACE2 receptor. *Omicron* is thought to combine various mutations (we know some of them from other variants), some of which simultaneously help it escape the immune response and bind to ACE2 [43]. The mutations have affected the mechanism of viral entry into the cell. Unlike other variants, which use the mechanism of fusion with the cytoplasmic membrane of the host cell, *omicron* uses another mechanism of entry, namely the uptake by the endosome. According to one hypothesis, this may at least partially explain *omicron*'s preference for the upper respiratory tract (nose and throat) [42]. The mutations have also affected the spectrum of hosts—it is known

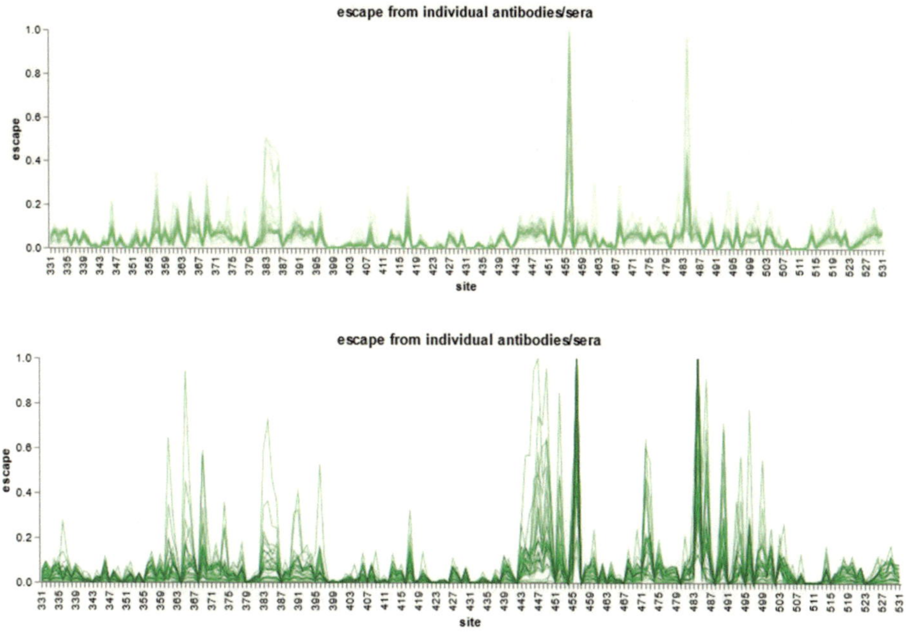

Figure 5.
Bloom plots (https://jbloomlab.github.io/SARS2_RBD_Ab_escape_maps/) top: Moderna's vaccine serum and bottom: Convalescent serum; on 2022-05-31 [45].

that SARS-CoV-2 can infect a wide range of domestic and wild animals, including cats, dogs, ferrets, hamsters, leopards, minks, deer, etc., but not mice and rats. However, unlike "conventional" SARS-Cov-2 variants, *omicron* can bind to the ACE2 receptor in turkeys, chickens and mice, as well as rats (linked to N501Y and Q498R mutations) [1, 45].

All in all, *omicron* consists of several genome sublines / subvariants (BA.1, BA.2, BA.3, BA.4, BA.5), some of which (BA.1, BA.2) have already been established worldwide, while the growth of the others (BA.4, BA.5) is increasing at the moment. BA4 and BA5 appeared in late December 2021 and early January 2022, they are better transmissible than earlier versions of *omicron* (BA2 and especially BA1) and may partially escape the immune protection provided by infection with previous variants or vaccination. At the beginning of May 2022, infections with BA.4 and BA.5 were 60–75% of the cases in South Africa, and have been registered in a number of other countries in Europe and North America [42, 46]. According to the European Centre for Disease Prevention and Control (ECDC; https://www.ecdc.europa.eu/en/news-events/epidemiological-update-sars-cov-2-omicron-sub-lineages-ba4-and-ba5), as of May 13, 2022, BA.5 represents already 37% of the cases in Portugal, and the expectation is to become dominant by May 22, 2022. *Omicron* has a large number of mutations (50 as compared to the original variant of SARS-CoV-2 isolated in Wuhan in the end of 2019). Its origin is not yet fully established. Clarifying it is extremely important not only from a theoretical point of view, but also because it will help us to be better prepared to manage with future variants [42]. Among the more recognized hypotheses, we can distinguish four: First, accumulation of mutations during its transmission from person to person. It is known that, unlike other RNA viruses, coronaviruses, including SARS-CoV-2, carry an editing enzyme system that helps it to correct errors occurring during in RNA molecule synthesis [47, 48]; Second, the appearance of such large number of mutations can be facilitated by infecting immunosuppressed individuals in whose body the virus persists for a long time, which creates conditions for its continuous reproduction and selection of mutations that avoid the immune response; Third, the emergence can be related to its circulation (and consequent accumulation of mutations) in animal organisms. This shows that we need to monitor the fate of the virus also in the animal kingdom [42]; and Fourth, the changes in coronaviruses can be induced through a process of recombination—in this case, the formation of the next vital generation may be the result of combining genetic information. It has been reported that this process takes place not only in bats, but in humans as well and can lead to the emergence of new variants and strains [49, 50].

4. In silico comprehensive mutagenesis

We can postulate new viral variants along with key (canonical) mutations, especially at the receptor binding domain (RBD) of the Spike protein (Spro), improve the ability of the virus to recognize relevant host receptor (ACE2) via steric adaptation and new interactions with the binding partner. In order to inspect all possible mutations at the Spro RBD we performed a comprehensive *in silico* mutagenesis study using FoldX [46]. 3D complexes of Spro wild type along with Spro FoldX mutants were iteratively used for ΔΔG prediction. All possible mutations of RBD binding domain of SARS-CoV-2 S protein (PDB ID: 6M0J) with sequence from K417 towards Y505 (length of 89; *KIADYNYKLPDDFTGCVIAWNSNNLDSKVGGNYNYLYRLFRKSNLKPFERD ISTEIYQAGSTPCNGVEGFNCYFPLQSYGFQPTNGVGY*) for a total of 1780 point mutations were calculated and the resulting heatmap is presented in **Figure 6** [49]. Individual point mutation calculations were repeated once and mutations with no structural change left for validation purposes where all no-change mutation produced ΔΔG energies below 0.1 kcal/mol.

Upon structural inspection and superimposition (PDB ID: 6M0J, 7DK3), the Spro RBD-ACE2 interface was identified as: 417 LYS, 445 VAL, 446 GLY, 449 TYR, 453 TYR, 455 LEU, 456 PHE, 473 TYR, 475 ALA, 476 GLY, 484 GLU, 486 PHE, 487 ASN, 489 TYR, 493 GLN, 496 GLY, 498 GLN, 500 THR, 501 ASN, 502 GLY, 503 VAL, 505 TYR. Reference key mutations were placed on this interface such as E484K, Q493N, Q493Y, and N501Y with ample experimental data for validation. Namely, N501Y confers increased binding affinity to human ACE2 while N501T shows reduced host ACE2-binding affinity *in vitro* all according to P0DTC2 Uniprot reference [47, 48].

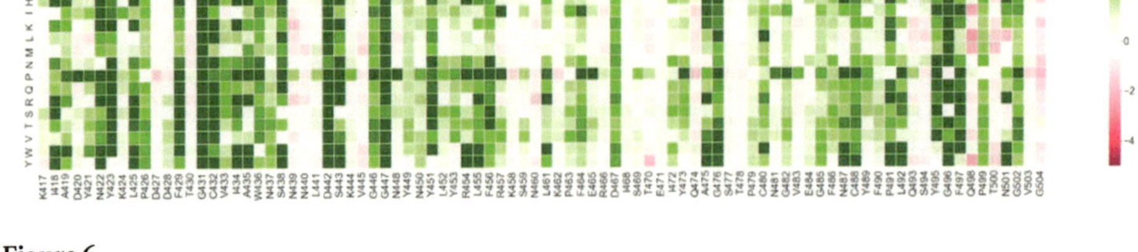

Figure 6.
We conducted a full RBD 417–505 mutagenesis study using FoldX in order to assess the key mutations and their effects on the stability of the system; in total 1780 point mutations.

We observed FoldX total energies of 0.37, 0.62, and −0.95 kcal/mol upon point mutations E484K, Q493N, and Q493Y respectively in accordance with literature [50]. Furthermore, canonical *delta* L452R, and E484Q displayed insignificant FoldX force field Δ energies of 0.04, 0.09 kcal/mol, respectively [51]. If we focus on *omicron* variant, it possesses the following mutations at the Spro RBD not in contact with ACE2 binding partner: G339D, S371L, S373P, and S375F. In the ACE2 PPI, however the following mutations are present with calculated FoldX Δ energies in kcal/mol: K417N: −0.34, G446S: 2.99, N440K: −0.61, S477N: 0.14, T478K: −0.18, E484A: 1.31, Q493K: −1.20, G496S: −0.06, Q498R: −0.93, N501Y: 6.18 and Y505H: 1.62. The results confirm the observed ensemble of mutations substantially modify the resulting PPI in accordance with the literature [52–60]. It should be stressed, that FoldX evaluations are single-point only and detailed binding energetics should be further studied by experiment supported MD. We postulate however such *in silico* interaction profiling approaches could be further developed to quickly assess key mutations or mutation ensembles for further study in the future.

5. Conclusions

One of the most interesting questions is undoubtedly in which direction the evolution of the SARS-CoV-2 will continue. Viruses strive for a successful dissemination and more intensive replication, which means that they evade the immune response and bypass the effects of antiviral agents. The omicron variant (and especially its subvariants) represents one of the fastest spreading viruses known. In addition, it is more successful at evading the immune response triggered by previous variants and/or available vaccines. What would be the profile of the next variant(s) to replace omicron? It is clear that the new variant must outperform the old one in order to prevail—this is achieved by bypassing the immune response and spreading efficiently, as evidenced by the evolution of new (sub)variants. From a public health perspective, the most important question is how severe the disease pattern of the next variant(s) will be and how effectively we can study the evolution of viral variants along with their impact on the drug/vaccine development in the future, with the final goal of preventing such future pandemics.

Funding

This study is supported by the National Science Fund, Bulgarian Ministry of Education and Science—Grant No. КП-06-КОСТ/16 from 16.12.2020 (AR) as well as by the Slovenian Research Agency (ARRS) through the research programs P1-0201 (CP), P1-0403, P2-0046 and the research project J1-2471 (UB, MJ).

Conflict of interest

Authors declare no conflict of interest.

Author details

Črtomir Podlipnik[1*], Radostina Alexandrova[2], Sebastian Pleško[1,3], Urban Bren[4,5] and Marko Jukič[4,5*]

1 Faculty of Chemistry and Chemical Technology, University of Ljubljana, Ljubljana, Slovenia

2 Institute of Experimental Morphology, Pathology and Anthropology with Museum, Bulgarian Academy of Sciences, Sofia, Bulgaria

3 Reactor Physics Department, Jozef Stefan Institute, Ljubljana, Slovenia

4 Faculty of Chemistry and Chemical Engineering, University of Maribor, Maribor, Slovenia

5 Faculty of Mathematics, Natural Sciences and Information Technologies, University of Primorska, Koper, Slovenia

*Address all correspondence to: crtomir.podlipnik@fkkt.uni-lj.si; marko.jukic@um.si

References

[1] Alexandrova R, Beykov P, Vassilev D, Jukić M, Podlipnik Č. The virus that shook the world: Questions and answers about SARS-CoV-2 and COVID-19. Biotechnology and Biotechnological Equipment. 2021;**35**(1):74-102

[2] Kahn JS, McIntosh K. History and recent advances in coronavirus discovery. The Pediatric Infectious Disease Journal. 2005;**24**(11 SUPPL):S223-S227

[3] Zardecki C, Dutta S, Goodsell DS, Lowe R, Voigt M, Burley SK. PDB-101: Educational resources supporting molecular explorations through biology and medicine. Protein Science. 2022;**31**(1):129-140

[4] De Wit E, Van Doremalen N, Falzarano D, Munster VJ. SARS and MERS: Recent insights into emerging coronaviruses. Nature Reviews Microbiology. 2016;**14**(8):523-534

[5] Lu G, Wang Q, Gao GF. Bat-to-human: Spike features determining "host jump" of coronaviruses SARS-CoV, MERS-CoV, and beyond. Trends in Microbiology. 2015;**23**(8):468-478

[6] Hilgenfeld R, Peiris M. From SARS to MERS: 10 years of research on highly pathogenic human coronaviruses. Antiviral Research. 2013;**100**(1):286-295

[7] Li Q, Guan X, Wu P, Wang X, Zhou L, Tong Y, et al. Early transmission dynamics in Wuhan, China, of novel coronavirus–infected pneumonia. The New England Journal of Medicine. 2020;**382**(13):1199-1207

[8] Hui DS, Azhar EI, Madani TA, Ntoumi F, Kock R, Dar O, et al. The continuing 2019-nCoV epidemic threat of novel coronaviruses to global health—The latest 2019 novel coronavirus outbreak in Wuhan, China. International Journal of Infectious Diseases. 2020;**91**:264-266

[9] O'Driscoll M, Ribeiro Dos Santos G, Wang L, Cummings DAT, Azman AS, Paireau J, et al. Age-specific mortality and immunity patterns of SARS-CoV-2. Nature. 2021;**590**(7844):140-145

[10] Lu R, Zhao X, Li J, Niu P, Yang B, Wu H, et al. Genomic characterisation and epidemiology of 2019 novel coronavirus: Implications for virus origins and receptor binding. Lancet. 2020;**395**(10224):565-574

[11] Flanagan KL, Best E, Crawford NW, Giles M, Koirala A, Macartney K, et al. Progress and pitfalls in the quest for effective SARS-CoV-2 (COVID-19) vaccines. Frontiers in Immunology. 2020;**11**:579250

[12] Kyriakidis NC, López-Cortés A, González EV, Grimaldos AB, Prado EO. SARS-CoV-2 vaccines strategies: A comprehensive review of phase 3 candidates. NPJ Vaccines. 2021;**6**(1):28

[13] Jayk Bernal A, Gomes da Silva MM, Musungaie DB, Kovalchuk E, Gonzalez A, Delos Reyes V, et al. Molnupiravir for Oral treatment of Covid-19 in nonhospitalized patients. The New England Journal of Medicine. 2022;**386**(6):502-520

[14] Kabinger F, Stiller C, Schmitzová J, Dienemann C, Kokic G, Hillen HS, et al. Mechanism of molnupiravir-induced SARS-CoV-2 mutagenesis. Nature Structural & Molecular Biology. 2021;**28**(9):740-746

[15] Drożdżal S, Rosik J, Lechowicz K, Machaj F, Szostak B, Przybyciński J, et al. An update on drugs with therapeutic potential for SARS-CoV-2 (COVID-19)

treatment. Drug Resistance Updates. 2021;**59**:100794

[16] Mahase E. Covid-19: Pfizer's paxlovid is 89% effective in patients at risk of serious illness, company reports. BMJ. 2021;**375**:n2713

[17] Malik JA, Ahmed S, Mir A, Shinde M, Bender O, Alshammari F, et al. The SARS-CoV-2 mutations versus vaccine effectiveness: New opportunities to new challenges. Journal of Infection and Public Health. 2022;**15**(2):228-240

[18] Duan L, Zheng Q, Zhang H, Niu Y, Lou Y, Wang H. The SARS-CoV-2 spike glycoprotein biosynthesis, structure, function, and antigenicity: Implications for the Design of Spike-Based Vaccine Immunogens. Frontiers in Immunology. 2020;**11**:576622

[19] Tang X, Wu C, Li X, Song Y, Yao X, Wu X, et al. On the origin and continuing evolution of SARS-CoV-2. National Science Review. 2020;**7**(6):1012-1023

[20] Forster P, Forster L, Renfrew C, Forster M. Phylogenetic network analysis of SARS-CoV-2 genomes. Proceedings of the National Academy of Sciences of the United States of America. 2020;**117**(17):9241-9243

[21] Volz E, Mishra S, Chand M, Barrett JC, Johnson R, Geidelberg L, et al. Assessing transmissibility of SARS-CoV-2 lineage B.1.1.7 in England. Nature. 2021;**593**(7858):266-269

[22] Tegally H, Wilkinson E, Giovanetti M, Iranzadeh A, Fonseca V, Giandhari J, et al. Detection of a SARS-CoV-2 variant of concern in South Africa. Nature. 2021;**592**(7854):438-443

[23] Gu H, Chen Q, Yang G, He L, Fan H, Deng YQ, et al. Adaptation of SARS-CoV-2 in BALB/c mice for testing vaccine efficacy. Science. 2020;**369**(6511):1603-1607

[24] Wibmer CK, Ayres F, Hermanus T, Madzivhandila M, Kgagudi P, Oosthuysen B, et al. SARS-CoV-2 501Y. V2 escapes neutralization by south African COVID-19 donor plasma. Nature Medicine. 2021;**27**(4):622-625

[25] Voloch CM, da Silva Francisco R, de Almeida LGP, Cardoso CC, Brustolini OJ, Gerber AL, et al. Genomic characterization of a novel SARS-CoV-2 lineage from Rio de Janeiro, Brazil. Journal of Virology. 2021;**95**(10):e00119-21

[26] Cherian S, Potdar V, Jadhav S, Yadav P, Gupta N, Das M, et al. Sars-cov-2 spike mutations, L452R, T478K, E484Q and P681R in the second wave of covid-19 in Maharashtra, India. Microorganisms. 2021;**9**(7):1542

[27] Teng S, Sobitan A, Rhoades R, Liu D, Tang Q. Systemic effects of missense mutations on SARS-CoV-2 spike glycoprotein stability and receptor-binding affinity. Briefings in Bioinformatics. 2021;**22**(2):1239-1253

[28] Ledford H. Hundreds of COVID trials could provide a deluge of new drugs. Nature. 2022;**603**(7899):25-27

[29] Jackson CB, Farzan M, Chen B, Choe H. Mechanisms of SARS-CoV-2 entry into cells. Nature Reviews Molecular Cell Biology. 2022;**23**(1):3-20

[30] Xie Y, Karki CB, Du D, Li H, Wang J, Sobitan A, et al. Spike proteins of SARS-CoV and SARS-CoV-2 utilize different mechanisms to bind with human ACE2. Frontiers in Molecular Biosciences. 2020;**7**:591873

[31] Wrapp D, Wang N, Corbett KS, Goldsmith JA, Hsieh CL, Abiona O, et al. Cryo-EM structure of the 2019-nCoV spike in the prefusion conformation. Science. 2020;**367**(6483):1260-1263

[32] Choi YK, Cao Y, Frank M, Woo H, Park SJ, Yeom MS, et al. Structure, dynamics, receptor binding, and antibody binding of the fully glycosylated full-length SARS-CoV-2 spike protein in a viral membrane. Journal of Chemical Theory and Computation. 2021;**17**(4):2479-2487

[33] Watanabe Y, Allen JD, Wrapp D, McLellan JS, Crispin M. Site-specific glycan analysis of the SARS-CoV-2 spike. Science. 2020;**369**(6501):330-333

[34] Zhao X, Chen H, Wang H. Glycans of SARS-CoV-2 spike protein in virus infection and antibody production. Frontiers in Molecular Biosciences. 2021;**8**:629873

[35] Yin W, Xu Y, Xu P, Cao X, Wu C, Gu C, et al. Structures of the omicron spike trimer with ACE2 and an anti-omicron antibody. Science. 2022;**375**(6584):1048-1053

[36] Thakur S, Sasi S, Pillai SG, Nag A, Shukla D, Singhal R, et al. SARS-CoV-2 mutations and their impact on diagnostics, therapeutics and vaccines. Frontiers in Medicine. 2022;**9**:815389

[37] Shu Y, McCauley J. GISAID: Global initiative on sharing all influenza data – From vision to reality. Eurosurveillance. 2017;**22**(13):30494

[38] Sanjuán R, Nebot MR, Chirico N, Mansky LM, Belshaw R. Viral mutation rates. Journal of Virology. 2010;**84**(19):9733-9748

[39] Robson F, Khan KS, Le TK, Paris C, Demirbag S, Barfuss P, et al. Coronavirus RNA proofreading: Molecular basis and therapeutic targeting. Molecular Cell. 2020;**79**(5):710-727

[40] Harvey WT, Carabelli AM, Jackson B, Gupta RK, Thomson EC, Harrison EM, et al. SARS-CoV-2 variants, spike mutations and immune escape. Nature Reviews Microbiology. 2021;**19**(7):409-424

[41] Gribble J, Stevens LJ, Agostini ML, Anderson-Daniels J, Chappell JD, Lu X, et al. The coronavirus proofreading exoribonuclease mediates extensive viral recombination. PLoS Pathogens. 2021;**17**(1):e1009226

[42] Hadfield J, Megill C, Bell SM, Huddleston J, Potter B, Callender C, et al. Nextstrain: Real-time tracking of pathogen evolution. Bioinformatics. 2018;**34**(23):4121-4123

[43] Xiong C, Liu X, Xiong J, Sun Z, Hu W, Hu J, et al. Omicron: A chimera of two early SARS-CoV-2 lineages. 2022;**7**(1):90

[44] Shah M, Woo HG. Omicron: A heavily mutated SARS-CoV-2 variant exhibits stronger binding to ACE2 and potently escapes approved COVID-19 therapeutic antibodies. Frontiers in Immunology. 2022;**12**:838527

[45] Eguia RT, Crawford KH, Stevens-Ayers T, Kelnhofer-Millevolte L, Greninger AL, Englund JA, et al. A human coronavirus evolves antigenically to escape antibody immunity. PLoS Pathogens. 2021;**17**(4):e1009453

[46] Buß O, Rudat J, Ochsenreither K. FoldX as protein engineering tool: Better than random based approaches? Computational and Structural Biotechnology Journal. 2018;**16**:25-33

[47] Motozono C, Toyoda M, Zahradnik J, Saito A, Nasser H, Tan TS, et al. SARS-CoV-2 spike L452R variant evades cellular immunity and increases infectivity. Cell Host & Microbe. 2021;**29**(7):1124-1136

[48] Shang J, Ye G, Shi K, Wan Y, Luo C, Aihara H, et al. Structural basis of receptor recognition by SARS-CoV-2. Nature. 2020;**581**(7807):221-224

[49] Jukić M, Kralj S, Nikitina N, Bren U. Bioinformatic and MD analysis of N501Y SARS-CoV-2 (UK) variant. In: International Conference on Computer Science Protecting Human Society against Epidemics. Cham: Springer; 2021. pp. 1-13

[50] Wang WB, Liang Y, Jin YQ, Zhang J, Su JG, Li QM. E484K mutation in SARS-CoV-2 RBD enhances binding affinity with hACE2 but reduces interactions with neutralizing antibodies and nanobodies: Binding free energy calculation studies. Journal of Molecular Graphics and Modelling. 2021;**109**:108035

[51] Li Q, Wu J, Nie J, Zhang L, Hao H, Liu S, et al. The impact of mutations in SARS-CoV-2 spike on viral infectivity and antigenicity. Cell. 2020;**182**(5):1284-1294

[52] Lupala CS, Ye Y, Chen H, Su XD, Liu H. Mutations on RBD of SARS-CoV-2 omicron variant result in stronger binding to human ACE2 receptor. Biochemical and Biophysical Research Communications. 2022;**590**:34-41

[53] Hatmal MMM, Alshaer W, Al-Hatamleh MA, Hatmal M, Smadi O, Taha MO, et al. Comprehensive structural and molecular comparison of spike proteins of SARS-CoV-2, SARS-CoV and MERS-CoV, and their interactions with ACE2. Cell. 2020;**9**(12):2638

[54] Saville JW, Mannar D, Zhu X, Srivastava SS, Berezuk AM, Demers JP, et al. Structural and biochemical rationale for enhanced spike protein fitness in delta and kappa SARS-CoV-2 variants. Nature Communications. 2022;**13**(1):1-10

[55] Roy U. Comparative structural analyses of selected spike protein-RBD mutations in SARS-CoV-2 lineages. Immunologic Research. 2022;**70**(2):143-151

[56] Nie C, Sahoo AK, Netz RR, Herrmann A, Ballauff M, Haag R. Charge matters: Mutations in omicron variant favor binding to cells. Chembiochem. 2022;**23**(6):e202100681

[57] Mittal A, Khattri A, Verma V. Structural and antigenic variations in the spike protein of emerging SARS-CoV-2 variants. PLoS Pathogens. 2022;**18**(2):e1010260

[58] Gómez SA, Rojas-Valencia N, Gómez S, Cappelli C, Restrepo A. The role of spike protein mutations in the infectious power of SARS-COV-2 variants: A molecular interaction perspective. Chembiochem. 2022;**23**(7):e202100393

[59] Magazine N, Zhang T, Wu Y, McGee MC, Veggiani G, Huang W. Mutations and evolution of the SARS-CoV-2 spike protein. Viruses. 2022;**14**(3):640

[60] Kistler KE, Huddleston J, Bedford T. Rapid and parallel adaptive mutations in spike S1 drive clade success in SARS-CoV-2. Cell Host & Microbe. 2022;**30**(4):545-555

Chapter 14

Perspective Chapter: Real-Time Genomic Surveillance for SARS-CoV-2 on Center Stage

Mercedes Paz, Pilar Moreno and Gonzalo Moratorio

Abstract

The course of the COVID-19 pandemic depends not only on how the SARS-CoV-2 virus mutates but on the actions taken to respond to it. Important public health decisions can only be taken if we know viral dynamics, viral variants distribution, and whether new variants are emerging that may be more transmissible or/and more virulent, displaying evasion to vaccines or antiviral treatments. This situation has put the use of different approaches, such as molecular techniques and real-time genomic sequencing, to support public health decision-making on center stage. To achieve this, robust programs based on: (i) diagnostic capacity; (ii) high-throughput sequencing technologies; and (iii) high-performance bioinformatic resources, need to be established. This chapter focuses on how SARS-CoV-2 evolved since its discovery and it summarizes the scientific efforts to obtain genomic data as the virus spread throughout the globe.

Keywords: genomic surveillance, SARS-CoV-2, variant of concern, sequencing, PCR, genotyping, phylogenetic trees

1. Introduction

At the early stages of the COVID-19 pandemic, sequencing the full genome of SARS-CoV-2 was key to investigate the newly emerging outbreak of pneumonia in Wuhan, China. In addition, this fact provided evidence that it was being caused by a novel virus belonging to the family *Coronaviridae* [1–3]. The viral sequence became public very rapidly, permitting the scientific community to carry out analyses and pandemic preparedness to start promptly [4]. Back then, having available the full viral genomic sequence made possible the development of rapid and affordable molecular diagnostic tools to isolate infectious patients (symptomatic and asymptomatic). This was the first weapon to control the disease spread, given the lack of approved therapeutics and vaccines at that time [5, 6]. Later on, genomic surveillance of the virus played a center role in the prevention and control of the disease throughout the course of the pandemic [7]. In fact, it made it possible to study many different aspects of the disease, such as the transmission patterns of the virus, the time and from where the virus was introduced into a country, and local and superspreading events. Most notably, genomic surveillance was key to track virus evolution,

IntechOpen

evidencing the emergence of genomic variants worldwide. Those variants that are more transmissible or virulent, and/or can decrease the effectiveness of treatments, vaccines, and public health measures were defined, by the WHO - in consultation with the Technical Advisory Group on Virus Evolution - as variants of Concern (VOC) [8]. To date, five VOCs (named Alpha, Beta, Gamma, Delta, and Omicron) have emerged at different times and places as a result of viral evolution displaying different features compared to the first strain isolated from Wuhan. Among these, Alfa, Beta, Gamma, and Delta are now designated former VOCs as they appear to no longer circulate in the population. Omicron and its descendent sub-lineages are, at the time of writing this chapter, the only circulating VOCs [8]. The five VOCs have demonstrated to be able to act as 'game changers', reshaping infection dynamics and causing new waves of infections in many countries. Periodic genomic sequencing of viral samples kept the world informed in a global pandemic setting and facilitated proper public health measures to be made. Implementation of comprehensive real-time genomic surveillance programs is vital for monitoring, detecting, and characterizing new variants, helping sanitary authorities to better manage the crisis.

2. SARS-CoV-2 then

Whole-genome sequencing of specimens of an outbreak of pneumonia in Wuhan, China in December 2019, led to the discovery of a previously uncharacterized virus capable of infecting humans [2]. The first annotation of the complete 29,903 nucleotide-length genome of SARS-CoV-2 revealed it was a positive-sense, single-stranded RNA virus from the genus Betacoronavirus (β-CoVs). Comparative phylogenetic analysis shed light on the genomic organization of SARS-CoV proving that it shared key structural similarities with coronaviruses including SARS-CoV the causative agent of the severe acute respiratory syndrome outbreak in Asia in 2003. In addition, this novel virus, like many other members of the β-CoVs genus, had its evolutionary roots in viruses known to commonly infect bats [9, 10]. Yet, none of the SARS-CoV-2 related coronaviruses that can be found in public databases present more than 99% similarity to SARS-CoV-2 across the genome as a whole, suggesting that none of these viruses could be its direct ancestor. Efforts to find possible reservoirs and/or an intermediate host of the virus in wild animals' reservoirs, mostly bats and pangolins, had still not made clear the exact emergence event of the virus in the human population. The genome of SARS-CoV-2 has a rather mosaic pattern, to which different progenitors seem to contribute [11].

The closest related bat-borne virus at the whole-genome level identified so far is RaTG13 (from R. affinis, China, 2013), sharing 96.2% identity with SARS-CoV-2 [3]. Despite its apparent higher percentage of similarity, the receptor binding domain (RBD) sequence of the Spike (S) protein of SARS-CoV-2 shows a significant divergence from the RaTG13 strain. RaTG13 lacks the four-residue (PRRA) insertions at the furin cleavage site on the S protein, essential for viral binding to human cell receptors and infection [12, 13]. Furthermore, the authors referenced in [13] demonstrated the binding affinity between the RaTG13 RBD and human angiotensin-converting enzyme 2 (hACE2) to be approximately 70-fold lower than that between the SARS-CoV-2 RBD and hACE2. Further phylogenetic analysis identified pangolin-derived coronaviruses clustering with RaTG13 and SARS-CoV-2 and sharing a higher amino acid similarity to the RBD of SARS-CoV-2 (97.4%) [14]. This analysis raised the possibility that SARS-CoV-2 might have originated from a recombination event of a virus similar to pangolin-CoV with one similar to RaTG13 [15, 16]. Other groups have identified coronaviruses sampled from bats that shared higher similarity to the RBD of SARS-CoV-2, as STT182 and STT200 sampled from Cambodia [17] and BANAL-52 and BANAL-103 sampled from Laos [18]. Of note, comparative sequence analysis of the viruses sampled in Laos showed that those viruses have an RBD with only one or two amino acidic mismatches at the 17 residues that interact with the hACE2 receptor. Many more groups continued collecting genomic sequence data of coronaviruses and sampling animal reservoirs to better understand the exact spillover event and emergence process of SARS-CoV-2. These studies are of high importance due to the latent threat of the emergence and re-emergence of infectious diseases from animal origins.

3. Understanding SARS-CoV-2 long game: mechanisms for viral evolution and variant emergence

SARS-CoV-2 has acquired many mutations over the course of the pandemic, resulting in altered viral replication and transmission. One of the mechanisms that can explain the generation of new genomic variants is that, SARS-CoV-2 as well as all CoVs, rely on an error prone RNA-dependent RNA polymerase (RdRp) to replicate within the host's cells to produce more viral particles [19]. The errors that occurred during replication, however, are corrected by nsp14-ExoN, a 3′-to-5′ proofreading exoribonuclease that acts on both ssRNA and dsRNA, which helps the virus to reduce its error rate 100–1000-fold compared to other RNA viruses [20]. This repair mechanism however is not flawless, resulting in the retention of some of the mutations during replication. The error rate for SARS-CoV-2 replication has been estimated to be in the range of 10^{-4}–10^{-3} nucleotide substitutions per site per year, which means the viral genome can acquire approximately two mutations per month [21]. Although most acquired mutations are synonymous - producing a change in the ARN sequence but not the amino acid composition- some are non-synonymous, which allows the virus to acquire a different amino acid composition. When these mutations help the virus to reproduce and transmit better in the host, either by improving the virus intrinsic fitness, the interaction with key host cell components, or by permitting the virus to escape from the host immune system, they exert a positive selection force resulting in the appearance of new variants [22].

Another mechanism that has been proposed to drive SARS-CoV-2 variants' emergence is recombination [23–26]. For positive sense-RNA viruses, recombination can occur within a cell that was coinfected with more than one genomic species via a process known as 'strand switching' mediated by the viral RdRp, producing chimeric subgenomic RNA and proteins [27, 28]. Recombination has been commonly observed in β-CoVs, most notably in SARS-CoV and MERS-CoV [27, 29–31]. Unlike the mutations acquired due to errors occurring via the replication process, recombination allows the virus to acquire larger genome sections more quickly and causes dramatic changes in the SARS-CoV-2 phenotype [32, 33]. These recombination events have been identified throughout the genome, but most of them have been detected in the ORF1a and N-terminus regions of the S protein [25]. Mutations in the S protein have been of more attention as it plays a critical role in viral infection and immunity, although mutations in other genes can play a role in viral replication and fitness.

4. Tracking SARS-CoV-2 evolution worldwide

Tracking the evolution of SARS-CoV-2 was made possible by the state-of-the-art molecular and bioinformatic tools that were rapidly adapted for an efficient data-driven response against the COVID-19 pandemic. Although these tools are now used widely, they did not exist a couple of decades ago. SARS-CoV-2 is the first virus to which its evolution has been monitored and assessed in real time since its discovery, leading to the accumulation of an unprecedented volume of data - more than 11 million SARS-CoV-2 genomes have been sequenced up to the time of writing this chapter [34].

4.1 Whole-genome sequencing

Next-generation sequencing has been the major molecular tool to identify and study viral genomic variants. Its widespread application turned out to be possible thanks to the extensive collaborative efforts of the scientific community for developing standardized sequencing protocols and making public the bioinformatics workflows for consensus genome assembly. The main method used for the identification of SARS-CoV-2 variants relied on sequencing the whole genome of the virus. For this purpose, several sequencing technologies have been employed, including Illumina, Oxford Nanopore, Pacbio, Ion Torrent, BGI, Sanger and Qiagen; where the first two remain the most used platforms. The protocol for sequencing SARS-CoV-2 by these two technologies employs a tailed amplicon sequencing approach. The protocol for nanopore sequencing of tiled PCR-generated amplicon pools was developed by the ARTIC Network [35] in 2017 for sequencing Ebola, Zika, and Chikungunya viral genomes [36]. It has been adapted throughout the course of the pandemic in order to convert into a rapid and cost-effective method to acquire high-quality genomic data at a great scale [37]. This method proved to be helpful for obtaining whole viral genomes from clinical samples with limited viral genomic material promptly, as it is the only technology capable of sequencing in real-time long-read nucleic acid sequences. Other approaches like sequence capture methods, that enrich libraries by using sequence capture with a respiratory virus panel containing probes against SARS-CoV-2, have also been used particularly as a tool for recovering more data for low input samples [38].

Having the information on the entire viral genome not only permits us to identify viral variants, but it is also essential to perform phylogenetic analysis to study viral evolution. It has helped scientists to answer several questions, for example, understanding whether an outbreak was caused by imported viruses or by community transmission, through tracking when and where new mutations are introduced in a geographical region [39]. This information was particularly valuable at the beginning of the pandemic when there were no treatments available, as it provides evidence of high-risk transmission routes prompting enhanced public health control measures. Additionally, phylogenetics was also used to monitor the effectiveness of global travel restrictions and lockdowns. Later, with the appearance of the variants of concern harboring distinctive mutations, having their whole-genome sequence provided valued data for understanding their emergence and distribution across the globe and also to investigate the risk associated with specific mutations.

4.2 RT-qPCR

Another molecular tool that turned out to be extremely valuable to investigate the prevalence of emerging viral variants is multiplex real-time RT-qPCR [40]. This assay has been employed by different groups to identify genomic fingerprints associated with emerging VOCs. VOCs specific mutations, such as amino acid S deletion 69–70 (del69-70) found first in Alpha and later in Omicron BA.1, S deletion 241 in VOC Delta, and ORF1a nucleotide deletion 3675–3677 in VOC Gamma and Beta, generate a negative or a significantly weaker positive result in the PCR when the target probe is designed to align with the deletion. This failure of the amplification target caused by the specific mutation in a gene is known as gene target failure or gene dropout [41–43]. Choosing this method works perfectly for monitoring the introduction of a variant in a population when another one is already circulating at high prevalence, as it becomes evident very quickly when the two variants display a different PCR gene dropout pattern [44]. For example, this method was used to evidence the introduction of the VOC Gamma into Uruguay, as this VOC has the ORF1ab deletion which displaced the other lineages with no ORF1ab deletion circulating before Gamma introduction [45]. The use of this method is more convenient in resource-limited settings compared to sequencing, as the latter is time-consuming, costly, and requires extensive data processing [46]. RT-qPCR-based variant analysis of SARS-CoV-2 is rapid, low-cost, and does not require bioinformatics expertise. Another TaqMan-based RT-qPCR that was widely used to estimate VOC prevalence was an assay that can detect specific amino acid substitutions or single nucleotide polymorphisms (SNPs) present in VOCs, particularly in the S gene [47]. Ascertaining SNPs allowed certain countries to estimate the prevalence of the variants carrying specific mutations in a population.

Employing the methods mentioned above, genomics consortiums – networks of multidisciplinary workgroups with diverse expertise – were created in many countries around the world for real-time monitoring for SARS-CoV-2 genomic variants with public health implications. Following a sentinel strategy, samples that tested positive for SARS-CoV-2 are collected weekly from different regions within a country in order to adequately represent the geographic spread, to then send them for whole-genome sequencing to a laboratory that can perform molecular and bioinformatics analysis. As an example of this strategy, genomic surveillance of SARS-CoV-2 in Uruguay during the firsts months of 2021 was focused on a representative number of samples collected from all provinces of the country, as a need for detecting the imminent introduction of the VOC Gamma promptly, as this variant was circulating at great scale in neighbor countries (mostly Brazil and Argentina) by the time Uruguay was just starting to vaccinate its population. Phylogenetics analysis revealed that SARS-CoV-2 was introduced into Uruguay from multiple routes to then become the most prevalent variant in a matter of weeks, most likely causing the first wave of coronavirus in the country [45]. Later on, when Uruguay started to ease travel restrictions due to low positive cases and a high vaccination percentage, genomic surveillance started to focus mostly on the variants that could be imported by international travelers and their close contacts in the community. In this way, the introduction of the VOC Delta, Beta, and Alfa was detected in travelers, where only Delta surpassed the prevalence of Gamma that was previously circulating in great proportion.

4.3 Nomenclature schemas to explain SARS-CoV-2 phylogeny

Different standardized nomenclatures schemas have been developed by bioinformatic investigators in charge of tracking SARS-Cov-2 population dynamics to define and explain the divisions of the different viral genomes circulating globally.

There are currently mainly three schemas. Two are based on clade separation: the Nextstrain and GSAID [34, 48], where a clade is defined as a group of organisms that include a single ancestor in all its descendants. Both Nextstrain and GSAID aim to provide generic categorization of globally circulating diversity. The other schema, Phylogenetic Assignment of Named Global Outbreak Lineages (Pangolin) was developed to implement the dynamic nomenclature of SARS-CoV-2 lineages and to correspond to outbreaks [49]. Later on, the WHO recommended using letters of the Greek alphabet to designate viral variants in order to make the use of the nomenclature schemas easier for the general public without previous knowledge in bioinformatics and to ease the discussion about the topic [8].

5. Variants of concern

As of June 2022, there were five reported lineages defined as VOCs by the WHO [8]. Alpha, Beta, Gamma, and Delta were all first detected between late 2020 and January 2021. Omicron was the fifth emerging VOC, first reported in South Africa a year later in November 2021. Phylogenetic analysis of SARS-CoV-2 whole genomic sequences shows clearly that these variants did not emerge one from another but that they emerged from the ancestral SARS-CoV-2 genotype (Wuhan-Hu reference sequence) as shown in **Figure 1**.

VOCs have acquired many mutations independently by convergent evolution, which provided them with either enhanced transmissibility, higher severity of disease, or lower neutralization capacity by vaccine and/or sera from people who recovered from COVID-19. Most of these mutations are located at the subunit 1 (S1) of the spike protein, especially in the RBD and NTD domains. Interestingly, although VOCs are genetically divergent, they share many amino acid mutations at the S1 subunit as schematized in **Figure 2**, whereas they do not share mutations at the subunit 2 (S2). This phenomenon is hypothesized to have occurred most likely because the S1 subunit is the most immunodominant viral region and the one under a higher and constant selective pressure, as 90% of the neutralizing antibodies found in COVID-19 convalescent plasma were found to block the RBD [51].

5.1 Alpha

The VOC Alpha – defined as Pango lineage B.1.1.7 and Nextstrain clade 20I/V1– was the first VOC, identified by the COVID-19 Genomics UK Consortium (CoG-UK). It was first sampled in late September of 2020 [52] from a rapid rise in cases in the southeast of England during a national lockdown and caused a second wave of infections in December 2020 [44, 53]. It has 17 mutations located at the S, N, ORF1ab, and ORF8 genes and exhibited around a 50% increase in transmissibility over previously circulating lineages [44, 54]. The several amino acid mutations carried in S protein were proven to be of epidemiological concern as they play a crucial role in the infectivity and pathogenicity of the virus. The N501Y substitution (also found in

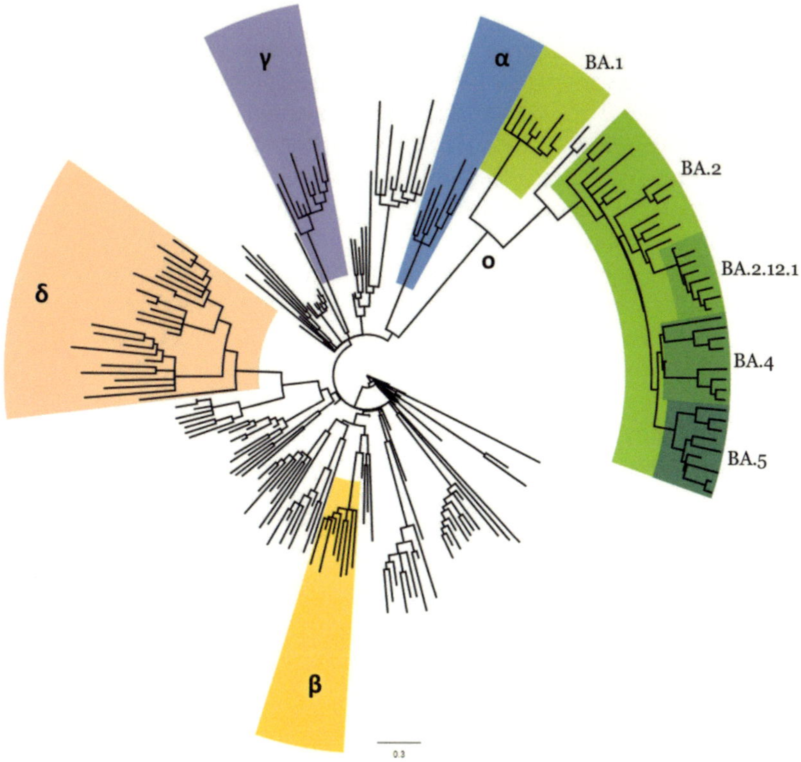

Figure 1.
Phylogenetic tree showing divergent SARS-CoV-2 VOCs emerging from the ancestral Wuhan Hu-1 strain sequence. Data was downloaded from Nextstrain [48] under a CC BY 4.0 license and corresponds to a subsampling of reference genomic sequences from GISAID [34]. The phylogenetic tree was edited with FigTree v1.4.4 [50].

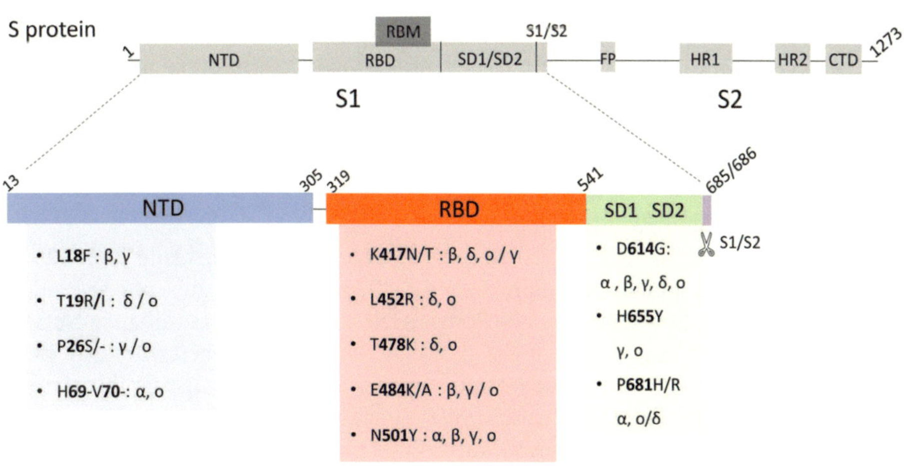

Figure 2.
Shared amino acid mutations of VOCs at the S protein S1 subunit. NTD, amino-terminal domain; RBD, receptor-binding domain; RBM, receptor-binding motif; SD, subdomain; S1/S2, the junction between the exposed S1 attachment domain and the partially buried S2 fusion domain; FP, fusion peptide; HR, heptad repeat; CTD, C-terminal domain.

Beta, Gamma, and Omicron) located at the RBD, increases the binding affinity to the human ACE2 receptor and improves transmissibility [55]. The authors referenced in [56] developed a mouse-adapted strain model (MASCp6) to evaluate the SARS-CoV-2 infectivity and virulence after intranasal inoculation and observed that the N501Y mutation favors interaction with ACE2 and promotes virus entry, and increases infectivity in mouse lung tissue. Recent studies have suggested that the N501Y mutation has a low impact on clinical outcomes and pathogenicity [53, 57] and on the immune response generated by monoclonal antibodies (mAbs), vaccines, or previous infections [58, 59]. Conversely, in the work referenced in [60], the group evaluated more than 2.2 million people with SARS-CoV-2 positive tests and 17,452 related deaths in England and observed a 61% higher mortality rate in those infected with the B.1.1.7 variant than other pre-existing variants. Likewise, another group that assessed the mortality rate of this variant showed Alpha appears to have a 30% higher mortality rate along with other variants of SARS-CoV-2 [61]. Moreover, an increased likelihood of hospitalizations was observed for Alpha cases compared to non-Alpha cases [62]. Thus, this variant presented increased transmissibility and virulence and increased the risk of contracting a more severe disease. The P618H substitution on the S protein is reported as a key determinant for efficient SARS-CoV-2 transmission. It is located immediately adjacent to the furin cleavage site, which is essential for viral entry into the host's cell [63]. Alpha also possesses two amino acid deletions (del69-70) in the S1 of the S protein. It was demonstrated that this variant requires this deletion for efficient cleaved S protein incorporation and infectivity, thus promoting cell entry and cell-to-cell fusion activity [64].

Several studies have demonstrated that existing vaccines remained protective of this variant. For example, the susceptibility of Alpha to mRNA vaccines, specifically the BNT162b from Pfizer Biontech has not been seen to be affected in great measure. Cohort studies from Israel and Qatar – which were the first countries to have a high vaccination rate at the time Alpha was spreading in the population – demonstrated that the vaccine retained more than 90% efficacy against Alpha after a second dose [65]. For the Novavax vaccine NVX-CoV2373, clinical trials showed that the vaccine efficacy against Alpha was 86.3% [66], proving that it could still retain a high efficacy. Regarding the susceptibility to neutralization by commercial mAbs or sera from patients that recovered from COVID-19, Alpha was shown to be susceptible to neutralization [67].

5.2 Beta

The VOC Beta – defined as Pango lineage B.1.351 and Nextstrain clade 20H/V2 – has the earliest clinical sample date of September 2020, and was the cause of a second wave of infections in South Africa. The South African Genomic Surveillance Network (NGS-SA) reported that it was the most prevalent variant sequenced from October 2020 to May 2020 and it was estimated to be around 50% more transmissible than the Wuhan strain [68]. Following its discovery, it was reported in at least 119 countries but it has not been detected since March 2022 [69]. Beta variant contains eight mutations in S protein: three are located at the RBD (mutations K417N, E484K, and N501Y) and five are located in the NTD (substitutions L18F, R246I, D80A, and D215G and three amino acid deletion 242–244). The N501Y mutation is associated with increased affinity to the hACE2 receptor as discussed above for Alpha. The amino acid substitution K417N, also found in Delta and Omicron, replaces a lysine (positively charged) for an asparagine (neutral charge), resulting in a reduced positive-positive charge repulsion between S protein and hACE2 receptor [70] which favors RBD-hACE2 interaction. The E484K substitution extends the amino acid side chain and creates a change in the charge of the amino acid from negative to positive. It was found also in Gamma and Alpha sub-lineages and was important for improving the association of the S protein with hACE2 and it was mostly associated with immune escape [71, 72]. Most of the antibody-based therapies for COVID-19 have shown to decrease the efficacy against Beta. Regarding immune escape from convalescent plasma, the group referenced in [73] showed in studies using a pseudovirus expressing Beta S protein that this variant had almost a complete escape from neutralization, but not binding, by convalescent plasma [73]. Another study showed that the neutralization titers were reduced 13.3-fold for Beta compared with an early Wuhan-related isolate viral strain in 34 convalescent plasma samples from a cohort of patients infected during the first wave of infections in the UK, where precisely 14 of 34 failing to reach the 50% neutralization titer (NT50) at a 1:20 dilution and some showing almost complete knockdown of activity [74]. Furthermore, it was shown that Beta-specific and cross-reactive RBD antibodies from the serum of Beta-infected patients had reduced neutralization of wild-type virus [75]. Regarding immune escape from mAb treatments, the VOC Beta has a widespread escape from mAb neutralization largely driven by E484K. This mutation interferes with the binding of several class 1 and 2 mAbs that target the receptor binding motive. The group referenced in [74] showed that Beta is much more difficult to neutralize than previous circulating viral strains, as the neutralization capacity of 14 out of 20 mAbs used in the study was seriously compromised and some of their neutralization was completely abolished [74]. Regarding vaccines, the immunity acquired by all the available vaccines (Pfizer-BioNTech, Moderna, AstraZeneca-Oxford, Johnson and Johnson, Novavax) has been shown to have reduced neutralization capacity against this variant [76] although vaccine effectiveness against fatal disease from Beta infections has been shown to remain high [77]. Furthermore, there is evidence that Beta may have caused increased disease severity as it was associated with in-hospital mortality increase in the second wave in South Africa compared to the first wave [78]; although the authors state these findings could be attributed to admissions in the second wave being more likely in older individuals and to an increment on the health system pressure.

5.3 Gamma

VOC Gamma – defined as Pango lineage P.1 and Nextstrain clade 20 J/V3 – was the third VOC identified. It was first detected in Japan in travelers returning from the Amazonas state in Brazil in January 2021 [79]. It originated in Brazil where the earliest documented samples are associated with an outbreak in Manaus, capital of the Amazonas state, in November 2020 which was preceded by a period of faster molecular evolution [80]. Its high transmissibility became rapidly evident after the observation of a short period between its emergence and its high prevalence in the reported cases from the Amazonas state [81]. Gamma introduction in Brazil and its neighboring countries in South America was followed by the displacement of previously circulating SARS-CoV-2 variants and a rapid increase in prevalence in the entire continent. As an illustration of this phenomenon, Uruguay, which shares 600 miles of dry border with Brazil, is a clear example of how Gamma worsened the COVID-19 pandemic as this country experienced an exponential increase in COVID-19 cases after the variant was introduced. By June 2021, Uruguay was among the countries with the highest number of daily cases and deaths per million persons [82] which could be attributed to an almost 100% Gamma prevalence. Also, Gamma accounted for the high number of infections in several South American and Caribbean countries by June 2021 - the most affected region by this VOC. It has been reported in more than 86 countries since its discovery but is no longer detected since December 2021. Gamma is characterized by mutations N501Y, E484K (also seen in VOCs Beta and Omicron), and K417T in the RBD. It also contains five mutations in the NTD, among which the substitution L18F has a known impact of interfering with the binding of neutralizing antibodies targeting NTD. There is also a mutation in nucleocapsid (N) protein P80R and the deletion in ORF1a(Nsp6) gene at positions 3675–3677 (also present in Alpha and Beta). Having the mutation N501Y confers Gamma with an increased affinity for the hACE2 receptor as mentioned before for Alpha and Beta [83]. Gamma was proved to be between 1.4 and 2.2 times more transmissible than the Wuhan strain [80]. The E484K mutation, associated with immune evasion, supports that this variant is able to infect and cause illness in persons previously infected with other variants, which explained the resurgence of COVID-19 cases in Manaus despite the high seroprevalence in its population [84, 85]. In addition, Gamma was associated with increased mortality risk and severity of COVID-19 cases in younger age groups – corresponding to the unvaccinated population at that time in Brazil [86]. The mortality rate associated with Gamma infections was estimated to be 1.1-fold to 1.8-fold higher than with earlier variants and people infected with Gamma showed to have approximately 3 to 4 times higher viral loads [80].

5.4 Delta

VOC Delta – defined as Pango lineage B.1.617.2 and Nextstrain clade 21A – is the fourth VOC identified. It was first detected in India during an uncontrollable surge of COVID-19 infections that hit the country in May 2021 [87] and spread rapidly worldwide causing a second global wave by mid-2021. Delta rapidly outcompeted Alpha and was determined to be approximately 60% more transmissible [88], leading the WHO to classify Delta as a Variant of Concern on May 11, 2021. It has a total of 10 amino acid mutations in the S protein: T19R, G142D, 156del, 157del, R158G, L452R, T478K, D614G, P681R, and D950N. Both L452R and T478K are located at the RBM of the S protein and have been shown to enhance the binding affinity of the virus to the host cell leading to increased infectivity [89] and reduce the neutralizing activity of monoclonal antibodies and convalescent plasma [90, 91]. The mutation L452R when present together with the T478K mutation was shown to increase the stability of the spike protein, which could alter the interaction capacity of neutralizing antibodies [92]. The T478K mutation substitutes the non-charged amino acid threonine with a positively charged lysine, which alters the electrostatic surface in the RBD, affecting the protein interaction with the cellular receptor [93]. The P618R is located adjacent to the polybasic furin cleavage site between S1 and S2 and makes the sequence less acidic. This alteration has been demonstrated to be key in enhancing Delta infectivity, as facilitates the cleavage by the furin protease giving the virus a higher fusogenicity and pathogenicity [91]. COVID-19 cases caused by Delta infections have been associated with a shorter incubation period before disease onset and with a viral load of about 1000 times greater compared to earlier infections by previous viral variants [94]. Regarding the impact on immunity, Delta exhibited some resistance to immunity acquired either by previous natural infection or by first-generation vaccines. The neutralizing ability of convalescent serum from unvaccinated individuals was shown to be significantly decreased against Delta, by four-fold when compared to Alpha and by six-fold when compared to B.1 strains [91] Other studies conducted using data collected by the Scotland-wide COVID-19 surveillance platform have shown that the vaccines from Oxford-AstraZeneca and Pfizer-BioNTech could still reduce the risk of infection or hospitalizations, although this reduction was considerably less when compared to infections with Alpha [95]. Importantly, two doses of these vaccines can still safeguard their effectiveness, as it was shown to decrease only from 87.5% with the Alpha variant to 79.6% with the Delta variant.

The accumulation of more mutations overtime gave rise to 133 Delta sub-lineages, identified with the AY alias by Pangolin nomenclature (Delta AY.1 to AY.133) [96]. One of these sub-lineages was reported to be more transmissible, referred to by the media as 'Delta plus', which was first identified in Nepal. It carried an additional K417N mutation which is also found in Beta and has been related to decrease neutralization by antibodies.

5.5 Omicron

Omicron was the fifth VOC to emerge in late 2021, undermining all predictions about where the next variant would come from. Most scientists believed it would descend out of Delta or one of its sub-lineages, but instead it evolved to a completely different lineage from previous ones as it is shown in **Figure 1**. Omicron currently refers to a larger group of descendent variants of the Pango lineage B.1.1.529 or Nextstrain clade 21 M. They are currently classified as VOC-Linages Under Monitoring (LUM) by the WHO due to their high prevalence of transmission in the population and concomitant increase in viral sequence diversity. This large group consist of variants BA.1 (clade 21 K), BA.2 (clade 21 L) and its descendent lineages BA.4 (clade 22A), BA.5 (22B), BA.2.12.1 (22C), BA.2.9.1, BA.2.11, BA.2.13, and BA.2.75 [8].

The first identification of Omicron (BA.1) was on November 24, 2021 from an immunocompromised individual in South Africa. It caused a sharp increase in daily cases, which rose rapidly from 273 on November 16 to more than 1200 by November 25, more than 80% of which were in the northern province of Gauteng, where the first cases were seen. Genomic sequencing revealed it acquired an astounding number of 62 amino acid mutations, where 36 of them are located in the S protein, particularly at the N-terminal and RBD as shown in **Figure 3**. The BA.1 sub-lineage was the first variant to displace Delta, becoming the most prevalent variant worldwide by December 2021. BA.2 variant gradually replaced BA.1, becoming the most prevalent worldwide by May 2022. BA.1 and BA.2 have 21 amino-acid mutations in common at the S protein, with BA.1 having 12 additional unique mutations and BA.2 having 7 (including a three amino acid deletion) which is shown in **Figure 3**. BA.4 and BA.5 arose in mid-January 2022 displacing BA.2, have an identical S protein amino acid composition (**Figure 3**), and are differentiated only by mutations in the following positions: BA.4 has the mutation L11F at the ORF7b gene and the mutation P151S at the N gene whereas BA.5 has the mutation D3N at the membrane (M) protein [97]. Both have estimated growth advantages over BA.2 and can also display immune evasion acquired after a previous infection with Omicron sub-lineages. BA.2.12.1 is a sub-lineage of BA.2 that differs from it only for the mutations in S protein L452Q at the RBD and the S704F at the S2 (**Figure 3**), but it continues to be closely monitored due to its high prevalence and its capacity to evade the immunity acquired by vaccines and previous infection with other Omicron sub-lineages [98]. Although Omicron possesses high transmissibility, it was the first VOC to show signs of viral attenuation which helped to decrease the disease burden [78].

S protein

	NTD	RBD	SD1/SD2	S2 subunit
BA.1 (21K)	A67V; H69-; V70-; T95I; G142-; V143-; Y144-; Y145D; N211-; L212I; ins214EPE	G339D; S371L; S373P; S375F; K417N; N440K; G446S; S477N; T478K; E484A; Q493R; G496S; Q498R; N501Y; Y505H	T547K; D614G; H655Y; N679K; P681H	N764K; D796Y; N856K; Q954H; N969K
BA.2 (21L)	T19I; L24-; P25-; P26-; A27S; G142D; V213G	G339D;371F; S373P; S375F; T376A; D405N; R408S; K417N; N440K; S477N; T478K; E484A; Q493R; Q498R; N501Y; Y505H	D614G; H655Y; N679K; P681H	N764K; D796Y; Q954H; N969K
BA.4 (22A) BA.5 (22B)	BA.2- like mutations + H69- and V70-	BA.2- like mutations + L452R; F486V and Q493 reversion	BA.2- like mutations	BA.2- like mutations
BA.2.12.1 (22C)	BA.2 - like mutations	BA.2- like mutations + L452Q	BA.2- like mutations	BA.2- like mutations + S704F

Figure 3.
Spike amino acid mutations in the most prevalent Omicron sub-lineages circulating during the first half of 2022.

6. Conclusion

Since its discovery in 2020, the SARS-CoV-2 virus has been circulating in the human population evolving in genomic variants with distinct evolutionary advantages, such as increased transmissibility, immune evasion, and increased virulence, causing outbreaks and new waves of infections worldwide. By monitoring the evolution of SARS-CoV-2 scientists provided valuable information about newly emerging variants over the course of the COVID-19 pandemic. Thus, the implementation of comprehensive real-time genomic surveillance programs is vital for monitoring, detecting, and characterizing new variants, helping sanitary authorities to better manage the crisis.

Author details

Mercedes Paz[1,2,3*], Pilar Moreno[1,2,3] and Gonzalo Moratorio[1,2,3]

1 Center for Innovation in Epidemiological Surveillance, Institut Pasteur of Montevideo, Montevideo, Uruguay

2 Experimental Evolution of Viruses, Institut Pasteur of Montevideo, Montevideo, Uruguay

3 Laboratory of Molecular Virology, Faculty of Science, University of the Republic UdelaR, Montevideo, Uruguay

*Address all correspondence to: moratorio@pasteur.edu.uy

References

[1] Zhu N, Zhang D, Wang W, et al. A novel coronavirus from patients with pneumonia in China, 2019. The New England Journal of Medicine. 2020;**382**:727-733

[2] Wu F, Zhao S, Yu B, et al. A new coronavirus associated with human respiratory disease in China. Nature. 2020;**579**:265-269

[3] Zhou P, Yang X-L, Wang X-G, et al. A pneumonia outbreak associated with a new coronavirus of probable bat origin. Nature. 2020;**579**:270-273

[4] Novel 2019 coronavirus genome - SARS-CoV-2 coronavirus. Virological. 2020. Available from: https://virological.org/t/novel-2019-coronavirus-genome/319 , [Accessed: June 28, 2022]

[5] Lai C-C, Shih T-P, Ko W-C, et al. Severe acute respiratory syndrome coronavirus 2 (SARS-CoV-2) and coronavirus disease-2019 (COVID-19): The epidemic and the challenges. International Journal of Antimicrobial Agents. 2020;**55**:105924

[6] Deng S-Q, Peng H-J. Characteristics of and public health responses to the coronavirus disease 2019 outbreak in China. Journal of Clinical Medicine. 2020;**9**:E575

[7] Seemann T, Lane CR, Sherry NL, et al. Tracking the COVID-19 pandemic in Australia using genomics. Nature Communications. 2020;**11**:4376

[8] Tracking SARS-CoV-2 variants. Available from: https://www.who.int/activities/tracking-SARS-CoV-2-variants. [Accessed: June 28, 2022]

[9] Gorbalenya AE, Baker SC, et al. The species Severe acute respiratory syndrome-related coronavirus: Classifying 2019-nCoV and naming it SARS-CoV-2. Nature Microbiology. 2020;**5**:536-544

[10] Lu R, Zhao X, Li J, et al. Genomic characterisation and epidemiology of 2019 novel coronavirus: Implications for virus origins and receptor binding. The Lancet. 2020;**395**:565-574

[11] Temmam S, Vongphayloth K, Baquero E, et al. Bat coronaviruses related to SARS-CoV-2 and infectious for human cells. Nature. 2022;**604**:330-336

[12] Wrobel AG, Benton DJ, Xu P, et al. SARS-CoV-2 and bat RaTG13 spike glycoprotein structures inform on virus evolution and furin-cleavage effects. Nature Structural & Molecular Biology. 2020;**27**:763-767

[13] Liu K, Pan X, Li L, et al. Binding and molecular basis of the bat coronavirus RaTG13 virus to ACE2 in humans and other species. Cell. 2021;**184**:3438-3451.e10

[14] Xiao K, Zhai J, Feng Y, et al. Isolation of SARS-CoV-2-related coronavirus from Malayan pangolins. Nature. 2020;**583**:286-289

[15] Wong MC, Javornik Cregeen SJ, Ajami NJ, et al. Evidence of recombination in coronaviruses implicating pangolin origins of nCoV-2019. BioRxiv Preprint Server for Biology. 2020:939207

[16] Chaw S-M, Tai J-H, Chen S-L, et al. The origin and underlying driving forces of the SARS-CoV-2 outbreak. Journal of Biomedical Science. 2020;**27**:73

[17] Delaune D, Hul V, Karlsson EA, et al. A novel SARS-CoV-2 related coronavirus in bats from Cambodia. Nature Communications. 2021;**12**:6563

[18] Wacharapluesadee S, Tan CW, Maneeorn P, et al. Evidence for SARS-CoV-2 related coronaviruses circulating in bats and pangolins in Southeast Asia. Nature Communications. 2021;**12**:972

[19] Smith EC, Denison MR. Coronaviruses as DNA Wannabes: A new model for the regulation of RNA virus replication fidelity. PLoS Pathogens. 2013;**9**:e1003760

[20] RNA 3′-end mismatch excision by the severe acute respiratory syndrome coronavirus nonstructural protein nsp10/nsp14 exoribonuclease complex. Proceedings of the National Academy of Sciences of the United States of America. Available from: https://www.pnas.org/doi/10.1073/pnas.1201130109. [Accessed: June 28, 2022]

[21] Domingo E, García-Crespo C, Lobo-Vega R, et al. Mutation rates, mutation frequencies, and proofreading-repair activities in RNA virus genetics. Viruses. 2021;**13**:1882

[22] Gordon DE, Jang GM, Bouhaddou M, et al. A SARS-CoV-2 protein interaction map reveals targets for drug repurposing. Nature. 2020;**583**:459-468

[23] Ou J, Lan W, Wu X, et al. Tracking SARS-CoV-2 Omicron diverse spike gene mutations identifies multiple inter-variant recombination events. Signal Transduction and Targeted Therapy. 2022;**7**:1-9

[24] RDS FJ, LGP d A, Lamarca AP, et al. Emergence of Within-Host SARS-CoV-2 Recombinant Genome After Coinfection by Gamma and Delta Variants: A Case Report. Front Public Health. 2022:10. Available from: https://www.frontiersin.org/article/10.3389/fpubh.2022.849978. [Accessed: June 29, 2022]

[25] Boni MF, Lemey P, Jiang X, et al. Evolutionary origins of the SARS-CoV-2 sarbecovirus lineage responsible for the COVID-19 pandemic. Nature Microbiology. 2020;**5**:1408-1417

[26] Wertheim JO, Wang JC, Leelawong M, et al. Detection of SARS-CoV-2 intra-host recombination during superinfection with Alpha and Epsilon variants in New York City. Nature Communications. 2022;**13**:3645

[27] Simon-Loriere E, Holmes EC. Why do RNA viruses recombine? Nature Reviews. Microbiology. 2011;**9**:617-626

[28] Lai MM. RNA recombination in animal and plant viruses. Microbiological Reviews. 1992;**56**:61-79

[29] Hu B, Zeng L-P, Yang X-L, et al. Discovery of a rich gene pool of bat SARS-related coronaviruses provides new insights into the origin of SARS coronavirus. PLoS Pathogens. 2017;**13**:e1006698

[30] Memish ZA, Perlman S, Van Kerkhove MD, et al. Middle East respiratory syndrome. Lancet (London, England). 2020;**395**:1063-1077

[31] MERS coronaviruses from camels in Africa exhibit region-dependent genetic diversity. Proceedings of the National Academy of Sciences of the United States of America. Available from: https://www.pnas.org/doi/full/10.1073/pnas.1718769115. [Accessed: June 29, 2022]

[32] Dudas G, Rambaut A. MERS-CoV recombination: Implications about the reservoir and potential for adaptation. Virus Evolution. 2016;**2**:vev023

[33] Evidence of the recombinant origin of a bat severe acute respiratory syndrome (SARS)-like coronavirus and its implications on the direct ancestor of SARS coronavirus. Journal of Virology. DOI: 10.1128/JVI.01926-07. [Accessed: June 29, 2022]

[34] GISAID – Initiative. Available from: https://www.gisaid.org/. [Accessed: June 29, 2022]

[35] Artic Network. Available from: https://artic.network/ [Accessed: June 29, 2022]

[36] Multiplex PCR method for MinION and Illumina sequencing of Zika and other virus genomes directly from clinical samples. Nature Protocols. Available from: https://www.nature.com/articles/nprot.2017.066. [Accessed: June 29, 2022]

[37] Freed NE, Vlková M, Faisal MB, et al. Rapid and inexpensive whole-genome sequencing of SARS-CoV-2 using 1200 bp tiled amplicons and Oxford Nanopore Rapid Barcoding. Biology Methods and Protocols. 2020;**5**:bpaa014

[38] Rehn A, Braun P, Knüpfer M, et al. Catching SARS-CoV-2 by sequence hybridization: A comparative analysis. mSystems. 2021;**6**:e0039221

[39] Tessema SK, Inzaule SC, Christoffels A, et al. Accelerating genomics-based surveillance for COVID-19 response in Africa. Lancet Microbe. 2020;**1**:e227-e228

[40] Bustin SA, Nolan T. RT-qPCR testing of SARS-CoV-2: A primer. International Journal of Molecular Sciences. 2020;**21**:E3004

[41] Brown KA, Gubbay J, Hopkins J, et al. S-gene target failure as a marker of variant B.1.1.7 among SARS-CoV-2 isolates in the greater toronto area, December 2020 to March 2021. JAMA;**2021**(325):2115-2116

[42] Vogels CBF, Breban MI, Ott IM, et al. Multiplex qPCR discriminates variants of concern to enhance global surveillance of SARS-CoV-2. PLoS Biology. 2021;**19**:e3001236

[43] Boršová K, Paul ED, Kováčová V, et al. Surveillance of SARS-CoV-2 lineage B.1.1.7 in Slovakia using a novel, multiplexed RT-qPCR assay. Scientific Reports. 2021;**11**:20494

[44] Volz E, Mishra S, Chand M, et al. Assessing transmissibility of SARS-CoV-2 lineage B.1.1.7 in England. Nature. 2021;**593**:266-269

[45] Rego N, Costábile A, Paz M, et al. Real-time genomic surveillance for SARS-CoV-2 variants of concern, Uruguay. Emerging Infectious Diseases. 2021;**27**:2957-2960

[46] Gwinn M, MacCannell D, Armstrong GL. Next generation sequencing of infectious pathogens. JAMA. 2019;**321**:893-894

[47] Neopane P, Nypaver J, Shrestha R, et al. SARS-CoV-2 variants detection using TaqMan SARS-CoV-2 mutation panel molecular genotyping assays. Infection and Drug Resistance. 2021;**14**:4471-4479

[48] Hadfield J, Megill C, Bell SM, et al. Nextstrain: Real-time tracking of pathogen evolution. Bioinformatics. 2018;**34**:4121-4123

[49] Rambaut A, Holmes EC, O'Toole Á, et al. A dynamic nomenclature proposal for SARS-CoV-2 lineages to assist genomic epidemiology. Nature Microbiology. 2020;**5**:1403-1407

[50] FigTree. Available from: http://tree.bio.ed.ac.uk/software/figtree/. [Accessed: July 22, 2022]

[51] Piccoli L, Park Y-J, Tortorici MA, et al. Mapping neutralizing and immunodominant sites on the Sars-Cov-2 spike receptor-binding domain by structure-guided high-resolution serology. Cell. 2020;**183**:1024-1042.e21

[52] Preliminary genomic characterisation of an emergent SARS-CoV-2 lineage in the UK defined by a novel set of spike mutations - SARS-CoV-2 coronavirus / nCoV-2019 Genomic Epidemiology. Virological. 2020. Available from: https://virological.org/t/preliminary-genomic-characterisation-of-an-emergent-sars-cov-2-lineage-in-the-uk-defined-by-a-novel-set-of-spike-mutations/563. [Accessed: July 15, 2022]

[53] Conti P, Caraffa A, Gallenga CE, et al. The British variant of the new coronavirus-19 (Sars-Cov-2) should not create a vaccine problem. Journal of Biological Regulators and Homeostatic Agents. 2021;**35**:1-4

[54] Leung K, Shum MH, Leung GM, et al. Early transmissibility assessment of the N501Y mutant strains of SARS-CoV-2 in the United Kingdom, October to November 2020. Euro Surveill Bull Eur Sur Mal Transm Eur Commun Dis Bull. 2021:26. DOI: 10.2807/1560-7917.ES.2020.26.1.2002106

[55] Liu Y, Liu J, Plante KS, et al. The N501Y spike substitution enhances SARS-CoV-2 infection and transmission. Nature. 2022;**602**:294-299

[56] Gu H, Chen Q, Yang G, et al. Adaptation of SARS-CoV-2 in BALB/c mice for testing vaccine efficacy. Science. 2020;**369**:1603-1607

[57] Graham MS, Sudre CH, May A, et al. Changes in symptomatology, reinfection, and transmissibility associated with the SARS-CoV-2 variant B.1.1.7: An ecological study. Lancet. Public Health. 2021;**6**:e335-e345

[58] Neutralization of SARS-CoV-2 lineage B.1.1.7 pseudovirus by BNT162b2 vaccine–elicited human sera. DOI: 10.1126/science.abg6105. [Accessed: July 15, 2022]

[59] Focosi D, Maggi F. Neutralising antibody escape of SARS-CoV-2 spike protein: Risk assessment for antibody-based Covid-19 therapeutics and vaccines. Reviews in Medical Virology. 2021;**31**:e2231

[60] Davies NG, Jarvis CI, Edmunds WJ, et al. Increased mortality in community-tested cases of SARS-CoV-2 lineage B.1.1.7. Nature. 2021;**593**:270-274

[61] Iacobucci G. Covid-19: all non-urgent elective surgery is suspended for at least three months in England. BMJ. 2020;**368**:m1106

[62] Vusirikala A, Flannagan J, Czachorowski M, et al. Impact of SARS-CoV-2 Alpha variant (B.1.1.7) on prisons, England. Public Health. 2022;**204**:21-24

[63] Hoffmann M, Kleine-Weber H, Pöhlmann S. A multibasic cleavage site in the spike protein of SARS-CoV-2 is essential for infection of human lung cells. Molecular Cell. 2020;**78**:779-784.e5

[64] Meng B, Kemp SA, Papa G, et al. Recurrent emergence of SARS-CoV-2 spike deletion H69/V70 and its role in the Alpha variant B.1.1.7. Cell Reports. 2021;**35**:109292

[65] Chemaitelly H, Yassine HM, Benslimane FM, et al. mRNA-1273 COVID-19 vaccine effectiveness against the B.1.1.7 and B.1.351 variants and severe

COVID-19 disease in Qatar. Nature Medicine. 2021;**27**:1614-1621

[66] Heath PT, Galiza EP, Baxter DN, et al. Safety and efficacy of NVX-CoV2373 Covid-19 vaccine. The New England Journal of Medicine. 2021;**385**:1172-1183

[67] Yaqinuddin A, Shafqat A, Kashir J, et al. Effect of SARS-CoV-2 mutations on the efficacy of antibody therapy and response to vaccines. Vaccines. 2021;**9**:914

[68] Anthes E. The Beta Variant: What Scientists Know. The New York Times; 2021. Available from: https://www.nytimes.com/2021/07/19/health/beta-variant-covid-19.html. [Accessed: July 15, 2022]

[69] Available from: outbreak.info. outbreak.info, https://outbreak.info/. [Accessed: July 15, 2022]

[70] Yang J, Zhang P, Cheng WX, et al. Exposing structural variations in SARS-CoV-2 evolution. Scientific Reports. 2021;**11**:22042

[71] Andreano E, Piccini G, Licastro D, et al. SARS-CoV-2 escape from a highly neutralizing COVID-19 convalescent plasma. Proceedings of the National Academy of Sciences of the United States of America. 2021;**118**:e2103154118

[72] Starr TN, Greaney AJ, Hilton SK, et al. Deep mutational scanning of SARS-CoV-2 receptor binding domain reveals constraints on folding and ACE2 binding. Cell. 2020;**182**:1295-1310.e20

[73] Wibmer CK, Ayres F, Hermanus T, et al. SARS-CoV-2 501Y.V2 escapes neutralization by South African COVID-19 donor plasma. Nature Medicine. 2021;**27**:622-625

[74] Zhou D, Dejnirattisai W, Supasa P, et al. Evidence of escape of SARS-CoV-2 variant B.1.351 from natural and vaccine-induced sera. Cell. 2021;**184**:2348-2361.e6

[75] SARS-CoV-2 Beta variant infection elicits potent lineage-specific and cross-reactive antibodies. DOI: 10.1126/science.abm5835. [Accessed: July 15, 2022]

[76] Garcia-Beltran WF, Lam EC, St. Denis K, et al. Multiple SARS-CoV-2 variants escape neutralization by vaccine-induced humoral immunity. Cell. 2021;**184**:2372-2383.e9

[77] Duong D. Alpha, beta, delta, gamma: What's important to know about SARS-CoV-2 variants of concern? Canadian Medical Association Journal. 2021;**193**:E1059-E1060

[78] Jassat W, Karim SSA, Mudara C, et al. Clinical severity of COVID-19 in patients admitted to hospital during the omicron wave in South Africa: A retrospective observational study. The Lancet Global Health. 2022;**10**:e961-e969

[79] Fujino T, Nomoto H, Kutsuna S, et al. Novel SARS-CoV-2 variant in travelers from Brazil to Japan. Emerging Infectious Diseases. 2021;**27**:1243-1245

[80] Faria NR, Mellan TA, Whittaker C, et al. Genomics and epidemiology of the P.1 SARS-CoV-2 lineage in Manaus, Brazil. Science. 2021;**372**:815-821

[81] Naveca FG, Nascimento V, de Souza VC, et al. COVID-19 in Amazonas, Brazil, was driven by the persistence of endemic lineages and P.1 emergence. Nature Medicine. 2021;**27**:1230-1238

[82] Ritchie H, Mathieu E, Rodés-Guirao L, et al. Coronavirus pandemic (COVID-19). Our World Data. 2020. Available from: https://ourworldindata.org/covid-deaths [Accessed: July 15, 2022]

[83] Tian F, Tong B, Sun L, et al. N501Y mutation of spike protein in SARS-CoV-2 strengthens its binding to receptor ACE2. eLife;**10**:e69091

[84] Estofolete CF, Banho CA, Campos GRF, et al. Case study of two post vaccination SARS-CoV-2 infections with P1 variants in CoronaVac vaccinees in Brazil. Viruses. 2021;**13**:1237

[85] Sabino EC, Buss LF, Carvalho MPS, et al. Resurgence of COVID-19 in Manaus, Brazil, despite high seroprevalence. The Lancet. 2021;**397**:452-455

[86] Banho CA, Sacchetto L, Campos GRF, et al. Impact of SARS-CoV-2 Gamma lineage introduction and COVID-19 vaccination on the epidemiological landscape of a Brazilian city. Communication & Medicine. 2022;**2**:1-11

[87] SARS-CoV-2 variants of concern are emerging in India. Nature Medicine. Available from: https://www.nature.com/articles/s41591-021-01397-4. [Accessed: July 16, 2022]

[88] Liu Y, Liu J, Johnson BA, et al. Delta spike P681R mutation enhances SARS-CoV-2 fitness over Alpha variant. Cell Reports. 2022;**39**:110829

[89] Tchesnokova V, Kulasekara H, Larson L, et al. Acquisition of the L452R mutation in the ACE2-binding interface of spike protein triggers recent massive expansion of SARS-CoV-2 variants. Journal of Clinical Microbiology;**59**:e00921-e00921

[90] Deng X, Garcia-Knight MA, Khalid MM, et al. Transmission, infectivity, and neutralization of a spike L452R SARS-CoV-2 variant. Cell. 2021;**184**:3426-3437.e8

[91] Planas D, Veyer D, Baidaliuk A, et al. Reduced sensitivity of SARS-CoV-2 variant Delta to antibody neutralization. Nature. 2021;**596**:276-280

[92] Kumar V, Singh J, Hasnain SE, et al. Possible link between higher transmissibility of alpha, kappa and delta variants of SARS-CoV-2 and increased structural stability of its spike protein and hACE2 affinity. International Journal of Molecular Sciences. 2021;**22**:9131

[93] Di Giacomo S, Mercatelli D, Rakhimov A, et al. Preliminary report on severe acute respiratory syndrome coronavirus 2 (SARS-CoV-2) Spike mutation T478K. Journal of Medical Virology. 2021;**93**:5638-5643

[94] Li B, Deng A, Li K, et al. Viral infection and transmission in a large, well-traced outbreak caused by the SARS-CoV-2 Delta variant. Nature Communications. 2022;**13**:460

[95] SARS-CoV-2 Delta VOC in Scotland: Demographics, risk of hospital admission, and vaccine effectiveness. The Lancet. Available from: https://www.thelancet.com/journals/lancet/article/PIIS0140-6736(21)01358-1/fulltext. [Accessed: July 16, 2022]

[96] New AY lineages and an update to AY.4-AY.12. Pango Network. Available from: https://www.pango.network/new-ay-lineages-and-an-update-to-ay-4-ay-12/. [Accessed: July 16, 2022]

[97] CoVariants: 22A (Omicron). Available from: https://covariants.org/variants/22A.Omicron. [Accessed: July 16, 2022]

[98] Cao Y, Yisimayi A, Jian F, et al. BA.2.12.1, BA.4 and BA.5 escape antibodies elicited by Omicron infection. Nature. 2022:1-3

Chapter 15

Perspective Chapter: Emergency COVID-19 Guidelines Impacts on the Human Microbiome and Immune System

Josphert N. Kimatu

Abstract

There have been over sixty microbiome scientific studies involving populations in Europe, Asia and America which have enabled researchers to be able to map the human microbiome. There have been also over hundred publications on the effects of skin cosmetic conditions on the dynamism of the human microbiome. The human body naturally has its own ecosystem of microbiome population which further studies have shown that they are associated and communicate with the human immune system. Recent studies have shown that there are benefits which are derived from a healthy microbiome which is composed of a balanced microbial diversity. Advances in technologies, and increased WHO guidelines due to the COVID-19 pandemic are increasingly being found to be impacting this long-standing human-microbiome synergy. The skin surface microbes and their interactions with other organisms have a significant capacity of influencing health by being immune modulators through either their cell components or other cellular metabolites. This Book Chapter shall discuss and propose microbiome targeted therapeutics strategy as a rationale to involve the role of immune system dynamics and human microbiome in the fight against COVID-19 pandemic and other pandemics.

Keywords: SARS CoV-2, WHO, sanitization, antibodies, vaccination, biota

1. Introduction

There is need to have a universal language on how practitioners can trace and treat the progression of a pandemic. This need has been highlighted by the COVID-19 outbreak. Furthermore, the long-term effects on the immune system need to be investigated. The impact of the WHO guidelines on the immune system should be determined at all ages of the human population as they were postulated to have contributed to the reduction of the spreading of the SARS CoV-2 [1]. This book chapter examines the rationale and impacts of wearing of masks, hand sanitization and social distancing as measures of containing COVID-19. The analysis gives possible advices on retaining a functioning immune system in the midst of contradicting forces. Recent studies have shown the role of microbiome in influencing health as a therapeutic strategy via modulation of the immune system. This modulation occurs through cell components and cellular metabolites.

Although the SARS CoV-2 is regarded as a new contagious corona virus, the human body has encountered, the family of coronaviruses for ages [2]. The common human pet called dog, usually hosts many corona viruses. Even with such advances in knowledge on corona viruses, we are still not sure about the origin of SARS CoV-2. Some speculations of natural SARS mutation or laboratory synthesized virus origins have been suggested.

If the SARS CoV-2 is a new virus, then the human immune system might take time to develop antibodies immediately. However, if it is not new, past ideas from similar virus can be give the body a strategic advantage over the new mutation called SARS CoV-2. This strategic immunity can be related to a possible innate kind of immunity which can provide protection from coronaviruses without the need for a preconditioning of the body from the current new virus in the environment. The need for a new diverse vaccine can also be argued on the same understanding. Various people will react to SARS CoV-2 exposure mainly depending on how their bodies respond to inbuilt immune defenses against specific past exposures on corona viruses. An individual health and locational responses to corona viruses can determine the outcome of the health status of an exposure. However, this expectation is not as straight forward as we expect if the SARS CoV-2 is a man made and new inserted genome sequences of a synthesized corona virus. The adaptability of the immune system can also circumvent the human induced mutation as it has been doing before naturally.

The joint ecosystem between the human body and microorganisms is referred to as holobiont. It is made of persistent microorganism communities [3]. At the cell level our bodies are also interacting with microorganisms. This interaction has physiological impacts in development, immunity, adaptation and general health. This microecology is maintained at particular balance because disturbance of their equilibrium can cause diseases. The microorganisms in our bodies have been found to be transferable from one body to another. A host and its microbiota constitute a holobiont [4]. This phenomenon has become more important in the spread of COVID-19 and the place and value of the immune system health. This microbiome has the ability to remain silent until when disturbed. Microbial activity is necessary for life on earth. The microbiota composition in humans in built in the early years of a new born before reaching a more stable adult-like configuration at the age of ~3 years [5–7]. Henceforth, studies have shown that the host-microbiota equilibrium in humans is important and that a perturbation of such homeostasis may lead to shifts from healthy to pre-disease and disease states [8]. It is amazing how diseases like obesity, which is lifestyle related can be linked to microbiome dynamics. The shift from a healthy microbiota to pathobiota is influenced by modern civilization which does not consider its impact on the microbiome [9, 10]. Therefore, the holobiont concept highlights the complexity of host–microbiota interactions as a challenge and as a new venture for research for the scientific community [11, 12].

2. The immune system and the microbiota

In a broad sense, we have the adaptive and innate immunity. The body has a mechanism that enables living organisms to distinguish its own cells and substances or humors from foreign ones. This ability is called adaptive immunity. It has the ability to generate a specific cellular response to new pathogens [13]. The innate immune system is made up of cells and organs which are distributed throughout the body. The blood and the lymph usually distribute the immune cells throughout the body. The Innate immune cells react fast and nonspecifically when foreign cells are detected. The adaptive immune cells usually have a delay in their response. However, they later end up forming specific immunological memories of the intruding proteins. Researchers have suggested several ways to boost the immune system. These include the following three ways; The increase of immune system cells circulation to do their functions by doing moderated exercises to increase blood circulation, The boosting of the endocrine system functions by reducing stress and thirdly by eating balanced foods that are rich in vitamins and minerals [14]. The interactions between microbiota and host immunity are complex, dynamic and context-dependent [15].

3. Diseases and the microbiome

Diseases that affect humanity mostly thrive on a dysregulated or disturbed immune systems. Human beings have over the years developed mechanisms to coexist with microorganism [16]. Furthermore, this microbiome inhabitants are in constant interactions with the immune system either on the body surface or on the inside. The role of this human-microbe interaction is to train and empower the immune system [17]. In other words, the human body produces natural antimicrobial substances like tears, saliva, mucus and acids that inhibit or kill pathogens. These natural are supposed to be maintained for the proper functioning of the body immune system. Surprisingly, the same pathogens are the ones which stimulate the body to produce these useful antimicrobial substances. The phenomenon has helped the immune system to be maintained strong. There are critical roles which the microbiome plays in the training and development of the host's innate and adaptive immune system major components [15].

4. Microorganisms' role in training and boosting the immune system

In general, adaptive immunity is described as a mechanism that enables living organisms to distinguish its own cells and humors from foreign ones. It then generates a specific cellular response to the new pathogen [13]. The Immune cells in the body are distributed throughout the body by the blood and the lymph. In comparison, the innate immune cells usually react fast and are nonspecific when foreign cells are detected. The adaptive immune cells usually have a delay in their response, however, they end up forming a specific intrusion protein immunological memory.

If we carefully assume that the SARS cov-2 is natural mutation of the SARS corona virus then we can trust the human body to fight and overcome its invasion. However, a human synthesized source can be different. We can try to envisage the effects of the inserted sequences by the symptoms and signs from patients or from the sequences bases available. In our studies we assume that the immune system is not being influenced by other environmental factors causing similar symptoms. However, we are aware of major emerging environmental factors like climate change and human factors including chemical pollutions, nano particles or electromagnetic waves including mobile phone radiations.

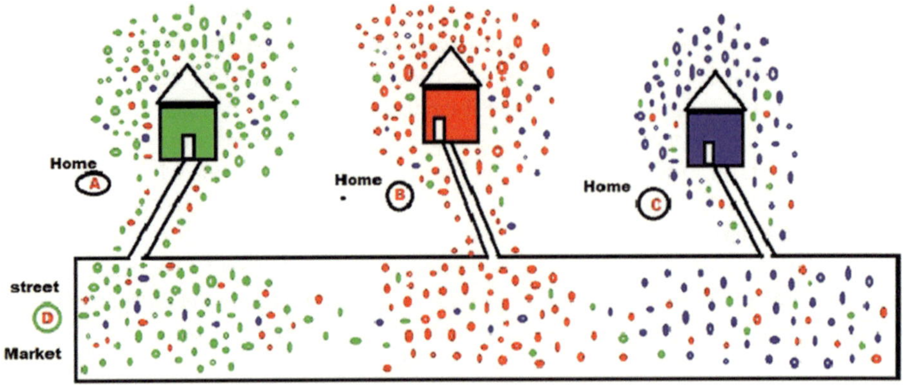

Figure 1.
The expected microbiome equilibrium around homes, and markets. It is worthy to note that each location has its own unique microbes which are also constantly being invaded by other microbes from other places and individuals. However, a new equilibrium is usually established after sometime due the law of the survival of the fittest due to competition or due to factors that enhance aggressive adaptation in changing environments.

Ref., [14], showed that the immune system can be boosted via reduction of stress, eating of balanced diet inclusive of vitamins and minerals. There are other ways of increasing the capacity of the immune system like doing moderate exercises which make the distribution of immune system cells to be faster and wider. A disturbed and dysregulated immune system have been shown to be the ground for diseases to be established in humanity. The earth biosphere is full of microbes as shown in **Figure 1**. Living bodies have over the years developed mechanisms to enable them to coexist and survive in the midst of microbes [16]. These microbes interact with the immune system on various levels. It can be very specific or non-specific. These interactions are very important in strengthening and training the immune system [17]. Furthermore, there is growing evidence of microbes influencing the peripheral cells of immune and thus consequently influencing cells at other distal sites [18].

5. The microbiome acting as a layer of defense

The normal body flora is composed of large community of microbes which associate with body cells. The association can be on the surface of on internal organs like in the digestive system. The layer of microbes can act as a physical barrier for cells and reduces the available surface for intruding pathogens. It also increases their survival competition, see.

Figure 2, The human microbiome is furthermore reinforced by the production of natural antimicrobial substances that act by inhibiting or killing invading pathogens. These natural body antimicrobial substances in animals include tears in eyes, saliva in the mouth, mucus in the respiratory surface and acids in the stomach. The body has to be stimulated to produce these useful antimicrobial substances. This is in many cases done by the same or similar pathogens. This scenario is developed and maintained continuously and is very important for the strengthening of the immune system. Pathogens that mutate have to fight the

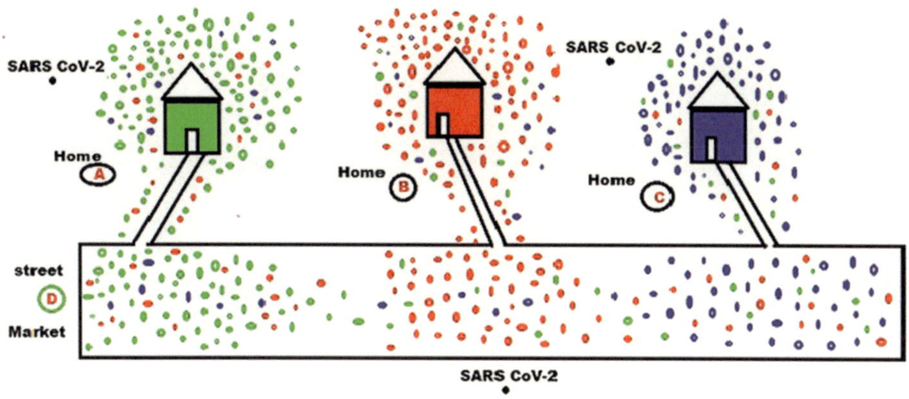

Figure 2.
The scenario of an invasion new microbes like in the current situation; the immune system is being attacked by the novel SARS CoV-2. The body will try to develop a new equilibrium. This is usually done easily and effectively if human external factors and extreme mutations in gene sequences are not added.

same microbial defense barrier. The body is only diseased if microbes overcome and pass this barrier.

6. Relooking at the WHO guidelines

Three main COVID-19 guidelines were issued by the world health organization (WHO) in the fight against the novel SARS CoV-2. One of them was the proper hand-washing of hands. This is based on the idea that the coronavirus is killed by proper handwashing of hands for 20 seconds with soap or by using hand sanitizer that has an alcohol concentration of more than 60%. The microbial envelop is assumed to be effectively being affected by the soap.

7. The implications of washing hands on the immune system

Normally, the human hand has a high concentration of microbial community. However, studies on the hand microbiome showed that there are some factors that can impact the hand microbiome composition. These factors include, temporal and biogeographical changes, age and intrinsic gender. Others are extrinsic product use, extrinsic cohabitants and extrinsic pet-ownership variables. Further studies have shown that the hand microbiome is always in constant changes. Therefore, hands are a critical factor in transmitting microbes between people, animals, inanimate objects and our environments see **Figure 3**). This transmission and establishment of microbes stimulates our immune system and prevents harmful microbes from colonizing the hands. Consequently, the WHO guideline seems to be enhancing the reduction of hand microbes and can contributing to the weakening the immune boosting abilities and opening the hand to new pathogens including novel viruses like SAR CoV-2. Washing hands with a sanitizer also makes it more difficult for the normal body flora to reoccupy their habitats due to changes of pH. It is like a reset of the microbiome. The touching eyes, skin, nose and mouth and other body parts after

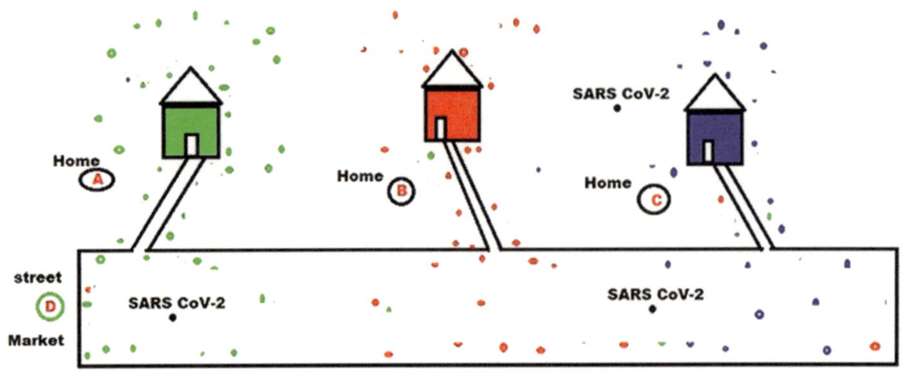

Figure 3.
The continuing wearing of face masks reduces the distribution of natural microbes to other places. Keeping interactive social distancing reduces the transfer of natural microbes from one person to another and from one region to another. This transfer of microbes from one source to another is crucial for the training and development of the immune system in children and boosting and strengthening the same immune system in adults. The current invasion of SARS CoV-2 into an intact and dynamic microbiome and its establishment is not possible. However, these studies show that it can be reinforced by a systematic destruction of the microbiome community or by having a novel synthetic virus which is more aggressive.

touching other places and people assist in boosting the strength of the immune system as a natural process.

8. The implications of social distance on the immune system

The maintenance of social distance or physical distance of at least 1 metre (3 feet) distance between one person and another has been used as a measure of preventing the spread of SARS CoV-2. This was to reduce the spray of contaminated droplets from nose and mouth to uninfected people. Moreover, people with symptoms like coughing, headache and fever were advised to self-isolate. However, the implication of the social distancing practice is that there shall be little person to person exchange of microbes. This if practice is coupled with the washing of hands and continuous sanitizing shall make it very difficult to recover the normal flora populations. This shall be another reset of normal body flora. It shall cause a weakening of the immune system and might most likely open an opportunity for new pathogens to attack the body including making the new SARS CoV-2 more virulent. Furthermore, in the face of the global climate change and increased migrations we might end up with a reset of the current human microbiome population.

9. The implications of wearing face masks on the immune system

In another the precaution of wearing face masks in crowded places is not natural to the body. It can increase mental stress in the body on people who are already bombarded with economic burden and frequent pandemic information. Immunological studies show that stressed bodies might have malfunctioning of the endocrine system and the weakening of the immune system. The use of a mask increases the intake of the respiratory carbon dioxide from the body which makes metabolism to be lower. This affects negatively people with other under laying conditions like diabetes, mental health and high blood pressure.

10. Discussions and conclusions

The diversity, abundance and functionality of the microbiome is still being deciphered. It is worthy to note that the microbiome role in health is of paramount importance. Much studies on microbiomes and microbiota have been done in bacteria. Less studies have been done in fungi, with only less than 400 fungal species so far having been isolated [19–21].

The training and development of the host immune system is promoted by natural body and environmental microbes. These interactions have been occurring to keep invading pathogens at bay. Some of these microbes are commensals and hence they promote the development of the immune system B cells that assist the body to produce Immunoglobulin A (IgA) which is a protective antibody. The role of the IgA is to neutralize pathogens and exotoxins. This promotes the development of the immune system. Deviations from this natural mechanism can have short term effects but after sometime it can produce new waves of disease out breaks and pandemics. The natural microbiome populations have been known to prevent the growth of harmful pathogens by using various parameters like altering pH, effectively consuming nutrients required for pathogen survival, and by even secreting toxins and antibodies that inhibit growth and competition of pathogens [16].

This Chapter has examined some of the potential effects of WHO guidelines in relation to microbiome and the human immune system. Suggestions have been made on how to have a balance between having a healthy immune system and not exposing it to pathogenic attacks when weakened. Microbes have a significant capacity in influencing health by being immune modulators through either their cell components

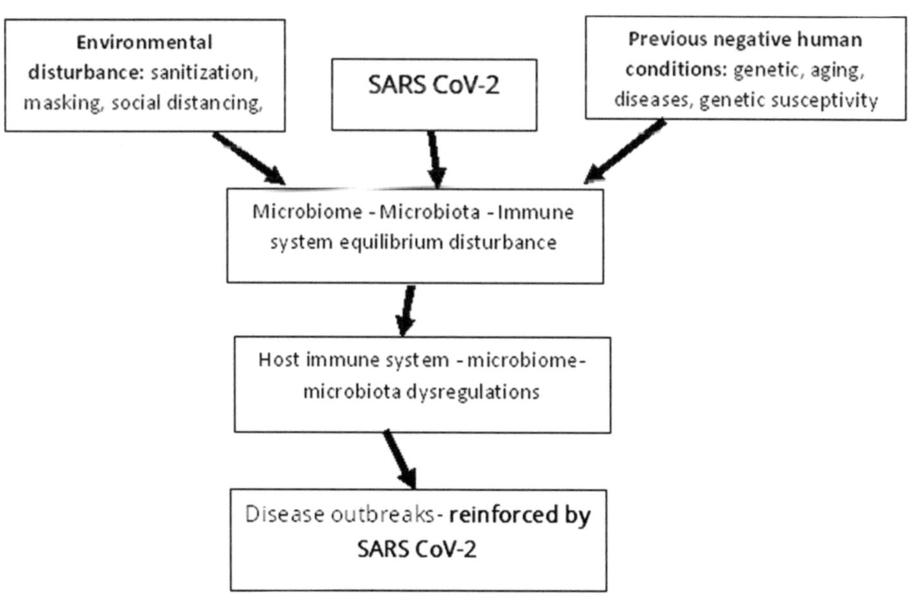

Figure 4.
The effects of the WHO guidelines of social distancing, sanitization of hands, streets and markets and homes is gradually reducing the protective microbiome barrier in human populations. The invasion of SARS CoV-2 into an intact and dynamic microbiome is being reinforced by destroying the microbiome community if a synthetic and more competitive, mutating virus which destroys the immune system is introduced in the equilibrium. This can lead to another pandemic due to the altering, replacing or editing the time proven human-microbiome interactions.

or other cellular metabolites including hormone production. We propose the development of microbiome targeted therapeutics strategy in order to involve the role of immune system dynamics in the fight against COVID-19 pandemic (**Figure 4**).

11. Impact of WHO guidelines on COVID-19 to the immune system

The COVID-19 outbreak caused the world health organization (WHO) to issue three major guidelines in the fight against the spread of the novel SARS CoV-2. These were washing of hands, wearing of masks and keeping physical distances. Careful examination of each of these guidelines show that they have a negative effect on the immune system.

The sanitization of hands or hand washing was based on the idea that the SARS CoV-2 was killed by proper hand washing for 20 seconds with soap or by using an alcohol-based hand sanitizer of more than 60% concentration. However, the implications of this washing hands guideline to the immune system are that the human hand which has a high amount of microbial abundance and diversity was being transformed to another composition gradually. Studies have shown that there is an intimate relationship between microbiomes and the immune system that requires a healthy host immunity to prevent commensals from overexploitation of the host resources while maintaining immune tolerance to innocuous stimuli [22, 23]. The hand microbiome is influenced by temporal and biogeographical dynamics, intrinsic age, intrinsic gender and extrinsic product use, extrinsic cohabitants and extrinsic pet-ownership variables. This microbiome is constantly changing as the hand involved in transmitting microbes between people, objects and environments. This transmission is crucial in stimulating the immune system and preventing harmful microbes from colonizing the hands. However, the WHO guidelines of sanitizing the hands just because of one virus has the potential of weakening the immune boosting abilities and opening the hand to new pathogen colonization. This could actually be the virulent SARS CoV-2 itself. Furthermore, the washing of hands with a sanitizer makes it more difficult for the normal body flora to reoccupy their natural habitat because of the new pH.

The second WHO guideline of keeping a physical distance of about 1.5 m between one person and another. This regulation is based on the idea that if somebody coughs or sneezes, the droplets with the virus will not be able reach the nose of another person. People are also advised to stay home and to self-isolate when they notice symptoms like coughing, headache and fever. This means that shall be little exchange of microbes from one individual to another. Therefore, if all these guidelines are implemented it might be very difficult to recover the normal microbiome of healthy individuals. Could this trigger a bigger pandemic?

The third major WHO guideline is the wearing face masks in crowded places or if one would like to go out so as to avoid infecting others. The idea is that contaminated droplets shall not be able to find their way to other people or land on surfaces to contaminate them. The wearing of masks is not natural to the body. This can stress the body who are already under economic and social burdens. This stress can impact the endocrine system and the immune system. This is more so on old peoples and people with chronic illnesses like diabetes. The later studies did sent caution that people with underlying conditions should not be vaccinated.

Studies have shown that human disease and therapeutic interventions affect microbial communities' abundance, diversity and functionality [24]. There are two drivers of the human microbiome composition: one is the genetic and immunological factors and two is the environmental, notably diet and environmental biodiversity. Human beings display a substantial loss of microbiome in comparison to chimpanzees and gorillas. This loss is attributed to much diet modification and environmental changes [25–27].

12. Microbiome-immunity crosstalk mechanisms and COVID-19

The microbiome is composed of a great number of microorganisms which in the human body are found in the gut and also on the skin and other mucosal microenvironments. Studies have shown that microbiome is active participant in a host functions like immunity and other metabolism activities. Other functions which have a microbiome impact are nutrition end products and the circadian clock operation [28–30]. Studies have shown that lung microbiome can modify the risk and consequences of COVID-19 by activating the immune response. On the same line, other suggestions show that bacterial co-infections as well as the gut-lung cross talk may be important players in COVID-19 disease prognosis. Recent studies have established that COVID-19 patients with GI complications experience more respiratory distress when compared to the patients without GI complications [31, 32]. Interestingly, obesity, *diabetes mellitus*, cardiovascular diseases and old age-related disorders have been related to weak microbiome communities and the same category of patients have also been more vulnerable to COVID-19 and SARS CoV-2 attacks [33–36]. Even in gut microbiome, COVID-19 patients were found to be deficient to beneficial commensals like *Eubacterium ventriosum, Faecalibacterium prausnitzii,* and *Roseburia* these microbes highly correlate to disease severity [37–39].

13. Recommendations

The recommendations from this crucial evaluation of the immune system role of the microbiome is that in future we should not over look natural mechanisms which have established an equilibrium with the immune system. This should also involve the educating of masses on how to cultivate the natural human microbiome defense systems as physical barriers. The training and boosting of the immune system both in children and adults respectively should regionally be evaluated. This is because increased traveling and climate change cannot be assumed to be of little consequences in pandemic control strategies in light of the microbiome roles.

Author details

Josphert N. Kimatu
Department of Life Sciences, South Eastern Kenya University, School of Pure and Applied Sciences, Kitui, Kenya

*Address all correspondence to: jkimatu@seku.ac.ke

References

[1] Li Q, Guan X, Wu P, Wang X, Zhou L, Tong Y, et al. Early transmission dynamics in Wuhan, China, of novel coronavirus-infected pneumonia. The New England Journal of Medicine. 2020

[2] Guarner J. Three emerging coronaviruses in two decades. American Journal of Clinical Pathology. 2020. DOI: 10.1093/ajcp/aqaa029

[3] Gilbert SF. Holobiont by Birth. Multilineage individuals as the concretion of cooperative processes. In: Tsing A, Swanson H, Gan E, Bubandt N, editors. Arts of Living in a Damaged Planet. Minneapolis – London: University of Minnesota Press; 2017

[4] Simon J-C, Marchesi JR, Christophe M, Marc-André S. Host-microbiota interactions: From holobiont theory to analysis. Microbiome. 2019;7:5

[5] Backhed F et al. Dynamics and stabilization of the human gut microbiome during the first year of life. Cell Host & Microbe. 2015;**17**:690-703

[6] Koenig JE et al. Succession of microbial consortia in the developing infant gut microbiome. Proceedings of the National Academy Science USA. 2011;**108**(Suppl 1):4578-4585

[7] Yatsunenko T et al. Human gut microbiome viewed across age and geography. Nature. 2012;**486**:222-227

[8] van de Guchte M, Blottière HM, Doré J. Humans as holobionts: Implications for prevention and therapy. Microbiome. 2018;**6**(1):81

[9] Broberg M, Doonan J, Mundt F, Denman S, McDonald JE. Integrated multiomic analysis of host-microbiota interactions in acute oak decline. Microbiome. 2018;**6**(1):21

[10] Hassani MA, Durán P, Hacquard S. Microbial interactions within the plant holobiont. Microbiome. 2018;**6**(1):58

[11] McFall-Ngai M, Hadfield MG, Bosch TC, Carey HV, et al. Animals in a bacterial world, a new imperative for the life sciences. Proceedings of the National Academy Science USA. 2013;**110**:3229-3236

[12] Vandenkoornhuyse P, Quaiser A, Duhamel M, Le Van A, Dufresne A. The importance of the microbiome of the plantholobiont. New Phytologist. 2015;**206**:1196-1206

[13] Takeuchi O, Akira S. Innate immunity to virus infection. Immunological Reviews. 2009;**227**(1):75-86

[14] Scher B. Boosting your immune system to fight the coronavirus: What you need to know. Diet Doctor 2020 https://www.dietdoctor.com/coronavirus. [Accessed: March 24, 2020]

[15] Zheng D, Timur L, Eran E. Interaction between microbiota and immunity in health and disease. Cell Research. 2020;**30**:492-506. DOI: 10.1038/s41422-020-0332-7

[16] Lozupone CA. Unraveling interactions between the microbiome and the host immune system to decipher mechanisms of disease., mSystems. 2018;**3**:e00183-e00187

[17] Olszak T, An D, Zeissig S, Vera MP, Richter J, Franke A, et al. Microbial exposure during early life has persistent

effects on natural killer T cell function. Science. 2012;**336**:489-493

[18] Cerf-Bensussan N, Gaboriau-Routhiau V. The immune system and the gut microbiota: Friends or foes? Nature Reviews. Immunology. 2010;**10**:735-744

[19] Gouba N, Drancourt M. Digestive tract mycobiota: A source of infection. Médecine et Maladies Infectieuses. 2015;**45**:9-16

[20] Oever JT, Netea MG. The bacteriome-mycobiome interaction and antifungal host defense. European Journal of Immunology. 2014;**44**:3182-3191

[21] Seed PC. The human mycobiome. Cold Spring Harbor Perspectives in Medicine. 2014;**5**:a019810

[22] Chu H, Mazmanian SK. Innate immune recognition of the microbiota promotes host-microbial symbiosis. Nature Immunology. 2013;**14**:668-675

[23] Macpherson AJ, Geuking MB, McCoy KD. Immune responses that adapt the intestinal mucosa to commensal intestinal bacteria. Immunology. 2005;**115**:153-162

[24] Mezouar S, Yannick C, Justin M, Alexandre F, Jean-Christophe D, Marc L, et al. Microbiome and the immune system: From a healthy steady-state to allergy associated disruption. Human Microbiome Journal. 2018;**10**:11-20

[25] Groussin M, Mazel F, Sanders JG, Smillie CS, Lavergne S, Thuiller W, et al. Unraveling the processes shaping mammalian gut microbiomes over evolutionary time. Nature Communications. 2017;**8**:14319

[26] Gupta VK, Paul S, Dutta C. Geography, ethnicity or subsistence-specific variations in human microbiome composition and diversity. Frontiers in Microbiology. 2017;**8**:1162

[27] Moeller AH, Caro-Quintero A, Mjungu D, Georgiev AV, Lonsdorf EV, Muller MN, et al. Co-speciation of gut microbiome with hominids. Science. 2016;**353**:380-382

[28] Hacquard S et al. Microbiota and host nutrition across plant and animal kingdoms. Cell Host & Microbe. 2015;**17**:603-616

[29] Lynch JB, Hsiao EY. Microbiomes as sources of emergent host phenotypes. Science. 2019;**365**:1405-1409

[30] Sender R, Fuchs S, Milo R. Are we really vastly outnumbered? Revisiting the ratio of bacterial to host cells in humans. Cell. 2016;**164**:337-340

[31] Wan Y et al. Enteric involvement in hospitalized patients with COVID-19 outside Wuhan. The Lancet Gastroenterology & Hepatology. 2020;**5**:534-535

[32] Wang D, Hu B, Hu C. Clinical characteristics of 138 hospitalized patients with 2019 novel coronavirus—Infected pneumonia in Wuhan China. JAMA. 2020

[33] Du RH et al. Predictors of mortality for patients with COVID-19. The European Respiratory Journal. 2020;**55**:2000524

[34] Durack J, Lynch SV. The gut microbiome: Relationships with disease and opportunities for therapy. The Journal of Experimental Medicine. 2018;**216**:20-40

[35] Mehra MR, Desai SS, Kuy S, Henry TD, Patel AN. Cardiovascular disease, drug therapy, and mortality in

Covid-19. The New England Journal of Medicine. 2020;**382**:e102

[36] Zhou F et al. Clinical course and risk factors for mortality of adult inpatients with COVID-19 in Wuhan, China: A retrospective cohort study. Lancet. 2020;**395**:1054-1062

[37] Khatiwada S, Subedi A. Lung microbiome and coronavirus disease 2019 (COVID-19): Possible link and implications. Human Microbes Journal. 2020;**17**:100073

[38] Halwachs B, Madhusudhan N, Krause R, Nilsson RH, Moissl-Eichinger C, Högenauer C, et al. Critical issues in mycobiota analysis. Frontiers in Microbiology. 2017;**8**:180

[39] Kamada N. Control of pathogens and pathobionts by the gut microbiota. Nature Immunology. 2013;**14**(7):685-690. DOI: 10.1038/ni.2608. PMC 4083503. PMID 23778796

Section 4

Trials and Studies

Chapter 16

Perspective Chapter: Ethics of Using Placebo Controlled Trials for Covid-19 Vaccine Development in Vulnerable Populations

Lesley Burgess, Jurie Johannes Jordaan and Matthew Wilson

Abstract

When clinical trials are conducted in vulnerable communities such as those found within low-to-middle-income-countries (LMICs), there is always the risk of exploitation or harm to these communities during the course of biomedical research. Historically, there have been multiple instances where significant harm was caused. Various organisations have proposed guidelines to minimise the risk of this occurring, however, questionable clinical trials are still conducted. Research Ethics Committees have an additional duty of care to protect these vulnerable populations. During the Covid-19 pandemic the ongoing use of placebo-controlled trials (PCTs), even after approval of a safe and efficacious vaccine, is a topic of great debate and is discussed from an ethical and moral perspective.

Keywords: Covid-19, research ethics, clinical trials, equity, placebo, randomisation

1. Introduction

Randomised control trials have existed in medicine since the 1940s [1]. Many iterations of guidelines to govern their use in research to protect vulnerable populations that have historically been abused for the betterment of science. Unfortunately, with a concept as abstract as ethics in clinical research, there is no universal consensus, and one may argue for or against their use with equal vigour depending on the specific circumstances of the trial [1–5].

Ethics of conducting clinical trials, particularly placebo-controlled trials (PCTs) in low-to-middle-income-countries (LMICs), is controversial. The emergence of placebo-controlled vaccine clinical trials against severe acute respiratory syndrome coronavirus 2 (SARS-CoV-2), the causative agent of coronavirus disease 2019 (COVID-19), has renewed interest in the debate. According to the World Bank Group (2021) [6], LMICs are defined as countries in the developing world with a gross national income per capita of $1046–$4095. The need for clinical trials to be conducted in LMICs is paramount to bridging the health gap, a concept so starkly highlighted in the recent pandemic.

Medical research in these countries requires proper adjudication and protection to maximise benefits and deter potential harm [7].

Pharmaceutical companies tend to pursue these communities, capitalising on lower costs, fewer restrictions, and weaker local standards [8]. In 2008, the United States Food and Drug Administration (FDA) published its decision to abandon the Declaration of Helsinki (DoH) as an ethical guideline when conducting and reviewing data from clinical trials conducted outside the United States of America (USA). As a result, there is limited protection for LMICs where USA-based companies conduct clinical trials [9]. The responsibility to uphold moral ethics thus shifts to the local investigators and review boards [9]. The limited protection referenced above pertains to the Good Clinical Practices of the Conference of International Harmonisation (ICH-GCP) being more flexible when choosing comparator drugs in clinical trials [10]. Article 33 in the DoH outlines stricter criteria for using placebo as an alternative to best proven intervention [7]. ICH-GCP, however, has no enforceable article guiding the choice of comparator leaving the decision to the study designer and review board's discretion [10]. Consequentially, this avenue is open for exploitation in LMICs where scientific knowledge and ethics are comparatively weaker [8]. Together, the DoH and ICH-GCP should govern the impact clinical trials have in vulnerable communities, however, there is more nuance to the situation [1–3].

To ensure exploitation does not occur, participants must not be exposed to excessive risk and must understand the difference between clinical trials and clinical medicine [1, 5–7]. To participate in a trial, you willingly join an experimental process rather than have a therapy tailored to your medical needs [2–3, 11–17]. We will discuss the aspects of trials as a whole and why LMICs are vulnerable to this exploitation, explore the concept of clinical equipoise, and discuss PCTs in the setting of COVID-19 vaccine trials during the pandemic.

2. What makes LMICs so vulnerable?

All manner of ethical research necessitates non-use of undue influence to garner research participant compliance [7, 8, 10]. However, what may seem negligible to cause undue influence in developed countries, could very well double or even be whole income for a household in LMICs that suffer from poverty, poor living conditions and no access to running water. For these reasons, it's imperative to consider the medical benefits of clinical trials [9].

In LMICs, there is a prevailing lack of access to healthcare [11]. Clinical trials offer the opportunity for recruited participants to receive healthcare not otherwise available to them [1–4, 8]. The DoH states: "medical research within a vulnerable group is only justified if the research is responsive to the health needs..." [7]. This highlights an obvious gap in the protection of these populations which is easily exploited if not appropriately safeguarded. The argument for choice of comparator weighs heavily on this point. Internationally, there is a call for using "best available standard" when designing clinical trials. However, in LMICs, there is no legal basis enforcing an international gold standard over a locally available comparator choice [1–5, 8–12]. Problems arise when conducting clinical trials in LMICs where there is no "locally available standard". In vaccine trials, specifically where cold chain continuation is paramount, there's advocation against use of the international gold standard should the target country have insufficient infrastructure to ensure preservation of drug.

Multiple publications reference the lack of ethics conducting clinical trials in LMICs [7, 18–21]. Major challenges noted include: incomplete ethical regulations and guidance, limited knowledge of science, language barriers between researchers, sponsors and communities, and insufficient financial and material resources of local authorities to govern the conduct of clinical trials. Exploitation of LMICs is well documented throughout history. In 1994, the ACTG 076 trial involved in reviewing low-cost regimes of antiretroviral drugs to prevent mother to child transmission of human immunodeficiency virus (HIV), was rife with controversy. Placebo was administered despite having proven knowledge that zidovudine is effective in prevention of vertical transmission of HIV [8, 22]. Another example was a rotavirus vaccine trial conducted in India from 2011 to 2012. The use of placebo as comparator, despite availability of two internationally registered vaccines recommended by the World Health Organisation (WHO), and one locally registered vaccine. As a result, more than 3000 out of 7500 randomised children were exposed to rotavirus and associated risks [23]. Such use of placebo would be unacceptable in developed countries and the expectation that LMICs should carry this burden is unjust.

3. Principles of medical ethics and how they apply to LMICs

The cardinal pillars of medical ethics are autonomy, beneficence, non-maleficence, and justice. All manner of clinical research takes heed of these pillars and can be described and applied in a myriad of ways [24].

3.1 Social and clinical value

Risk exposure must be justified; any resulting scientific knowledge gains should be significant enough to warrant inconveniencing and risking the population of unknown health outcomes for the greater good [1, 8]. There are certain areas of research that are better conducted in LMICs based on the endemic nature of diseases such as HIV and tuberculosis (TB) [19]. Populations are thus able to benefit directly from the trial as participants. The common shortfall is post-trial access to the tested intervention. There is massive debate on the responsibility of stakeholders to provide post-trial access to drugs. Some cite reciprocal justice to participants, while others cite practicality of large-scale rollouts being the jurisdiction of government entities [19]. Clinical trials in LMICs need to account for these factors during study design to ensure value.

3.2 Scientific validity

Studies should be designed to answer specific questions, using research methods that are valid, and feasible [8]. Poor scientific reasoning and application of research trials damages the perception of clinical research. In the realm of LMICs it can be deleterious to future relationships in garnering support for clinical trials. Standards in LMICs may permit approval of fallacious studies by local authorities without better knowledge or insight. It is the responsibility of sponsors to ensure this avenue of exploitation is protected to the level of the country of origin [1–5, 18].

3.3 Favourable risk-benefit ratio

Uncertainty about the degree of risks and benefits associated with a treatment is implicit in clinical research [8, 13–17]. Clinical research is not conducted to provide health care though it is often a beneficial by-product [1–4, 8]. When looking to conduct trials in LMICs and other vulnerable populations, there needs to be increased emphasis on these benefits [7]. Maintaining a favourable ratio requires the use of interim reviews during a study to timeously detect whether an intervention arm (active or control) is associated with increased risk. Should this occur, research should be stopped to allow the protection of participants [24].

3.4 Independent review

An independent review panel, with no vested interest in the outcome of the trial, should review proposal validity and ensure its integrity [8]. This is generally done by Institutional Review Boards (IRBs) and Research Ethics Committees (RECs). In high income countries, these committees comprise of highly qualified and experienced individuals who are well-suited to manage complex ethical issues. Their role serves to make sound, consistent and ethical decisions on matters related to patient safety. There is trepidation that IRBs and RECs in LMICs may not be adequately equipped to protect the human rights of clinical trial participants, due to lack of financial and material resources, inadequate training of members, lack of diversity of membership, lack of independence and inability to monitor approved protocols [21]. As a result, there may be inconsistencies in the review process outcomes thus compromising patient safety. Some countries intentionally weaken their regulatory framework to encourage foreign investment through externally sponsored research [24]. These shortcomings are historically exploited to conduct research in LMICs that would never pass the review process in the country of origin [24].

3.5 Informed consent

Participants must decide, independently and without duress, to take part in research [8, 24]. Subjects must be appropriately informed of the purpose, method, risks, benefit, and alternatives to research [24]. Furthermore, subjects must be made to understand these factors and how they apply to their situation. In LMICs, a common roadblock is language and minimum level of education [18, 21]. At times it is difficult to know the degree of participants understanding especially when translators are used [21]. Even in developed countries, the understanding of what a PCT is can be lacking.

3.6 Respect for subjects

Confidentiality and ensuring informed voluntary participation are the hallmarks of respecting autonomy of subjects [8]. Abiding by a subject's wishes to withdraw consent and discontinue from a trial without consequence is important [24]. Sharing information that arises from interim review of previously unknown adverse events is the responsibility of research staff, even though it may change the subject's opinion on the risks and benefits of participation [24]. In LMICs there is a role for Community Advisory Boards (CABs) to advocate for trial participants and promote the ethical conduct of clinical trials [20]. In South Africa, CABs are used to protect the interests of participants on HIV and TB drug trials. Their main roles have been preventing exploitation and building capacity for research in communities. By consisting of community members and encouraging interest in research by the individual in a community, CABs bring the value of research to the home country. Assisting in advancing research goals, their use has had positive benefit in information distribution and recruitment for trials [25].

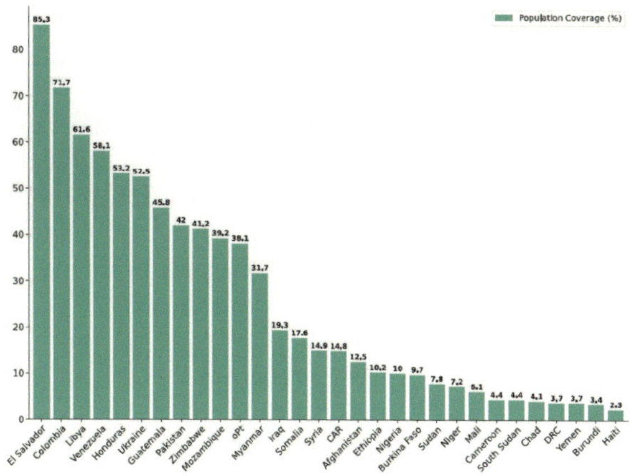

Figure 1.
Estimated percent of population covered by delivered vaccines to HRP countries (based on two doses), as of 31 December 2021 [27].

4. Effects of Covid-19 on LMICs

The Covid-19 pandemic augmented the effects of resource deficiency in LMICs. In such countries, where healthcare access is limited under normal circumstances, the added burden of a pandemic will and has caused vast morbidity and mortality. In India alone, there was an estimated 30,000–50,000 ventilators available to service a projected 1 million people with severe disease requiring ventilation during the peak of their first COVID-19 wave [26]. Access to oxygen in LMICs has been a challenge, with many hospitals running out of oxygen amidst a massive surge in patients due to COVID-19. During these periods, many hospitals in LMICs had an additional shortage of beds and staff [26]. The development of life saving vaccines against Covid-19 can mitigate this devastation, by preventing severe disease completely and limiting hospitalisation. With development and initial distribution of vaccines occurring predominantly in the western world's high-income countries, a potentially faster way for LMICs to receive any form of Covid-19 vaccination is through clinical trials. While controversial, it cannot be overstated (especially given the critical nature of the pandemic), that there is a need for clinical trials to collaborate with communities in LMICs and involve them in research of novel and affordable versions of these vaccines. This will provide them all the benefits of early access and equip their governments with tools to advance a vaccine rollout plan, while the scientific world benefits from the data they provide.

Figure 1 [27] is from the United Nations Office for the Coordination of Humanitarian Affairs, showing countries with inter-agency humanitarian response plan (HRP). This graph depicts the vaccine coverage of population, provided by developed countries to HRP countries. This clearly depicts the health gap, the inequity of vaccine rollouts on a global scale.

5. Ethics of trial design in Covid-19 vaccines

The genetic sequence of SARS-CoV-2 was published early in January of 2020. A global research and development effort followed to develop a safe and efficacious vaccine. Human clinical testing of the first vaccine candidate started in March 2020 [28]. At that time there was no doubt that PCTs were ethical and the preferred trial design to test potential Covid-19 vaccines.

A global pandemic is a highly dynamic situation and regular change in the clinical landscape can be expected. Ethical and moral considerations will also change as new developments unfold and new information becomes available. These considerations will be influenced by existing global inequality and a lack of resources in LMICs. The moment a safe and efficacious Covid-19 vaccine became available, it opened the ethical debate as to how long it will stay ethical to continue using PCTs.

5.1 Advantages of using PCTs in Covid-19 vaccines

Most of the arguments in favour of continuing the use of PCTs in Covid-19 vaccines stems from a document published in The New England Journal of Medicine by the WHO Ad Hoc Expert Group on the Next Steps for Covid-19 Vaccine Evaluation in January 2021 [29]. More than a year later, one could argue that this information is now outdated, but even though the global vaccine situation has changed dramatically, the WHO has not released any new guidelines.

The WHO Ad Hoc Expert Group stated that initial vaccine roll-out will be slow and in limited quantities. This would provide an opportunity to ethically obtain socially valuable data. Data could then be used to improve regulatory and public health decision making. Better data would lead to increasing public and professional confidence in vaccines [29].

Rapid vaccination of large numbers of people will inevitably cause the vaccine to seem temporarily associated with some uncommon side effects. A large, simple PCT could identify any rare short-term side-effects or show the absence of such side-effects. These probably unrelated events occurring by chance after vaccination, may incorrectly be attributed to the vaccine [29]. Groups opposed to vaccination may deliberately spread these anecdotes and cause vaccine hesitancy [29, 30].

Randomised, noninferiority trials can provide clinically relevant data but according to the WHO, "at considerable cost to efficiency". PCTs would assist with earning broad public confidence required for widespread vaccine acceptance. A PCT is still the scientific gold standard for testing any new intervention and alternative designs could yield inferior data [29–35]. Even following the availability of the first vaccines, it is still crucial to further evaluate candidate vaccines to meet the global needs. Observational data obtained from non-randomised studies after vaccine deployment could yield inaccurate answers and suffer from substantial biases [29].

The obligations researchers have to participants are not the same as those clinicians have towards patients [32, 33]. Proper informed consent would allow participants to voluntarily enrol in a trial and accept some risks to collect socially valuable data. In this unparalleled global crisis, billions of individuals might benefit from finding a new safe and efficacious vaccine, and thus some participants might enrol in PCTs because of altruistic reasons [29].

Those in favour of continuing to use PCTs in Covid-19 vaccines, argue that research-ethics guidelines such as the DoH and the Council for International Organizations of Medical Science (CIOMS) Guidelines were not written with Emergency Use Designation (EUD) of vaccines in mind [29]. A vaccine approved under EUD does not render it "best proven intervention" or an "established effective intervention" [29].

In January 2020 the WHO stated verbatim that trial sponsors are not ethically obligated to unblind participants who desire to obtain a different investigational vaccine [29].

As with any clinical trial, participants would still have the option to withdraw from the trial and the WHO did not comment on this probability when engaging with participants who request unblinding.

5.2 Ethical shortcomings of using PCTs in Covid-19 vaccines

Several Covid-19 vaccines have been approved for emergency use, with some vaccines already receiving full approval from various regulatory authorities across the world. These vaccines have been proven to have high levels of efficacy and safety [36].

Once there is an available vaccine, with high level of safety and efficacy, new candidate vaccines should be tested against approved vaccines. Ongoing PCTs of Covid-19 vaccine candidates should be unblinded [37]. Continuation of PCTs of new vaccines in conditions where efficacious vaccines already exist, contravenes the bio-ethics principle of beneficence. It will be in direct conflict with the participants' best interests. It puts them at a disadvantage compared to people who are not on the trial.

Researchers have a duty not to harm participants in clinical trials. In using placebo, researchers fail to provide protection against a deadly pandemic, as various Covid-19 vaccines have been proven to be safe, efficacious, and available [36]. The harm participants in the control group are exposed to is not minor [38]. There are limitations in current treatment options, thus it is in everyone's own interest to take the first vaccine found to be safe, instead of participating in a PCT.

Ravinetto [39] stated that an ethical strategy cannot be built on an unethical premise. In this case it is the inequitable allocation of vaccines between countries which is in essence unethical. This is a prime example of so-called "ethics dumping": undertaking research in LMIC settings, which would not be permitted in high income settings. This reverses the principle of benefit sharing in global research. The burden of the research is much higher for the most vulnerable communities, while the benefits are available only to the higher income countries.

In social justice terms, global health research should generate knowledge that improves the health and well-being of disadvantaged and marginalised communities [39, 40]. In the context of Covid-19 these communities are mostly in LMICs, those who lack access to vaccines due to unequal global distribution. Research involving this group should be based on health and social justice, rather than building on the existing structural injustice and exploitation of these groups.

Clinical equipoise can be defined as a state of uncertainty or true ambivalence toward the efficacy of a novel therapy in the medical or scientific community [41–43]. Based on the principle of beneficence if any novel therapy is believed, by consensus, to be efficacious, research subjects should not be denied access to that therapy. Similarly, if the novel therapy is found to cause harm, then it would go against the principle of nonmaleficence to continue that specific candidate as investigational product.

The ethical loophole that supporters of continuing PCTs in Covid-19 vaccine trials in LMICs are using, is based on the fact the so-called local "standard of care" in many LMICs would be no vaccine or very restricted access to a vaccine [40]. Arguing equipoise between placebo and local standard, in settings where vaccines are not yet available, due only to vaccines nationalism and lack of equity, would be unethical. One could argue that the ethical standards applied in the LMICs should be the same as if the research were carried out in the sponsoring country. People should be treated fairly, regardless of where they live.

The WHO states that if vaccines are not properly tested (with continuing PCTs), it might lead to public distrust [29]. However, in the authors' opinion, using a different set of ethical standards for certain countries just because they are poor, disadvantaged and cannot afford vaccines, could lead to even more distrust and scepticism around how the WHO is dealing with global inequality during a deadly pandemic.

Although those who argue in favour of continuing to use PCTs in Covid-19 vaccines state that randomised control trial is the golden standard for modern clinical decision making [29–35], there are various other study designs that could yield good data without endangering or leaving any participants unprotected [37–40, 44–48]. Non-inferiority blinded active control trials can be done to compare trial vaccines to an established vaccine, without leaving any participants unvaccinated [39]. If research can be conducted in several ways, the method that minimises morbidity and loss of human life should be prioritised above a method that supposedly gives scientific results more efficiently, but at a greater risk to the participants.

Various authors have commented on the WHO's call to altruism aimed at communities in LMICs [39, 40, 44]. To quote the WHO document: "people who enrol in clinical trials would probably understand the value of gathering data that will further elucidate the safety and efficacy of these vaccines and their appropriate use" [29]. This seems to underestimate the complex nature of decision-making regarding participating in a clinical trial by people living in LMICs [49]. The WHO is expecting the people from poor, marginalised and disadvantaged communities to accept that their sacrifice will be for the greater good. Firstly, this sacrifice is per definition not expected from their counterparts in higher income countries. Secondly, the "value of gathering of data" will directly benefit the sponsor country long before it benefits the general population of the LMIC where the trial was conducted.

Ironically, Dr Ghebreyesus, the WHO Director-General, in relation to global vaccine inequity, stated "The world is on the brink of a catastrophic moral failure—and the price of this failure will be paid with lives and livelihoods in the world's poorest countries" [50]. Now it is the WHO Ad Hoc Expert Group that is essentially giving researchers free reign to continue using PCTs in countries that are too poor to afford vaccines by misusing the clinical equipoise argument and thus further marginalising these vulnerable communities that they are meant to protect.

When conducting trials in LMICs there are certain specific considerations regarding informed consent [33–34]. The level of literacy in LMICs is lower than in high income countries and thus it is more likely that a participant will have a diminished understanding of what a PCT entails [34]. The authors can reflect on several cases where despite extensive counselling and a thorough informed consent process, participants in various Covid-19 vaccine PCTs, when coming back for subsequent visits, could not recall that they were told of the possibility of having a salt-water injection. This caused great confusion for many participants and highlights the ethical challenges of conducting clinical trials in LMICs.

In many LMICs, some participants are more likely to trust a clinician blindly as it is seen as a sacred profession [40]. The clinician is supposed to act in the patient's best interest and the participants cannot be expected to always know the subtle difference between a clinician and an investigator. In some cultures, the clinician is seen as an authority figure and participants find it difficult to say no [40]. Medical care is often limited in LMICs and joining a clinical trial is a way for a participant to gain access to a scarce resource. In many LMICs there is still great uncertainty about the access to vaccines and the people are vulnerable and desperate for any type of help.

The Covid-19 pandemic has led to a massive socio-economic crisis with countless jobs lost. The exact economic effect of Covid-19 on LMICs, will not be discussed in this chapter, but in summary all can agree that the economic situation of many people living in LMICs is worse than ever. The monetary gain involved in being part of a clinical trial, when converted into the currency of the sponsor nation, is often seen as negligible and not considered a formal payment. For a participant in a LMIC, there is a higher probability that this payment might be a very strong motivator to join a clinical trial even if there are substantial risks. If the participant joins the trial as the only way to feed himself and his family, one could argue that it is not truly informed consent.

The WHO stated that sponsors are not ethically obliged to unblind subjects as soon as a different investigational vaccine becomes available [29, 31]. In South Africa, the vaccine roll-out for health care workers was via the Sisonke open label clinical trial. Outside of a clinical trial setting, there was no other way for a health care worker to get vaccinated. A small group of these health care workers were already participating in Covid-19 vaccine PCTs. This is another example of how participants in LMICs are motivated to participate in PCTs, because a 50% chance of getting the vaccine is still better than no chance at all. Even though, according to the WHO, sponsors were not obliged to unblind these participants, it would have caused a great ethical scandal if they were not given the option. In the author's experience, many participants made it clear that if they were denied unblinding, when they have a 100% chance of getting a vaccine elsewhere that is already authorised in several other countries, they would certainly withdraw from the PCT.

Ahmad and Dhrolia posed the following comparison. The question "Should we continue or permit placebo controlled vaccine trials for Covid-19 disease, when available vaccines have been found safe, efficacious and in use in many countries?" sounds very similar to "Should West African HIV-positive pregnant women receive placebo in HIV placebo-controlled trials when Zidovudine was found safe and efficacious for the prevention of vertical transmission of HIV infection elsewhere in the world?" or "Should African American men of Tuskegee, Alabama remain untreated even when penicillin was found safe and efficacious for the treatment of syphilis?" [40].

Any researcher who has attended training in Good Clinical Practice, should be familiar with these historical events, which serve as extreme examples of what should not happen during a clinical trial. They involve vulnerable, disadvantaged, poor populations with potentially life-threatening diseases. These populations do not have access to the standard of care that is available in higher income countries. They are trying to access interventions which the sponsors are able to provide, but deliberately chose not to do so.

Multiple Covid-19 vaccines have been found to be safe, efficacious and one of the only lifesaving interventions that would be able to end a pandemic. Over ten billion doses of vaccines have been administered globally [35]. The vaccine is freely available in high income countries, but only 9.5% of people in low-income countries have received at least one dose [51]. It could easily be argued that continuing to use PCTs in Covid-19 vaccines, and thus further exploiting the vulnerable pollution in LMICs, is no different to the West Africa or Tuskagee trials, and thus grossly unethical and a violation of human rights.

6. Conclusions

PCTs for a COVID-19 vaccine in vulnerable populations need to be reviewed with the above in mind. The onus of patient safety when looking to conduct clinical trials in vulnerable populations, which LMICs certainly are, should remain with the sponsor and country of origin that will benefit most from the data. Emphasis must be placed on autonomy; subjects need to understand what they are doing by participating. Cultural differences make this difficult and the need for community engagement is paramount. We have highlighted weakness in the ethical review process of LMICs, the lack of resources being a major factor. The COVID-19 pandemic has strained these resources further in all aspects, creating a need for investment in the health of LMICs by sponsors conducting clinical research. Necessary in these countries to bridge the health gap and provide healthcare access to the most impoverished of the world. We cannot however use this fact to exploit LMICs, the fact they are so desperate is more reason for sponsors to protect the communities, not less. The debate continues and each case will have its own nuance. The major points to take away are who benefits from the research, how will the local government use that research to generate national programs, are the communities adequately engaged throughout the process of clinical trials and what ethical frameworks, enforceable or otherwise, exist in the designated country where the trial will take place. Answering these questions will assist sponsors in maintaining ethical practice and protection of research participants in LMICs.

Conflict of interest

The authors declare no conflict of interest.

Author details

Lesley Burgess*, Jurie Johannes Jordaan and Matthew Wilson
TREAD Research, Cardiology Division, Department of Medicine, Tygerberg Hospital, Stellenbosch University, South Africa

*Address all correspondence to: lesley@treadresearch.com

References

[1] Miller FG, Brody H. What makes placebo-controlled trials unethical? The American Journal of Bioethics. 2002;**2**(2):3-9

[2] Millum J, Grady C. The ethics of placebo-controlled trials: Methodological justifications. Contemporary Clinical Trials. 2013;**36**(2):510-514. DOI: 10.1016/j.cct.2013.09.003

[3] Amdur RJ, Biddle CJ. An algorithm for evaluating the ethics of a placebo-controlled trial. International Journal of Cancer. 2001;**96**(5):261-269. DOI: 10.1002/ijc.1026

[4] Chiodo GT, Tolle SW, Bevan L. Placebo-controlled trials: Good science or medical neglect? The Western Journal of Medicine. 2000;**172**(4):271-273. DOI: 10.1136/ewjm.172.4.271

[5] Streiner DL. Placebo-controlled trials: when are they needed? Schizophrenia Research. 1999;**35**(3):201-210. DOI: 10.1016/s0920-9964(98)00126-1

[6] World Bank Official Definition of Low- and Middle-Income Countries. [Internet]. 2021. Available from: https://datahelpdesk.worldbank.org/knowledgebase/articles/906519-world-bank-country-and-lending-groups. [Accessed: 15 January 2022]

[7] World Medical Association. Declaration of Helsinki – Ethical Principles for Medical Research Involving Human Subjects. [Internet]. 2013. Available from: https://www.wma.net/policies-post/wma-declaration-of-helsinki-ethical-principles-for-medical-research-involving-human-subjects/. [Accessed: 20 January 2022]

[8] Bittker BM. The ethical implications of clinical trials in low- and middle-income countries; Human Rights Magazine; Vol. 46(4). The truth about science; 14 June 2021

[9] Burgess LJ, Pretorius D. FDA abandons the Declaration of Helsinki: The effect on the ethics of clinical trial conduct in South Africa and other developing countries. South African Journal of Bioethics and Law. 2012;**5**(2):87-90. DOI: 10.7196/SAJBL.222

[10] International Council for Harmonisation of Technical Requirements for Pharmaceuticals for Human Use (ICH). [Internet]. 2013. Available from: https://database.ich.org/sites/default/files/E6_R2_Addendum.pdf. [Accessed: 24 January 2022]

[11] Vieta E, Cruz N. Head to head comparisons as an alternative to placebo-controlled trials. European Neuropsychopharmacology. 2012;**22**(11):800-803. DOI: 10.1016/j.euroneuro.2011.11.011

[12] Miller FG. Placebo-controlled trials in psychiatric research: An ethical perspective. Biological Psychiatry. 2000;**47**(8):707-716. DOI: 10.1016/s0006-3223(00)00833-7

[13] Tramèr MR, Reynolds DJ, Moore RA, McQuay HJ. When placebo controlled trials are essential and equivalence trials are inadequate. British Medical Journal. 1998;**317**(7162):875-880. DOI: 10.1136/bmj.317.7162.875

[14] Christakis NA. Ethics are local: Engaging cross-cultural variation in the ethics for clinical research. Social Science and Medicine. 1992;**35**(9):1079-1091. DOI: 10.1016/0277-9536(92)90220-k

[15] Simon R. Are placebo-controlled clinical trials ethical or needed when

alternative treatment exists? Annals of Internal Medicine. 2000;**133**(6):474-475. [published correction appears in Ann Intern Med 2000 Nov 7;133(9):754]. DOI: 10.7326/0003-4819-133-6-200009190-00017

[16] Temple R, Ellenberg SS. Placebo-controlled trials and active-control trials in the evaluation of new treatments. Part 1: Ethical and scientific issues. Annals of Internal Medicine. 2000;**133**(6):455-463. DOI: 10.7326/0003-4819-133-6-200009190-00014

[17] Ellenberg SS, Temple R. Placebo-controlled trials and active-control trials in the evaluation of new treatments. Part 2: Practical issues and specific cases. Annals of Internal Medicine. 2000;**133**(6):464-470. DOI: 10.7326/0003-4819-133-6-200009190-00015

[18] Moodley K, Myer L. Health Research Ethics Committees in South Africa 12 years into democracy. BMC Medical Ethics. 2007;**8**:1. Published 2007 Jan 25. DOI: 10.1186/1472-6939-8-1

[19] Millum J. Post-trial access to antiretrovirals: Who owes what to whom? Bioethics. 2011;**25**(3):145-154. DOI: 10.1111/j.1467-8519.2009.01736.x

[20] Zhao Y, Fitzpatrick T, Wan B, Day S, Mathews A, Tucker JD. Forming and implementing Community Advisory Boards in low- and middle-income countries: A scoping review. BMC Medical Ethics. 2019;**20**(1):73. Published 2019 Oct 17. DOI: 10.1186/s12910-019-0409-3

[21] Davies SEH. The introduction of research ethics review procedures at a university in South Africa: Review outcomes of a social science research ethics committee. Research Ethics. 2020;**16**(1-2):1-26. DOI: 10.1177/1747016119898408

[22] de Zulueta P. Randomised placebo-controlled trials and HIV-infected pregnant women in developing countries. Ethical imperialism or unethical exploitation? Bioethics. 2001;**15**(4):289-311. DOI: 10.1111/1467-8519.00240

[23] Kulkarni P, Desai S, Tewari T, et al. A randomized Phase III clinical trial to assess the efficacy of a bovine-human reassortant pentavalent rotavirus vaccine in Indian infants. Vaccine. 2017;**35**(45):6228-6237. DOI: 10.1016/j.vaccine.2017.09.014

[24] Avasthi A, Ghosh A, Sarkar S, Grover S. Ethics in medical research: General principles with special reference to psychiatry research. Indian Journal of Psychiatry. 2013;**55**(1):86-91. DOI: 10.4103/0019-5545.105525

[25] Reddy P, Buchanan D, Sifunda S, James S, Naidoo N. The role of community advisory boards in health research: Divergent views in the South African experience. Journal of Social Aspects of HIV/AIDS. 2010;**7**(3):2-8. DOI: 10.1080/17290376.2010.9724963

[26] Carter C, Lan Anh NT, Notter J. COVID-19 disease: perspectives in low- and middle-income countries. Clinics in Integrated Care. 2020;**1**:1-9. DOI: 10.1016/j.intcar.2020.100005

[27] United Nations Office for the Coordination of Humanitarian Affairs, COVID-19 Data Explorer: Global Humanitarian Operations. Monthly Report, 31 December 2021 [Internet]. https://data.humdata.org/visualization/covid19-humanitarian-operations/. [Accessed: 31 March 2022]

[28] Thanh Le T, Andreadakis Z, Kumar A, et al. The COVID-19 vaccine development landscape. Nature Reviews Drug Discovery. 2020;**19**(5):305-306. DOI: 10.1038/d41573-020-00073-5

[29] WHO Ad Hoc Expert Group on the Next Steps for Covid-19 Vaccine Evaluation, Krause PR, Fleming TR, et al. Placebo-controlled trials of Covid-19 vaccines - Why we still need them. The New England Journal of Medicine. 2021;**384**(2):e2. DOI: 10.1056/NEJMp2033538

[30] Grady C, Shah S, Miller F, et al. So much at stake: Ethical tradeoffs in accelerating SARSCoV-2 vaccine development. Vaccine. 2020;**38**(41):6381-6387. DOI: 10.1016/j.vaccine.2020.08.017

[31] World Health Organisation Access to COVID-19 Tools Accelerator Ethics and Governance Working Group, Singh J. Emergency Use Designation of COVID-19 candidate vaccines: Ethical considerations for current and future COVID-19 placebo-controlled vaccine trials and trial unblinding Policy brief. 2020. DOI: 10.13140/RG.2.2.14560.30728

[32] Wendler D, Ochoa J, Millum J, Grady C, Taylor HA. COVID-19 vaccine trial ethics once we have efficacious vaccines. Science. 2020;**370**(6522):1277-1279. DOI: 10.1126/science.abf5084

[33] Sisa I, Noblecilla E, Orozco F. Rationale to continue approving placebo-controlled COVID-19 vaccine trials in LMICs. Lancet. 2021;**397**(10277):878. DOI: 10.1016/S0140-6736(21)00357-3

[34] Singh JA, Kochhar S, Wolff J, WHO ACT-Accelerator Ethics & Governance Working Group. Author Correction: Placebo use and unblinding in COVID-19 vaccine trials: Recommendations of a WHO Expert Working Group. Nature Medicine. 2021;**27**(5):925. DOI: 10.1038/s41591-021-01360-3

[35] Lenzer J. Covid-19: Should vaccine trials be unblinded? British Msedical Journal. 2020;**371**:m4956. Published 2020 Dec 29. DOI: 10.1136/bmj.m4956

[36] Covid 19 Vaccine Tracker: Approved Vaccines [Internet]. 2022. Available from: https://covid19.trackvaccines.org/vaccines/approved/ [Accessed: 07 February 2022]

[37] Ortiz-Millán G. Placebo-controlled trials of Covid-19 vaccines - Are they still ethical? Indian Journal of Medical Ethics. 2021;**VI**(2):1-8. DOI: 10.20529/IJME.2021.015

[38] Wiesing U, Ehni HJ. Placebo control in Covid-19 trials: A missed opportunity for international guidance. Indian Journal of Medical Ethics. 2021;**VI**(2):1-7. DOI: 10.20529/IJME.2021.022

[39] Ravinetto R. Problematic Covid-19 vaccine trials in times of vaccine nationalism. Indian Journal of Medical Ethics. 2021;**VI**(2):1-7. DOI: 10.20529/IJME.2021.014

[40] Ahmad A, Dhrolia MF. "No" to placebo-controlled trials of Covid-19 vaccines. Indian Journal of Medical Ethics. 2021;**VI**(2):1-7. DOI: 10.20529/IJME.2021.019

[41] Freedman B. Equipoise and the ethics of clinical research. The New England Journal of Medicine. 1987;**317**(3):141-145. DOI: 10.1056/NEJM198707163170304

[42] London AJ. Social value, clinical equipoise, and research in a public health emergency. Bioethics. 2019;**33**(3):326-334. DOI: 10.1111/bioe.12467

[43] Friesen P, Caplan AL, Miller JE. COVID-19 vaccine research and the trouble with clinical equipoise. Lancet. 2021;**397**(10274):576. DOI: 10.1016/S0140-6736(21)00198-7

[44] Alqahtani M, Mallah SI, Stevenson N, Doherty S. Vaccine trials during a pandemic: Potential approaches to ethical dilemmas. Trials.

2021;**22**(1):628. Published 2021 Sep 15. DOI: 10.1186/s13063-021-05597-8

[45] van der Graaf R, Cheah PY. Ethics of alternative trial designs and methods in low-resource settings. Trials. 2019;**20**(Suppl. 2):705. Published 2019 Dec 19. DOI: 10.1186/s13063-019-3841-2

[46] Bonati M. Restrictions on the use of placebo in new COVID-19 vaccine trials. European Journal of Clinical Pharmacology. 2022;**78**(1):147-148. DOI: 10.1007/s00228-021-03203-z

[47] Knottnerus JA. New placebo-controlled Covid-19 vaccine trials are ethically questionable; it's now about comparative effectiveness and availability of registered vaccines. Journal of Clinical Epidemiology. 2021;**133**:175-176. DOI: 10.1016/j.jclinepi.2021.03.006

[48] Hunt A, Saenz C, Littler K. The global forum on bioethics in research meeting, "ethics of alternative clinical trial designs and methods in low- and middle-income country research": Emerging themes and outputs. Trials. 2019;**20**(Suppl. 2):701. Published 2019 Dec 19. DOI: 10.1186/s13063-019-3840-3

[49] Browne JL, Rees CO, van Delden JJM, et al. The willingness to participate in biomedical research involving human beings in low- and middle-income countries: A systematic review. Tropical Medicine & International Health. 2019;**24**(3):264-279. DOI: 10.1111/tmi.13195

[50] WHO Vaccine Equity Declaration [Internet]. 2022. Available from: https://www.who.int/campaigns/vaccine-equity/vaccine-equity-declaration. [Accessed: 23 January 2022]

[51] Coronavirus (COVID-19) Vaccinations [Internet]. 2022. Available from: https://www.bloomberg.com/graphics/covid-vaccine-tracker-global-distribution/ [Accessed: 23 January 2022]

Chapter 17

Perspective Chapter: Tracking Trails of SARS CoV-2 – Variants to Therapy

Ankur Kumar, Manju O. Pai, Gaurav Badoni, Arpana Singh, Ankit Agrawal and Balram Ji Omar

Abstract

A virus when replicates itself from one generation to another, tends to change a little bit of its structure. These variations are called mutations. History says that SARS CoV-2 originated from the virus reservoirs of animals, specifically non-human mammals like bats and minks. Since then, there are evolutionary changes in its genome due to recombination in divergent strains of different species. Thus, making the virus more robust and smarter to sustain and evade immune responses in humans. Probably, this has led to the 2019 SARS CoV-2 pandemic. This chapter tracks the evolutionary trails of the virus origin, its pathogenesis in humans, and varying variants with the coming times. Eventually, the chapter overviews the available vaccines and therapies to be followed for SARS CoV-2.

Keywords: evolution, pathogenesis, variant, SARS CoV-2, vaccine

1. Introduction

At the end of the year, 2019 a pandemic was caused by a new human infecting coronavirus, also called severe acute respiratory syndrome coronavirus 2 or SARS CoV-2. The first case of this novel virus was reported in Wuhan city of China and later it spread all over the globe. COVID-19 is the disease caused by SARS-CoV-2, which is characterized by different levels of severity and a range of signs and symptoms mainly fever, cough epidemic, sore throat, sudden onset of anosmia, shortness of breath, nausea, vomiting, and diarrhea [1]. This was announced a 'public health emergency of international concern' by the International Health Regulations (IHR) Emergency Committee of the World Health Organization (WHO) [2]. To date, more than 6 million deaths are caused by this disease around the globe (WHO, Coronavirus Disease COVID-19 Dashboard, accessed on 14/04/2022). Coronaviruses are positive-sense single standard RNA viruses that come under the family of *Coronaviridae* and *Orthocoronavirinae* subfamily. They are enveloped viruses having spherical, oval, or pleomorphic genomic shapes. The subfamily is further divided into four genera: Alpha, Beta, Gamma, and Deltacoronavirus [3]. Coronaviruses are not new to humans, and most of them cause minor respiratory infections in humans. They have also been known to infect domesticated animals for decades [4]. However, since the beginning of the twenty-first century, they have emerged as a major threat to the human population. There were six coronaviruses (CoV) known till now, among which severe acute respiratory syndrome CoV (SARS CoV) and Middle East respiratory syndrome CoV (MERS CoV) outbreaks took the life of a large number of people in 2002 and 2012, respectively. SARS CoV first appeared in China in 2002, infecting 8422 people followed by 916 deaths. MERS CoV afterward emerged in Arabian nations and infected around 1800 people. In 2019, the seventh CoV produced a large-scale outbreak that affected nearly every country on the planet. The new coronavirus was called SARS CoV-2 since it is closely related to SARS CoV. SARS CoV-2 is spreading quicker than SARS CoV and MERS CoV, with an increasing number of deaths [5].

2. History

Since the discovery of the virus in China in late 2019, the SARS CoV-2 pandemic has progressed through numerous stages. Patients with pneumonia-like symptoms were reported from various local health institutions in Wuhan city of China in December 2019. The reason was unknown, and the majority of the patients came from Wuhan's sea/wet food market. The pathogen was identified and confirmed in the laboratory using real-time polymerase chain reaction, and next-generation sequencing. Because its genome did not entirely match any previously sequenced viral genome and the clinical signs were distinct from other recognized viral diseases, the virus was named 2019-nCov, where "n" stands for "novel" [5], and the disease was called COVID-19. The novel virus was classified as a Beta coronavirus based on the highly conserved protein-encoding open reading frame (ORF) 1a/1b sequence. As a result, the International Committee on Taxonomy of Viruses changed the nomenclature to SARS CoV- 2 [6].

3. Evolution

Based on mutation research, Li et al. [7] proposed that the virus appears to have emerged in late summer 2019 in China, and it may have invaded the West as early as October 2019. According to Dorp CH et al. [8], the illness spread globally most likely from the start of the epidemic. By Chaw SM et al. [9], SARS-CoV-2 spread cryptically well before the late 2019 outbreak in China, and Gambaro et al. [10] suspect the same for France. It is known that the SARS CoV-2 infection started in China, however, it is assumed that the virus arose in a mine in China in 2012, was collected in a laboratory, that may have escaped during manipulations in 2018 or 2019 [11]. This explanation might account for the virus's circulation before the epidemic; during this early era, the virus could have undergone unnoticed mutations.

4. Structure

Coronaviruses are members of the Coronavirinae subfamily of the Coronaviridae family, which includes four genera as mentioned earlier. CoVs have a single-stranded Positive-sense RNA genome (27–32 kb) which is bigger than any other kind of RNA virus. The capsid was formed outside the genome by the nucleocapsid protein

(N), and the genome is further packed by an envelope that is associated with three structural proteins: membrane protein (M), spike protein (S), and envelope protein (E) [12]. After the virus was confirmed to be the member of the coronavirus family, the genome size of SARS CoV-2 which was sequenced which approximately was found to be 29.9 kb [13]. Other than the structural proteins, SARS-CoV-2 contains 16 non-structural proteins (nsp1 to nsp16). Majorly, to mention a few, Nsp1 mediates RNA processing and replication. Nsp2 modulates the survival signaling pathway of the host cell. Nsp3 is believed to separate the translated protein. Nsp4 is a transmembrane domain 2 (TM2) protein thus promotes alterations in the endoplasmic reticulum membranes. Nsp5 participates in the polyprotein process during replication. Nsp6 is a likely transmembrane domain. The presence of Nsp7 and Nsp8 boosted the combination of Nsp12 with template-primer RNA. Nsp9 is a protein that binds to ssRNA. Nsp10 is required for viral mRNA cap methylation. Nsp12 includes the RNA-dependent RNA polymerase (RdRp), which is required for coronavirus replication/translation. Nsp13 binds ATP and the zinc-binding domain for replication and transcription. Nsp14 is an exoribonuclease proofreading domain. Endoribonuclease activity of Nsp15 is Mn (2+) dependent. Nsp16 is a 2'-Oribose methyltransferase [14, 15]. According to one study, NSP-mediated effects on splicing, translation, and protein trafficking can suppress host defenses. When infected with SARS CoV-2, NSP16 binds to the mRNA recognition domains of the U1 and U2 snRNAs, suppressing mRNA splicing. NSP1 binds to 18S ribosomal RNA in the ribosome's mRNA entry channel, interfering with mRNA translation. NSP8 and NSP9 bind to the 7SL RNA, which is found at the Signal Recognition Particle, causing protein trafficking to the cell membrane to be disrupted [16].

SARS CoV-2 virus contains a series of spike proteins on the surface. Microscopically, this virus appears like a crown, which gives rise to its name *corona,* which in Latin means crown [16, 17]. The structural and spike proteins are responsible for allowing the virus to attach to the membrane of the host cell. It contains a receptor binding domain that recognizes a specific receptor ACE-2 (Angiotensin Converting Enzyme- 2 Receptor), which is expressed in the lungs, heart, kidneys, and intestines [5, 18]. These proteins bind to the ACE-2 receptor with at least the same affinity and potentially as much as 20 times greater affinity than the SARS CoV-2 virus [6].

5. Pathogenesis

The structural proteins of this virion has specific roles for virus adhesion and invasion. The S glycoprotein mediates the viral particle's entrance phases, which include adhesion to the host cell membrane and fusion. S protein is formed as a homotrimer and inserted in numerous copies into the virion membrane, giving it a crown-like appearance. Many viruses utilize these similar glycoproteins for host entry including HIV-1, Ebola virus, and avian influenza viruses. This is split into two subunits: extracellular and transmembrane in infected cells (that is, the cleavage happens before the virus is released from the cell that generates it). Similarly, some coronaviruses break their S protein into S1 and S2 subunits during biosynthesis in infected cells, whereas other coronaviruses cleave their S protein only when they reach the next host cell. SARS- CoV-2 and MERS- CoV, come under the first category: its S protein is cleaved in virus-producing cells by proprotein convertases such as furin [19, 20]. As a result, the mature virion's S protein is made up of two non-covalently linked subunits: the S1 subunit binds ACE2 and the S2 subunit fixes the S protein to the membrane. The S2 subunit also contains a fusion peptide and other machinery required to promote membrane fusion during new cell infection.

Receptor interaction by viral entry glycoproteins, generally in conjunction with other triggers, causes substantial conformational changes in both subunits, bringing the viral and cellular membranes together and eventually forming a fusion hole that allows the viral DNA to access the cell cytoplasm. The cleavage of a second site internal to the S2 subunit, known as the 'S2′ site, 'is one such trigger for SARS-CoV-2. The virus exposes the S2′ location by engaging ACE2. Cleavage of the S2′ site by an enzyme called transmembrane protease, serine 2 (TMPRSS2) [21–23] at the cell surface or by cathepsin L in the endosomal compartment releases the fusion peptide, beginning fusion pore development. Because the viral genome requires access to the cytoplasm and can only do so when this hole develops and the viral and cell membranes merge perfectly, where each step of the procedure is essential.

6. Evolution of viral variants

Viruses are complex molecular structures with simple-looking morphology. They are just single-cell microorganisms containing genetic material either DNA or RNA [1]. That genetic material is made up of molecules that can be represented as a series of deoxy-ribonucleotides in the form of A = T (DNA), A = U (RNA), and G = C. Each part of this code contains instructions for how to make one specific protein that allows the virus to function. A virus has one goal that is, to make more of itself. But because it's not so simple, it cannot do that on its own. So, it uses a host. Every time a virus infects a person, it uses its cells to make copies of itself replicating this complex code again and again [1, 24]. But eventually, it makes a mistake, sometimes it deletes or adds a letter. Sometimes it flips them around. This mistake is called a mutation, which changes the instructions for making a virus. This slightly altered virus is a variant. Since viruses are constantly going through this copying process, it's normal for them to change over time [2, 25]. Most of the time mutations are harmless or even make the virus weaker, and they quietly disappear without making any notable difference. But when a series of mutations occur it gives the virus a slight edge over us. If a particular set of mutations makes a variant more successful, it might become more prominent than others and that's when it gets noticed. That is how the scientists started to notice SARS CoV2, back in September of 2020 [3, 4]. oronaviruses are covered in spike proteins that they use to bind with and infect human cells. The thing is, that binding is not a perfect fit. So, it does not always get past the cell's defenses. But the B.1.1.7 variant, which scientists later renamed the "Alpha" variant, has multiple mutations on the spike protein: Mutations that make it easier for the virus to bind with cells [5, 6, 26],help make the virus more transmissible. Which led it to become a dominant strain in many places around the world. But SARS CoV2 has been mutating all along. It's important to remember that a virus does not make active decisions. It creates strategy within the cells [17]. Mutations are random errors. But the longer a virus is around, the more people it infects, the more it will change and the more those changes accumulate and the virus evolves into something more dangerous. Alpha, Beta, Gamma, Omicron, and Delta are five variants considered as "variants of concern" by the W.H.O. All have mutations on the spike protein [2–4]. Delta, the most recent addition to this list, has been referred to as a "double mutant," because, while it has many different mutations, it has two significant mutations (L452R & E484Q). These two mutations seem to make the virus more transmissible. Variant strains of the virus make it easier for the virus to re-infect people who have already had Covid-19, meaning that variants may have evolved to dodge natural immune responses [17, 27]. The Omicron variant of COVID-19 is spreading more rapidly in comparison to other strains because it has more mutations majority of them on the spike proteins. The new omicron variant BA-2 appears to be about 50% more transmissible in comparison to the original omicron BA-1 and causes same severity of disease [2, 3]. BA-1 strain of omicron is more infectious in younger people and according to reports several people have been infected with omicron BA-1 and within a month infection with omicron BA-2. It appeared that this version of omicron was either highly infectious that it could overcome vaccine load or previous infection immunity, or it can evade immunity due to the mutation that it has evolved with [5, 27]. It was also more contagious compared to the Delta variants, as it quickly became the dominant strain in the US. W.H.O said it expects that people can spread omicron even if they are vaccinated or do not have symptoms [3, 6, 26]. Viruses multiply by copying their genomes over and over, but as an old photocopier, these copies are not always perfect. Each of these imperfect copies is a variant. Normally the imperfections or mutations do not change how the virus behaves and they can often make it less successful than the original strain [25, 28]. But very rarely mutations can change the virus in some important ways. The more a virus is allowed to replicate unchecked, the more chance it has to accumulate these rare beneficial mutations [2, 18]. That can occur when viruses are allowed to spread quickly through a population, or if they encounter an immune compromised host.

7. Coronavirus and its new variants

Epidemiologists may even decide to label it as 'Variant of Concern' (VOC), like the examples identified in Brazil, South Africa, and the UK. For months, scientists have been striving to work out what's changed in these variants, and what those changes mean. Because a variant spreading does not necessarily mean that it has an advantageous mutation. For example, a small number of people could, by chance, move a variant from one region to another, like tourists traveling back from popular vacation spots. This could cause that variant to start spreading in a new location even though there may be no significant change to the biology of the virus. This is called the 'Founder Effect'. On November 5th, 2020, the United Kingdom went into lockdown [4, 18]. But, despite having the same lockdown measures, infections in Kent, an area outside of London, were still rising. In early December, the overall drop in cases led the country to relax restrictions anyway and then this happened [5]. It was not until around this time that researchers realized that somewhere in Kent, the virus itself had changed. It was a new variant. It was more contagious and it was spreading. By the time scientists gave it a name called B.1.1.7, it had spread to most of southeast England [18]. Two months later it was in 30 other countries. Five months later, it was the most common form of the virus found in the United States [6]. Lately, more and more variants are emerging in various places around the world. XE is a new variant of omicron and it is first detected in the UK. After successful detection of the XE variant, W.H.O has issued a warning against XE. It has been suggested that the variant could be more transmissible than any Covid-19 strain so far. XE is a combination of recombinants of both sub-variants (BA.1 and BA.2) of Omicron. Understanding why a variant has emerged requires a combination of studies. Epidemiology can help detect and trace new variants and flag new or worrying patterns of infection. Meanwhile, lab studies can start to pinpoint how the mutations are changing the properties of the virus [5, 18, 25]. Some variants are faster spreading like the D614G mutation, known to virologists as Doug. It spread widely in the early days of the pandemic and can be seen in almost all variants [2, 17]. It affects the spike protein that coronavirus particles use to penetrate cells. N501Y also known as Nelly, is another spike protein mutation that appears to be associated with increased transmissibility. This mutation has been detected in the B.1.1.7, B.1.351, and P.1 strains - all variants of concern [5, 26]. The worry of so-called 'immune escape' has also been indicated with another spike protein mutation, E484K or Eek. Eek has been spotted in B.1.351 and P.1, the variants detected in South Africa and Brazil. Lab studies early in 2021 showed that the variant could evade some virus-blocking antibodies, while trials in South Africa suggested that the variant reduced the efficacy of several vaccines [28, 29]. Despite these worries, the coronavirus is mutating very slowly compared to something like influenza and it seems like the vaccines developed so far will remain at least partly effective. It is very important to monitor and trace the emergence of variants and that is not always simple to do [3, 18]. Organizations like the COVID -19 genomics UK consortium or COG-UK, have stepped up their efforts to combine fast sequencing with efficient data sharing. COG-UK has already sequenced over 400,000 SARS-CoV-2 genomes [3–5]. Next step for researchers is the need to look forward to how these mutated strains of SARS CoV-2 could affect global vaccination efforts. Existing vaccines can be redesigned and combinations of vaccines are also being tested but it could be difficult to perform reliable clinical trials amid the ongoing vaccination programmes. Public health policies such as track and trace, social distancing, and vaccine rollouts are powerful tools to interrupt, transmit and keep tabs on new variants [17, 28, 30]. After all, every time the virus is prevented from spreading, it's also prevented from mutating, nipping new variants in the bud before they even have a chance to develop.

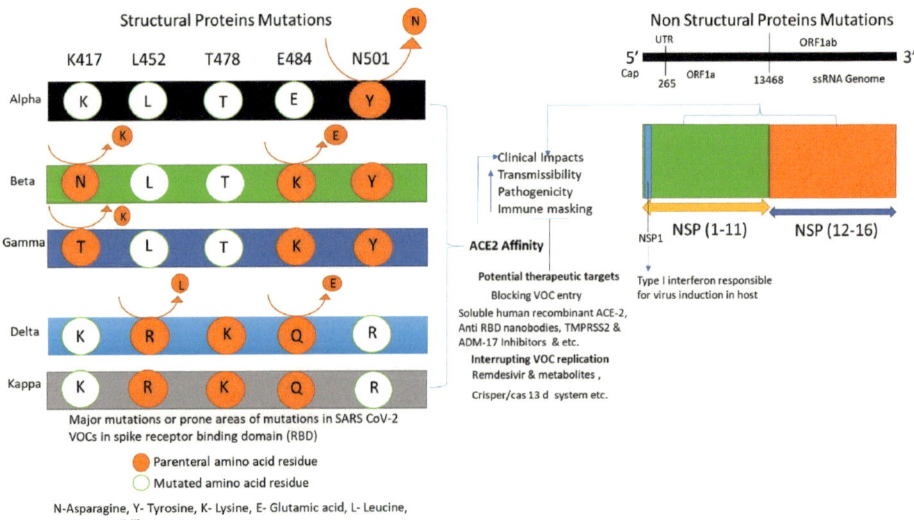

Figure 1.

Diagrammatic representation of mutations in different regions of SARS CoV-2 giving rise to different variants. Amino acid substitutions are depicted in both structural and non-structural proteins of SARS CoV-2, which modify their affinity to ACE2 receptors, thus making them VOC.

The hotspots and the mechanism of replacement of amino acids that bring about mutations at specific points in the SP's and NSP's have been shown in **Figure 1**. S1 and NSPs are thus considered hotspots for mutations that may have high clinical relevance in terms of virulence, transmissibility, and host immune evasion. NSPs are mostly biocatalyst or catalytic proteins or enzymes that induce viral replication and methylation and may play a critical role in host responses to infection. These genes are encoded in two important groups, namely ORF1a (NSP1-11), and ORF1b (NSP12-16). NSP1 is a principal protein to antagonizes type I interferon induction in the host and benefits the replication of the virus itself. The variants of concern (VOCs) have impacted the global health significantly, especially in the later year of 2020. The major ones are Alpha variant (B.1.1.7), Beta (B.1.351), Gamma (P.1), Kappa and Delta (B.1.617.1 and B.1.617.2) (**Table 1**). **Figure 1** also tries to depict the important mutations in these VOCs, for example, the Alpha variant has an N501 mutation, N asparagine has been replaced with Y tyrosine, as well as K417 where the lysine K is replaced with asparagine N (**Figure 1**). Another emerging variant derived from B.1.1.7 also carries E484 mutation where the glutamic acid E is replaced with lysine K. Both Beta and Gamma variants have more substitutions other than N501. The Beta variant has E484, while the Gamma variant has the E484 and the K417 mutations. The latest variants Delta, and Kappa share two mutations E484 (glutamic acid E substituted by glutamine Q) and L452 (leucine L altered by arginine R). Other than the two mutations above, Delta also harbors a unique mutation, T478 (threonine T replaced by lysine K) (**Figure 1**) [31].

Variants and their name according to W.H.O	Scientific Name	Canonical Mutations	Country, where first documented	References
Alpha	B.1.1.7	N501Y, 69/70 deletion, P681H	South-eastern England	[3, 6–8, 13]
Beta	B.1.351	K417N, N501Y, E484K	South Africa and Nigeria	[2–4, 7, 13]
Gamma	P.1	K417T, E484K, and N501Y	Brazil	[2, 5, 7, 13]
Delta	B.1.617.2	L452R, T478K, D614G and P681R	India	[3, 6–8, 13]
Omicron	B.1.1.529	N679K, H655Y, and P681H	South Africa	[4, 5, 10, 13]
Epsilon	B.1.427 and B.1.429	S13I, W152C, L452R. D614G	USA	[6, 7, 13]
Theta	P.3	—	Philippines	[7]
Zeta	P.2	—	Brazil	[7, 8]
Mu	B.1.621	—	Colombia	[5, 7]
Eta	B.1.525	—	Nigeria	[3, 7]
Iota	B.1.526	—	USA	[7]
XE	—	—	UK	—

Table 1.
Different variants of coronavirus with scientific names.

8. Variants and their effects on pathogenesis

Coronavirus is a large family of viruses, which are found in humans and animals [32, 33]. These viruses have had two large-scale outbreaks in the past two decades the SARS virus in 2002 and the MERS (Middle East Respiratory Syndrome) virus in 2012 [34–36]. It's generally been considered that these coronaviruses could cause future disease outbreaks because they are known to be able to evolve with animals and then jump to humans as an intermediate host in SARS. Palm civets and raccoon dogs were identified as the intermediate [37, 38]. According to the current mortality index total cases worldwide are found at 52.3 Cr and deaths confirmed at 62.7 L [34, 39]. The top five nations in terms of deaths in order are the US, India, Mexico, Brazil, and Russia. The UK has a much smaller number of deaths in comparison to these five countries. The highest number of cases are found in the US approximately 8.29 Cr and deaths confirmed 10 L. Coronavirus spreads mainly by respiratory droplets, cough, and sneezing. The aerosol-carrying virus allows it to travel into nasal or all cavities and it can live on surfaces for hours and even up to a few days on some surfaces [32, 35]. Infected touch can transfer the virus to mucous membranes in the eyes, mouth, nose, and upper airway [34, 35]. With that, symptoms arise like the common cold, stuffy nose, headache, sore throat, and fever [40, 41]. It is within the mucosal epithelium of the upper GI tract where primary viral replication is thought to occur similar to SARS CoV-2 is able to get further into the human respiratory system and lung's epithelial cells [38, 42]. ACE-2 receptor interaction with SARS CoV-2 binds S protein to the ACE-2 receptor, this mechanism of binding is followed t in the same way in airway epithelial cells [37, 43, 44]. The host cells have proteases that break down proteins and these cleave spike protein, this process activates a protein to trigger the process of membrane fusion before injecting the viral genome into the host cell [45, 46]. This mechanism is similar to direct cellular entry that facilitates cell entry in the influenza virus. The virus may also enter the cell via endocytosis, where it is engulfed and surrounded by an area of the cell membrane [39, 47]. Further down it forms a vesicle inside the host cell where specific RNA and proteins are synthesized within the cytoplasm [46, 48]. Viral proteins are assembled with the blueprint of information contained within viral RNA using hosts cellular machinery specifically ER and Golgi apparatus with specific processes to form envelope glycoproteins [40, 48]. New variants are assembled by fusing to plasma membranes and released as vesicles via exocytic secretory processes. The stress is placed on cells by a viral infection and the interaction of the immune system with viral antigens presented by infected host cells leads to cell death [47, 49, 50]. During this process of cell death, multiple inflammatory mediators are released and create an inflammatory response leading to a buildup of mucus. Thickening and hyperplasia of cells within airways this inflammation causes irritation of cells lining airways, which leads to cough [42, 51, 52]. In the lower respiratory tract, the virus acts within the lungs to get into the trachea or windpipe this branch is further bifurcated into the left and right main bronchi these bronchi branch into lobar bronchi. Bronchi have three sub-branches here one on the right and two on left, these branches are further segmented into segmental bronchi [49, 51, 53]. The segmental bronchi further branches into respiratory bronchiole and after that respiratory bronchiole culminate in tiny alveoli. COVID-19 infection may lead to inflamed alveolar walls, that get thickened and fill the alveolus with fluid, which can impair their ability to exchange gases [29, 40]. This can lead to the symptom of shortness of breath in some people infected with COVID-19 [38, 39].

DOI: http://dx.doi.org/10.5772/intechopen.106472

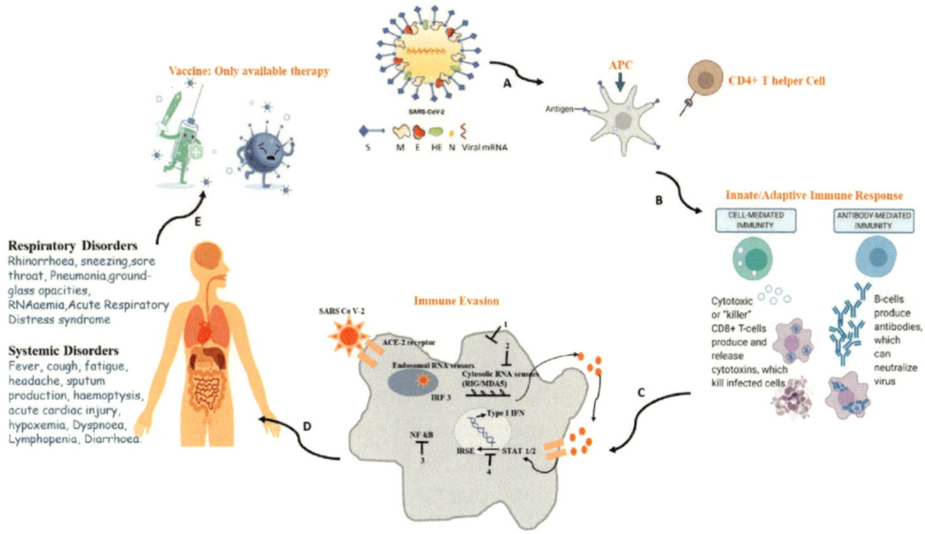

Figure 2.
A summarized cycle of SARS CoV-2 depicting (a) different parts of SARS CoV-2 virus (S = spike, M = membrane, E = envelope, viral mRNA, N = nuclear material) being represented on antigen presenting cells (APC) and T helper cells, (B) further initiating the immune responses in the human body that may be cell-mediated or antibody-mediated/innate or adaptive immunity (C) shows the potential immune evasion mechanisms. This shows a common evasion shared by all three respiratory viruses (SARS-CoV, MERS-CoV, and SARS-CoV-2). (1 and 2) shows hindrance created by coronaviruses during RNA sensing, starting the innate immune response and interferon (IFN-1) production. (3) shows the STAT1/2 activation leading to downstream activation of IFN/IFNAR (4) as sown by blocking marks. This blocking or oppression results in the decrease of interferon production thus impacting the adaptive immune response. Thus, helping the persistence of the virus in the host cells thus aggravates immune responses which may lead to immune exhaustion and immune suppression. (D) Shows the type and severity of disease manifestations inside the human host (E) indicates vaccine as the only available therapy which is helping in controlling this fatal viral infection.

Viruses can lead to an exaggerated immune response with a huge release of pro-inflammatory mediators causing, which is known as a cytokine storm or cytokine release syndrome. Cytokines are small proteins involved in cell signaling and crucial in mediating immune responses [39, 52]. The cascade of inflammatory mediators causes an uncontrolled systemic inflammatory response, which leads to acute respiratory distress syndrome or ARDS is the rapid and widespread inflammation of the lungs [47, 48]. ARDS causes epithelial and endothelial cells of the lungs to secrete inflammatory mediators, which fill the alveoli and allow these inflammatory signaling cells to recruit other cells of the immune system into the alveoli [50]. It further amplifies the problem and systemic inflammatory state causing increased capillary permeability, resulting in more fluid entering in alveoli causing pulmonary e dema [39, 50, 54]. Compounding the problem overall this pathological process severely impairs the ability of the lungs to exchange oxygen and carbon dioxide. This whole cycle of SARS CoV-2 invasion in general, pathogenesis, disease outcome, and current therapy has been illustrated in **Figure 2**.

9. Available therapy

COVID-19 is one virus that causes serious breathing difficulties other than common flu-like symptoms. Patients who have trouble breathing may be given supplemental oxygen, if the oxygen alone is insufficient to help the patient breathe then the patients are put on mechanical ventilation such as BiPAP, and in some situations, they may need to intubate and oxygenate the patient through conventional ventilators [37, 53]. Individual treatment depends heavily on their health condition and the resources available at a time. Remdesivir is an antiviral drug, which disrupts the virus's ability to replicate and spread within the body [55]. Remdesivir specifically is recommended for patients, who have been hospitalized and require oxygen but are not on mechanical ventilation. Globally remdesivir is in short supply and many health institutions have very limited quantities of it. Dexamethasone is a corticosteroid drug that makes adjustments to how the immune system regulates itself [55, 56]. Dexamethasone or other glucocorticoids similar to it can be used in patients, who need oxygen and can be used on patients who are on mechanical ventilation or non-mechanical ventilation [57]. However, patients who are not on supplemental oxygen are not recommended to take dexamethasone as the side effects of the drug may worsen their condition [41, 54, 58]. There have been some proposed treatment solutions like the use of blood plasma of patients, who have recovered from COVID-19 also called convalescent plasma [58, 59]. But this therapy could not find much success in seriously sick patients with COVID-19. In the spring of 2020, there was a lot of news coverage regarding the use of chloroquine and hydroxychloroquine to treat severe covid-19 patients [23, 60]. In August of 2020, the National Institute of Health issued a statement that recommended against using these drugs as initial trials in Covid-19 had either shown no benefit at all or had led to worst outcomes for patients due to drugs with dangerous side effects [59, 61, 62]. In 2021 India has begun to roll out an antibody cocktail drug therapy for COVID-19 patients and a similar therapy was used to treat former US president, Sir Donald Trump. This was a cocktail of two drugs, casirivimab and imdevimab [63]. The cocktail therapy claims to reduce hospitalization and death in Covid-19 patients by 70%. Each patient's dose is 1200 mg (600 mg of casirivimab and 600 mg of imdevimab) and the price of each patient's dose will be around 60,000 rupees [63–66]. Majority of these drugs are a recipe of monoclonal or artificial antibodies that are generated by cloning a unique white blood cell [67]. These amalgamated antibodies are designed in such a way that they can well bind to the spike protein of SARS CoV-2 and fight against the infection. But the effectiveness of these antibodies is limited to Covid-19 patients with mild to moderate symptoms [64, 65, 68]. Its effectiveness shows best when given during the first seven days of the infection when the virus is multiplying. Thus the viral entry at this time point is ceased. This therapy is not advised for severe Covid-19 patients, who require oxygen therapy [54, 56, 68].

10. Vaccine against SARS CoV-2 and its efficacy

Researchers are racing towards the goal of delivering a safe and effective vaccine that could curb COVID-19 [69]. Production and scale-up for some of the vaccines have already started. New technologies are genetic vaccines and viral vector vaccines [70]. A lot of investment in them has especially focused on their potential to combat emerging infectious diseases and COVID-19 is putting that potential to test [15, 71]. Scientists developed a successful influenza vaccine was in 1953 where they injected viruses into fertilized eggs, which were then incubated to allow viral replication within the eggs [72]. These replicated viruses are then explored for developing two classical vaccine formulations, where the virus is either weakened (Live attenuated virus) or killed (Whole inactivated virus) live attenuated and whole inactivated virus vaccines. These are [34, 70, 72]. These approaches are still in use today, although different cell cultures have replaced the use of eggs. At the current time, vaccinology has introduced multiple other approaches to develop vaccines [71]. This has been summarized in **Figure 3**. Major types of vaccines being deployed against COVID-19 are genetic vaccines, protein subunits, virus-like particles, viral vector vaccines, live attenuated viruses, and whole inactivated virus vaccines [70, 73]. Because of previous research on SARS and MERS, researchers only focus initial attention on the S protein of the SARS CoV-2 virus that is necessary for viral entry into human cells [35, 74]. So, a vaccine that exposes the immune system to just a spike should induce a protective response and that is the strategy behind the majority of COVID-19 vaccines. A comparison between conventional vaccines (that contain the whole virus) and genetic vaccines is interesting. Researchers can take genetic material either as m-RNA or DNA, that codes spike protein and explore this for vaccine development [75]. Two types of genetic vaccines are being investigated for COVID-19, i.e. m-RNA and DNA vaccines. mRNA needs to reach the cytoplasm of host cells, while DNA needs to enter the nucleus. Then this genetic material gets taken up by cell machinery, and cells express spike protein [74, 75]. These spike proteins are recognized by the immune system, hopefully stimulating a protective response. Naked mRNA cannot easily cross cell membranes passively, and it's very susceptible to degradation [32, 43]. In vaccines, mRNA coding for the spike is encased in small carrier molecules called lipid nanoparticles [44, 75]. The goal is to induce immunity against the target antigen, the added genetic cargo. But these vaccines may also induce immunity to the vector itself and viruses used as vectors are attenuated or weakened, so they cannot cause disease. A lot of different viruses have been developed as vectors, and they can be broadly categorized into two types, replication-defective and replication-competent [74, 76]. A very popular choice among potential COVID-19 vaccines is adenoviruses as these viruses are common pathogens that typically cause mild cold or flu-like symptoms [77].

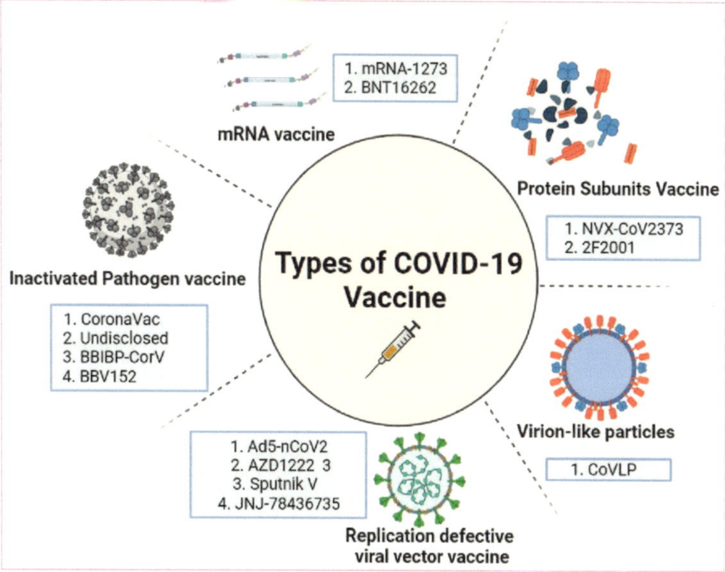

Figure 3.
The diagrammatical representation shows the different types of vaccines against COVID-19.

Lots of vaccines with adenovirus vector carries DNA coding for the spike to host cells., but it does not display on its surface. Once the virus infects a host cell, it delivers DNA to the nucleus, cells machinery expresses spikes using this DNA which is to genetic vaccines [77, 78]. Adenovirus vectors are replication defective, after the virus infects a cell no more viruses are produced [78]. Replication competent virus vectors used recombinant vesicular stomatitis virus. The wild-type VSV is usually asymptomatic in humans or it causes a mild flu-like illness. Scientists attempted to replace part of the RNA sequence with spike coding RNA of the virus genome [32, 40, 77]. Once the virus (rVSV) infects the host cell, cell machinery starts expressing a spike. This phenomenon mimics a real viral attack more closely [44, 78]. Adenovirus vectors, which are much further ahead in COVID-19 trials, have never been used in an FDA-approved vaccine and there are likewise no FDA-approved DNA or RNA vaccines.

11. Vaccines and their efficacy

A lot of viral evolution just comes down to statistics and a particular mutation that may confer the ability of the virus to make more copies of itself or to be stickier to cells. After that over time, it becomes more predominant in the population, because of that selective advantage it has and this is exactly what has happened with variants being detected around the globe [71, 79]. The variants reported are usually designated by their regions or locations where they were first found (B.1.17, B.1.351, P.1, and B.1.427/B.1.429). For example, some detected in California, South Africa, etc. [38, 80] (summarized in **Table 2**). But some variants were simultaneously found in

Vaccine Name	Clinical trial Number	Manufacture	Phage	Number of Participants	Immunity response	Efficacy
mRNA-1273	NCT04470427	MODERNA/ NIAID	3	30,000	CD4+ T-cell activation reported (Th1 skewed phenotype	94.10%
BNT 162b2	NCT04368728	BioNTech/Pfizer	3	44,000	Virus specific Th1 and CD8+ T cell responses reported	95%
Ad5-nCoV	NCT04526990	CanSino Biological	3	40,000	T-cell responses were observed in 88% of the participants	—
AZD1222	NCT04540393	AstraZeneca	3	30,000	T-cell responses were observed in all participants	62.10%

Vaccine Name	Clinical trial Number	Manufacture	Phage	Number of Participants	Immunity response	Efficacy
Sputnik V	NCT04530396	Gamaleya Research Institute	3	40,000	CD4+ and CD8+ T cell responses were observed in all participants	—
JNJ-78436735	NCT04505722	Janssen Pharmaceutical	3	90,000	CR4+ T cell responses in 80% of the participants	—
CoronaVac	NCT04456596	Sinovac Research & Development Co.	3	8870	Not Reported	—
BBIBP-CorV	NCT04560881	Beijing Institute of Biotechnology	3	63,000	Not Reported	79.38%
BBV152	CTRI/2020/11/028976	Bharat Biotech	3	26,000	Virus -specific CD4+ and CD8+ T cell responses Reported	—
NVX-CoV2373	NCT04611802	Novavax	3	45,000	CD4+ T cell activation in all tested participants	—
CoVLP	NCT04636697	Medicago	3	30,612	Not Reported	—

Table 2.
Advanced SARS-CoV-2 vaccine candidates.

many locations at the same time like a variant was first detected in the UK, South Africa, and Brazil which were already circulating in the US. This dilemma is still unanswered and may dampen the effectiveness of available vaccines [46, 66, 81]. When researchers talk about vaccine efficacy, a lot of attention is paid to antibodies, specifically neutralizing antibodies. The leading COVID-19 vaccines all induce neutralizing antibodies, which bind to the virus at a few different sites on spike proteins called epitopes [43, 81]. These neutralizing antibodies thus block the virus attachment to cells but to contrary, the evolving mutations in the virus are most worrisome in terms of vaccines, as they affect neutralizing antibody binding sites on spikes [81]. So, the first step in understanding how a variant will impact vaccine effectiveness is to analyze where the mutations are. But while this provides important clues, it does not give the full picture. **Table 2** below summarizes the available vaccines till now and their efficacy.

12. Testing variants against serum

Researchers and physicians have also explored different components of blood for imparting immunity to the Covid-19 affected patients. Serum, a component of blood that contains antibodies was taken from a vaccinated individual and combined with the virus in the lab, to see if antibodies contained in the serum block virus from infecting cells [82, 83]. There is currently no centralized system for testing all different vaccine sera against all different variants. Most studies have been small, and have primarily focused on mRNA vaccines [82, 84]. B.1.1.7 variant was first detected in the UK; and the B.1.351 variant was detected in South Africa, where serum testing showed a reduction of about six-fold in antibody sensitivity [85]. The other variants of concern currently identified by the CDC are P.1, which was first detected in travelers from Brazil, and two variants first detected in California B.1.427 and B.1.429 [85, 86]. Fewer studies are available on these variants, but current data indicate that the reduction in antibody sensitivity is somewhere between B.1.1.7 and B.1.351 [85]. Overall researchers need more laboratory data. But even when larger studies become available on all different variants and vaccine sera, these data may prove inconclusive [83]. Testing against serum samples has limitations. A big one is that antibodies are only one part of the immune response. In serum, the patient will not have our T cells, the patient will not even have our memory B cells or plasma cells that might be important just for antibody response [87, 88]. So, a lot is missing and that makes it hard to determine how a decrease in antibody sensitivity of 6 fold, in the lab, translates to vaccine effectiveness in the real world [86, 89]. Given these limitations to laboratory testing, it is of paramount importance to collect data on the ground. One example of such data would be sequencing variants infecting people, who become seriously ill with COVID-19 despite being vaccinated [84]. Another source of ground data is ongoing and recently completed vaccine clinical trials. ChAdOx1 nCoV-19 derived vaccine did not fare well in South Africa, where B.1.351 variant dominated, and South Africa halted its distribution in February [89, 90]. ChAdOx1 nCoV-19 derived vaccine is close to filling for authorization in the US and this vaccine is already being distributed elsewhere, including in the UK, and Europe by WHO [89]. Another vaccine that was tested in South Africa is from protein subunit vaccine, this vaccine is not yet being distributed, but it is getting close to filling for authorization in the UK, the US, and elsewhere. The most recent update read out of data suggests that while the protein subunit vaccine was almost 90% effective in the UK, it was much less effective in South Africa about 49 or 55% depending on whether or not people include participants infected with HIV [74, 90, 91]. A vaccine made by a piece of a modified virus is now being distributed in the US, reports a similar trend. This vaccine was 72% effective at preventing moderate to severe disease in US 28 days after vaccination. In South Africa, that number was only 64% [90]. But importantly this vaccine's efficacy against the severe disease was similarly high across regions [74, 84]. The currently available data indicate that while variants do pose a real threat to vaccine effectiveness, the available vaccines remain potent tools in fighting the pandemic. But researchers and public health experts also stress, that there will be more SARS- CoV-2 variants [92]. This underscores the importance of a global approach to surveillance, tracking, and vaccine development. But CDC Director Dr. Rochelle Walensky has emphasized the need to scale up surveillance across the US. In early January 2021, there were 250 samples a week that were being sequenced. In addition, CDC, NIH, vaccine procedures, and other groups are already discussing and collecting data on various vaccine strategies for combatting variants [92]. One potential strategy is a booster shot that would expose the human body to viral spike protein from the newer, resistant variant. This would stimulate the immune system to produce antibodies specific to the new variant in addition to an extra protective cushion for protection against other variants as well [88, 93, 94]. Studies evaluating both booster approaches have already started. Other strategies may also be like a bivalent vaccine, which induces an immune response to two different antigens with one shot. Such a vaccine could induce immunity to two different variants or two viral proteins from the same variant [79, 95]. But while such strategies are important to evaluate, the most significant way to mitigate the threat posed by variants is to reduce the community spread of SARS CoV-2. The way to decrease the amount of virus circulating is to get as many people vaccinated as possible, as quickly as possible, and to continue preventive measures like mask wearing and physical distancing [84, 95].

13. Future predictions of COVID-19

The continuous emergence of different variants of SARS CoV-2 has shown us that this coronavirus has high replication potential than other RNA viruses, due to which with every transmission and spread, the rate of mutation increases. Though predicting the future of an ongoing pandemic can never be explained with confidence and surety, still, possible future scenarios of COVID-19 can be explained [96–99].

1. The most important apprehension regarding this pandemic is that this will not end up with a sudden break in the coming times. Mini waves will keep coming, where we will face manifestations from severe disease, with high levels of infection to milder disease symptoms. Though the recent COVID-19 infection in the past 3 years and vaccination will provide herd immunity, still the diagnostic surveillance should go on.

2. As discussed earlier the other possible scenario of this pandemic in the near future can be its transition to the epidemic, where it will follow the story of the Influenza virus. It has been seen in the past years that 2% of the annual global deaths (out of which 2/3rd of the people above the age of 65) are because of respiratory illness which majorly includes flu. And if this is compared with SARS Co V-2 infection, the availability of vaccine and effective monoclonal antibody therapies (70–85% effective), gives an optimistic view of COVID-19 infections in the future. There is still high scope of more effective therapies against COVID-19 coming down the lane, thus keeping a positive approach towards decreasing SARS CoV-2 infections in the approaching times.

3. The other future scenario of SARS Co V-2 can be its transition from a pandemic to an endemic. As seen in the past with other coronaviruses like MERS and SARS, which got restricted to different pocket areas of the world and people of different ethnicity. Though there is limited data that supports the above information, it is therefore not possible to predict with confidence what adaptation SARS CoV-2 will take with time.

These future predictions of SARS CoV-2 virus spread and recurrence of COVID-19 will depend on one or all of these important facts: 1. Epidemiological tracking (updated data on continuous surveillance of the disease and its global spread); 2. Updated data on its pathogenicity, virulence, and variation in disease severity globally; 3. A continuous inflow of funds worldwide for more research in the development of efficient targeted therapies for COVID-19 [100].

14. Conclusion

The world has witnessed the recent pandemic of SARS CoV-2 and it is difficult to see that the world will return to pre-covid life any time soon. Although the global vaccination drive has brought this fatal respiratory infection under control, still SARS CoV-2 trajectory is yet to form a plateau. It is anticipated that with the transition of this pandemic to an endemic, uncertainties will remain with the human population. The persistence of this endemic virus in different pockets of the world may rise as a seasonal epidemic flu with some susceptible individuals who might succumb to its infection if immunocompromised or with waning levels of immunity.

We all share a beautiful world and as wisely said by "Sir Mahatma Gandhi", "Unity to be real must stand the severest strain without breaking". This pandemic has taught the world to be unanimous, be it in fighting against this disease by imposing national and international lockdowns to cease the spread of the disease or helping each other by providing daily bread and needs to the jobless migrants and affected people. Furthermore, the inflow of funds among different nations for rapid and continuous research led to the development of globally effective vaccines in the shortest time. The whole world stands together and looks forward to their respective contributions to keep an eye on the trajectory of COVID-19 so that we can reach the plateau with more effective strategies to combat COVID-19 and any more such pandemics in the near future if any.

Author details

Ankur Kumar[1], Manju O. Pai[1], Gaurav Badoni[1], Arpana Singh[1], Ankit Agrawal[2] and Balram Ji Omar[1*]

1 Department of Microbiology, AIIMS Rishikesh, India

2 Department of Anasthesia, AIIMS Rishikesh, India

*Address all correspondence to: balram.micro@aiimsrishikesh.edu.in

References

[1] World Health Organization. Naming the coronavirus disease (COVID-19) and the virus that causes it. Brazilian Journal of Implantology and Health Sciences. 2020;**2**(3):1-4

[2] Baj J, Karakuła-Juchnowicz H, Teresiński G, Buszewicz G, Ciesielka M, Sitarz E, et al. COVID-19: Specific and non-specific clinical manifestations and symptoms: The current state of knowledge. Journal of Clinical Medicine. 2020;**9**(6):1753

[3] Cui J, Li F, Shi ZL. Origin and evolution of pathogeniccoronaviruses. Nature Reviews. Microbiology. 2019;**17**:181-192

[4] Corman VM, Lienau J, Witzenrath M. Coronaviruses as thecause of respiratory infections. Internist (Berl). 2019;**60**:1136-1145

[5] Zhu N, Zhang D, Wang W, Li X, Yang B, Song J, et al. Anovel coronavirus from patients with pneumonia in China, 2019. The New England Journal of Medicine. 2020;**382**:727-733

[6] Gorbalenya AE, Baker SC, Baric RS, de Groot RJ, Gulyaeva AA, Haagmans BL, et al. The species and itsviruses—A statement of the coronavirus study group. bioRxiv. 2020. DOI: 10.1101/2020.02.07.937862

[7] Li W, Yang Y, Liu ZH, Zhao YJ, Zhang Q, Zhang L, et al. Progression of mental health services during the COVID-19 outbreak in China. International Journal of Biological Sciences. 2020;**16**(10):1732

[8] Dorp CH, Goldberg EE, Hengartner N, Ke R, Romero-Severson EO. Estimating the strength of selection for new SARS-CoV-2 variants. Nature Communications. 2021;**12**(1):1-3

[9] Chaw SM, Tai JH, Chen SL, Hsieh CH, Chang SY, Yeh SH, et al. The origin and underlying driving forces of the SARS-CoV-2 outbreak. Journal of Biomedical Science. 2020;**27**(1):1-2

[10] Gámbaro F, Behillil S, Baidaliuk A, Donati F, Albert M, Alexandru A, et al. Introductions and early spread of SARS-CoV-2 in France, 24 January to 23 march 2020. Eurosurveillance. 2020;**25**(26):2001200

[11] Sallard E, Lescure FX, Yazdanpanah Y, Mentre F, Peiffer-Smadja N. Type 1 interferons as a potential treatment against COVID-19. Antiviral Research. 2020;**178**:104791

[12] Brian DA, Baric RS. Coronavirus genome structure and replication. Current Topics Microbiology Immunology. 2005;**287**:1-30. DOI: 10.1007/3 540-26765-4_1

[13] Lu R, Zhao X, Li J, Niu P, Yang B, Wu H, et al. Genomic characterisation and epidemiology of 2019 novel coronavirus: Implications for virus origins and receptor binding. The lancet. 2020;**395**(10224):565-574

[14] Naqvi AA, Fatima K, Mohammad T, Fatima U, Singh IK, Singh A, et al. Insights into SARS-CoV-2 genome, structure, evolution, pathogenesis and therapies: Structural genomics approach. Biochimica et Biophysica Acta (BBA)-Molecular Basis of Disease. 2020;**1866**(10):165878. DOI: 10.1016/j.bbadis.2020.165878

[15] Wang MY, Zhao R, Gao LJ, Gao XF, Wang DP, Cao JM. SARS-CoV-2:

Structure, biology, and structure-based therapeutics development. Frontiers in Cellular and Infection Microbiology. 2020 Nov 25;**10**:587269. DOI: 10.3389/fcimb.2020.587269. PMID: 33324574; PMCID: PMC7723891

[16] Banerjee AK, Blanco MR, Bruce EA, Honson DD, Chen LM, Chow A, et al. SARS-CoV-2 disrupts splicing, translation, and protein trafficking to suppress host defenses. Cell. 2020;**183**(5):1325-1339. DOI: 10.1016/j.cell.2020.10.004

[17] Rambaut A, Loman N, Pybus O, Barclay W, Barrett J, Carabelli A, et al Preliminary Genomic Characterisation of an Emergent SARS-CoV-2 Lineage in the UK Defined by a Novel Set of Spike Mutations. 2020. Available at: https://virological.org/t/preliminary-genomic-characterisation-of-anemergent-sars-cov-2-lineage-in-the-uk-defined-by-a-novel-set-of-spikemutations/563.

[18] Atlanta GUSDoHaHS. Centers for Disease Control and Prevention. SARS-CoV-2 Variant Classifications and Definitions Centers for Disease Control and Prevention. Atlanta, Georgia: United States of America: Centers for Disease Control and Prevention; 2021

[19] Hoffmann M, Kleine-Weber H, Pöhlmann S. A multibasic cleavage site in the spike protein of SARS-CoV-2 is essential for infection of human lung cells. Molecular Cell. 2020;**78**(4):779-784

[20] Shang J, Wan Y, Luo C, Ye G, Geng Q, Auerbach A, et al. Cell entry mechanisms of SARS-CoV-2. Proceedings of the National Academy of Sciences. 2020;**117**(21):11727-11734

[21] Glowacka I, Bertram S, Müller MA, Allen P, Soilleux E, Pfefferle S, et al. Evidence that TMPRSS2 activates the severe acute respiratory syndrome coronavirus spike protein for membrane fusion and reduces viral control by the humoral immune response. Journal of Virology. 2011;**85**(9):4122-4134

[22] Matsuyama S, Nagata N, Shirato K, Kawase M, Takeda M, Taguchi F. Efficient activation of the severe acute respiratory syndrome coronavirus spike protein by the transmembrane protease TMPRSS2. Journal of Virology. 2010;**84**(24):12658-12664

[23] Shulla A, Heald-Sargent T, Subramanya G, Zhao J, Perlman S, Gallagher T. A transmembrane serine protease is linked to the severe acute respiratory syndrome coronavirus receptor and activates virus entry. Journal of Virology. 2011;**85**(2):873-882

[24] Plante JA, Liu Y, Liu J, Xia H, Johnson BA, Lokugamage KG, et al. Spike mutation D614G alters SARS-CoV-2 fitness. Nature. 2021;**592**(7852):116-121. DOI: 10.1038/s41586-020-2895-3

[25] Volz E, Mishra S, Chand M, Barrett JC, Johnson R, Geidelberg L, et al. Assessing transmissibility of SARS-CoV-2 lineage B. 1.1. 7 in England. Nature. 2021;**593**(7858):266-269. DOI: 10.1038/s41586-021-03470-x

[26] Mistry P, Barmania F, Mellet J, Peta K, Strydom A, Viljoen IM, et al. SARS-CoV-2 variants, vaccines, and host immunity. Frontiers in Immunology. 2021 Jan 3;**12**:809244. DOI: 10.3389/fimmu.2021.809244. PMID: 35046961. PMCID: PMC8761766

[27] Zhou B, Thao TT, Hoffmann D, Taddeo A, Ebert N, Labroussaa F, et al. SARS-CoV-2 spike D614G change enhances replication and transmission. Nature. 2021;**592**(7852):122-127. DOI: 10.1038/s41586-021-03361-1

[28] Legros V, Denolly S, Vogrig M, Boson B, Siret E, Rigaill J, et al.

A longitudinal study of SARS-CoV-2-infected patients reveals a high correlation between neutralizing antibodies and COVID-19 severity. Cellular & Molecular Immunology. 2021;**18**(2):318-327. DOI: 10.1038/s41423-020-00588-2

[29] Dhama K, Khan S, Tiwari R, Sircar S, Bhat S, Malik YS, et al. Coronavirus disease 2019–COVID-19. Clinical Microbiology Reviews. 2020;**33**(4):e00028-e00020

[30] Harari YN. The world after coronavirus. Financial Times. 2020;**20**(03):2020

[31] Griffiths E, Tanner J, Knox N, Hsiao W, Van Domselaar G. CanCOGeN interim recommendations for naming, identifying, and reporting SARS-CoV-2 variants of concern. SARS-CoV-2 variant classifications and definitions. CDC.gov. Centers for Disease Control and Prevention. 2021

[32] Koonin EV, Senkevich TG, Dolja VV. The ancient virus world and evolution of cells. Biology Direct. 2006 Dec;**1**(1):1-27

[33] Harapan H, Itoh N, Yufika A, Winardi W, Keam S, Te H, et al. Coronavirus disease 2019 (COVID-19): A literature review. Journal of Infection and Public Health. 2020;**13**(5):667-673

[34] Tang X, Wu C, Li X, Song Y, Yao X, Wu X, et al. On the origin and continuing evolution of SARS-CoV-2. National Science Review. 2020 Jun;7(6):1012-1023. DOI: 10.1093/nsr/nwaa036. Epub 2020 Mar 3. PMID: 34676127. PMCID: PMC7107875

[35] Koonin EV, Senkevich TG, Dolja VV. Compelling reasons why viruses are relevant for the origin of cells. Nature Reviews Microbiology. 2009;7(8):615

[36] Hu B, Guo H, Zhou P, Shi ZL. Characteristics of SARS-CoV-2 and COVID-19. Nature Reviews Microbiology. 2021;**19**(3):141-154

[37] Forster P, Forster L, Renfrew C, Forster M. Reply to Sánchez-Pacheco et al., Chookajorn, and Mavian et al.: Explaining phylogenetic network analysis of SARS-CoV-2 genomes. Proceedings of the National Academy of Sciences of the United States of America. 2020;**117**(23):12524

[38] Tao K, Tzou PL, Nouhin J, Gupta RK, de Oliveira T, Kosakovsky Pond SL, et al. The biological and clinical significance of emerging SARS-CoV-2 variants. Nature Reviews Genetics. 2021;**22**(12):757-773

[39] Witkowska D, Rabaan AA. Mass spectrometry and structural biology techniques in the studies on the coronavirus-receptor interaction. Molecules. 2020;**25**(18):4133

[40] Pal M, Berhanu G, Desalegn C, Kandi V. Severe acute respiratory syndrome coronavirus-2 (SARS-CoV-2): An update. Cureus. 2020 Mar 26;**12**(3):e7423. DOI: 10.7759/cureus.7423. PMID: 32337143. PMCID: PMC7182166

[41] Fung TS, Liu DX. Coronavirus infection, ER stress, apoptosis and innate immunity. Frontiers in Microbiology. 2014 Jun 17;5:296. DOI: 10.3389/fmicb.2014.00296. PMID: 24987391. PMCID: PMC4060729

[42] Masood N, Malik SS, Raja MN, Mubarik S, Yu C. Unraveling the epidemiology, geographical distribution, and genomic evolution of potentially lethal coronaviruses (SARS, MERS, and SARS CoV-2). Frontiers in Cellular and Infection Microbiology. 2020 Aug 27;10:499. DOI: 10.3389/fcimb.2020.00499. PMID: 32974224. PMCID: PMC7481402

[43] Dyson L, Hill EM, Moore S, Curran-Sebastian J, Tildesley MJ, Lythgoe KA,

et al. Possible future waves of SARS-CoV-2 infection generated by variants of concern with a range of characteristics. Nature Communications. 2021;**12**(1):1-3

[44] Wilton T, Bujaki E, Klapsa D, Majumdar M, Zambon M, Fritzsche M, et al. Rapid increase of SARS-CoV-2 variant B. 1.1. 7 detected in sewage samples from England between October 2020 and January 2021. Msystems. 2021;**6**(3):e00353-21

[45] Holmes EC, Goldstein SA, Rasmussen AL, Robertson DL, Crits-Christoph A, Wertheim JO, et al. The origins of SARS-CoV-2: A critical review. Cell. 2021;**184**(19):4848-4856

[46] Umakanthan S, Sahu P, Ranade AV, Bukelo MM, Rao JS, Abrahao-Machado LF, et al. Origin, transmission, diagnosis and management of coronavirus disease 2019 (COVID-19). Postgraduate Medical Journal. 2020;**96**(1142):753-758

[47] Mittal A, Khattri A, Verma V. Structural and antigenic variations in the spike protein of emerging SARS-CoV-2 variants. PLoS Pathogens. 2022;**18**(2):e1010260

[48] Habas K, Nganwuchu C, Shahzad F, Gopalan R, Haque M, Rahman S, et al. Resolution of coronavirus disease 2019 (COVID-19). Expert Review of Anti-infective Therapy. 2020;**18**(12):1201-1211

[49] Shang J, Ye G, Shi K, Wan Y, Luo C, Aihara H, et al. Structural basis of receptor recognition by SARS-CoV-2. Nature. 2020;**581**(7807):221-224

[50] Rabaan AA. Middle East respiratory syndrome coronavirus: Five years later. Expert Review of Respiratory Medicine. 2017 Nov;**11**(11):901-912. DOI: 10.1080/17476348.2017.1367288. Epub 2017 Aug 21. PMID: 28826284

[51] Zhang XY, Huang HJ, Zhuang DL, Nasser MI, Yang MH, Zhu P, et al. Biological, clinical and epidemiological features of COVID-19, SARS and MERS and AutoDock simulation of ACE2. Infectious Diseases of Poverty. 2020;**9**(04):10-20

[52] Zu ZY, Jiang MD, Xu PP, Chen W, Ni QQ, Lu GM, et al. Coronavirus disease 2019 (COVID-19): A perspective from China. Radiology. 2020 Aug;**296**(2):E15-E25. DOI: 10.1148/radiol.2020200490. Epub 2020 Feb 21. PMID: 32083985; PMCID: PMC7233368

[53] Liu Z, Xiao X, Wei X, Li J, Yang J, Tan H, et al. Composition and divergence of coronavirus spike proteins and host ACE2 receptors predict potential intermediate hosts of SARS-CoV-2. Journal of Medical Virology. 2020;**92**(6):595-601

[54] Burki TK. Coronavirus in China. The Lancet Respiratory Medicine. 2020;**8**(3):238

[55] Su S, Wong G, Shi W, Liu J, Lai AC, Zhou J, et al. Epidemiology, genetic recombination, and pathogenesis of coronaviruses. Trends in Microbiology. 2016;**24**(6):490-502

[56] Roser M, Ritchie H, Ortiz-Ospina E, Hasell J. Coronavirus disease (COVID-19)–statistics and research. Our World in data. WHO report. 2020;**4**

[57] Rutkowski S. Management challenges in chronic obstructive pulmonary disease in the COVID-19 pandemic: Telehealth and virtual reality. Journal of Clinical Medicine. 2021;**10**(6):1261

[58] Yang Y, Peng F, Wang R, Guan K, Jiang T, Xu G, et al. The deadly coronaviruses: The 2003 SARS pandemic and the 2020 novel coronavirus epidemic in China. Journal of Autoimmunity. 2020;**109**:102434

[59] Mason RJ. Pathogenesis of COVID-19 from a cell biology perspective. European Respiratory Journal. 2020 Apr 16;**55**(4):2000607. DOI: 10.1183/13993003.00607-2020. PMID: 32269085. PMCID: PMC7144260

[60] Sanders JM, Monogue ML, Jodlowski TZ, Cutrell JB. Pharmacologic treatments for coronavirus disease 2019 (COVID-19): A review. Journal of the American Medical Association. 2020;**323**(18):1824-1836

[61] Almeida JD, Berry DM, Cunningham CH, Hamre D, Hofstad MS, Mallucci L, et al. Coronaviruses. Nature. 1968;**220**(5168):650

[62] Forgie S, Marrie TJ. Healthcare-associated atypical pneumonia. In: Seminars in Respiratory and Critical Care Medicine. Vol. 30. Issue. 01. © Thieme Medical Publishers; 2009 Feb;**30**(1):67-85. DOI: 10.1055/s-0028-1119811. Epub 2009 Feb 6. PMID: 19199189

[63] Rabi FA, Al Zoubi MS, Kasasbeh GA, Salameh DM, Al-Nasser AD. SARS-CoV-2 and coronavirus disease 2019: What we know so far. Pathogens. 2020;**9**(3):231

[64] Zhu N, Zhang D, Wang W, Li X, Yang B, Song J, et al. China Novel Coronavirus Investigating and Research Team. A Novel Coronavirus from Patients with Pneumonia in China, 2019. The New England Journal of Medicine. 2020 Feb 20;**382**(8):727-733. DOI: 10.1056/NEJMoa2001017. Epub 2020 Jan 24. PMID: 31978945. PMCID: PMC7092803

[65] Chan JF, Yuan S, Kok KH, To KK, Chu H, Yang J, et al. A familial cluster of pneumonia associated with the 2019 novel coronavirus indicating person-to-person transmission: A study of a family cluster. The lancet. 2020;**395**(10223):514-523

[66] Livingston E, Bucher K. Coronavirus disease 2019 (COVID-19) in Italy. Journal of the American Medical Association. 2020;**323**(14):1335

[67] Lundgren JD, Grund B, Barkauskas CE, Holland TL, Gottlieb RL, Sandkovsky U, et al. ACTIV-3/TICO LY-CoV555 Study Group. A Neutralizing Monoclonal Antibody for Hospitalized Patients with Covid-19. The New England Journal of Medicine. Med. 2021 Mar 11;384(10):905-914. DOI: 10.1056/NEJMoa2033130. Epub 2020 Dec 22. PMID: 33356051. PMCID: PMC7781100

[68] Abduljalil JM, Abduljalil BM. Epidemiology, genome, and clinical features of the pandemic SARS-CoV-2: A recent view. New microbes and new infections. 2020;**35**:100672

[69] Li C, He Q, Qian H, Liu J. Overview of the pathogenesis of COVID-19. Experimental and Therapeutic Medicine. 2021;**22**(3):1-0

[70] Jean SS, Lee PI, Hsueh PR. Treatment options for COVID-19: The reality and challenges. Journal of Microbiology, Immunology and Infection. 2020;**53**(3):436-443

[71] Payne S. Viruses: From Understanding to Investigation. Elsiever, Academic Press; 2017

[72] Hossen M, Barek MA, Jahan N, Safiqul IM. A review on current repurposing drugs for the treatment of COVID-19: Reality and challenges. SN Comprehensive Clinical Medicine. 2020;**2**(10):1777-1789

[73] Chang J. Adenovirus vectors: Excellent tools for vaccine development. Immune Network. 2021 Feb 15;**21**(1)):e6. DOI: 10.4110/in.2021.21.e6. PMID: 33728099; PMCID: PMC7937504

[74] Burgos RM, Badowski ME, Drwiega E, Ghassemi S, Griffith N, Herald F, et al. The race to a COVID-19 vaccine: Opportunities and challenges in development and distribution. Drugs in Context. 2021 Feb 16;**10**:2020-12-2. DOI: 10.7573/dic.2020-12-2. PMID: 33643421. PMCID: PMC7889064

[75] Jin H, Lu L, Liu J, Cui M. COVID-19 emergencies around the globe: China's experience in controlling COVID-19 and lessons learned. International Journal for Quality in Health Care. 2021;**33**(1):mzaa143

[76] Bolze A, Cirulli ET, Luo S, White S, Cassens T, Jacobs S, et al. Rapid displacement of SARS-CoV-2 variant B. 1.1. 7 by B. 1.617. 2 and P. 1 in the United States. MedRxiv. 2021

[77] Taylor PC, Adams AC, Hufford MM, De La Torre I, Winthrop K, Gottlieb RL. Neutralizing monoclonal antibodies for treatment of COVID-19. Nature Reviews Immunology. 2021;**21**(6):382-393

[78] Marovich M, Mascola JR, Cohen MS. Monoclonal antibodies for prevention and treatment of COVID-19. Journal of the American Medical Association. 2020;**324**(2):131-132

[79] Mao L, Chen Z, Wang Y, Chen C. Design and application of nanoparticles as vaccine adjuvants against human corona virus infection. Journal of Inorganic Biochemistry. 2021;**219**:111454

[80] Majumder J, Minko T. Recent developments on therapeutic and diagnostic approaches for COVID-19. The AAPS Journal. 2021;**23**(1):1-22

[81] Alinia-Ahandani E, Sheydaei M. Overview of the introduction to the new coronavirus (Covid19): A review. Journal of Medicine Biology Science Research. 2020;**6**(2):14-20

[82] Kaur SP, Gupta V. COVID-19 vaccine: A comprehensive status report. Virus Research. 2020;**288**:198114

[83] Hajj Hussein I, Chams N, Chams S, El Sayegh S, Badran R, Raad M, et al. Vaccines through centuries: Major cornerstones of global health. Frontiers in Public Health. 2015 Nov 26;**3**:269. DOI: 10.3389/fpubh.2015.00269. PMID: 26636066. PMCID: PMC4659912

[84] Du L, Jiang S. Middle East respiratory syndrome: Current status and future prospects for vaccine development. Expert Opinion on Biological Therapy. 2015;**15**(11):1647-1651

[85] Thacker EE, Timares L, Matthews QL. Strategies to overcome host immunity to adenovirus vectors in vaccine development. Expert Review of Vaccines. 2009;**8**(6):761-777

[86] Li YD, Chi WY, Su JH, Ferrall L, Hung CF, Wu TC. Coronavirus vaccine development: From SARS and MERS to COVID-19. Journal of Biomedical Science. 2020;**27**(1):1-23

[87] Zhou P, Li Z, Xie L, An D, Fan Y, Wang X, et al. Research progress and challenges to coronavirus vaccine development. Journal of Medical Virology. 2021;**93**(2):741-754

[88] Chenchula S, Karunakaran P, Sharma S, Chavan M. Current evidence on efficacy of COVID-19 booster dose vaccination against the omicron variant: A systematic review. Journal of Medical Virology. 2022 Jul;**94**(7):2969-2976. DOI: 10.1002/jmv.27697. Epub 2022 Mar 14. PMID: 35246846. PMCID: PMC9088621

[89] Bartsch SM, O'Shea KJ, Ferguson MC, Bottazzi ME, Wedlock PT, Strych U, et al. Vaccine efficacy needed for a COVID-19 coronavirus vaccine to

prevent or stop an epidemic as the sole intervention. American Journal of Preventive Medicine. 2020;**59**(4):493-503

[90] Murali S, Sakthivel M, Kamaraj P, Venkataswamy V, Thangaraj JW, Shete A, et al. Effectiveness of ChAdOx1 nCoV-19 Corona virus vaccine (CovishieldTM) in preventing SARS-CoV2 infection, Chennai, Tamil Nadu, India, 2021. medRxiv. 2022

[91] Nowroozi A, Rezaei N. Severe acute respiratory coronavirus virus 2 (SARS-CoV-2) delta variant of concern breakthrough infections: Are vaccines failing us? Infection Control & Hospital Epidemiology. 2021 Aug 6:1-2. DOI: 10.1017/ice.2021.363. Epub ahead of print. PMID: 34353385. PMCID: PMC8387681

[92] Liang Q, Sun C, Liu H, Zhang X, Ahmed MA, Misra S, et al. Vaccination remains the first choice to control the spread of delta and other variants of severe acute respiratory coronavirus virus 2 (SARS-CoV-2). Infection Control & Hospital Epidemiology. 2021 Aug 6:1-2. DOI: 10.1017/ice.2021.361. Epub ahead of print. PMID: 34353390. PMCID: PMC8376837

[93] Zhou Y, Jiang S, Du L. Prospects for a MERS-CoV spike vaccine. Expert Review of Vaccines. 2018;**17**(8):677-686

[94] Tande AJ, Pollock BD, Shah ND, Binnicker M, Berbari EF. mRNA vaccine effectiveness against asymptomatic severe acute respiratory coronavirus virus 2 (SARS-CoV-2) infection over seven months. Infection Control and Hospital Epidemiology. 2022 Mar 43(3):393-395. DOI: 10.1017/ice.2021.399. Epub 2021 Sep 6. PMID: 34486511; PMCID: PMC8723985

[95] Luchsinger LL, Hillyer CD. Vaccine efficacy probable against COVID-19 variants. Science. 2021;**371**(6534):1116

[96] Ayoubkhani D, Bermingham C, Pouwels KB, Glickman M, Nafilyan V, Zaccardi F, et al. Trajectory of long covid symptoms after covid-19 vaccination: Community based cohort study. BMJ. 2022;**377**:e069676. DOI: 10.1136/bmj-2021-069676

[97] Fontanet A, Autran B, Lina B, Kieny MP, Karim SSA, Sridhar D. SARS-CoV-2 variants and ending the COVID-19 pandemic. Lancet. 2021;**397**(10278):952-954. DOI: 10.1016/S0140-6736(21)00370-6

[98] Thomson H. Two years of the coronavirus. New Scientist (1971). 2022;**253**(3368):10-13. DOI: 10.1016/S0262-4079(22)00003-3

[99] Gong W, Parkkila S, Wu X, Aspatwar A. SARS-CoV-2 variants and COVID-19 vaccines: Current challenges and future strategies. International Reviews of Immunology. 2022:1-22. DOI: 10.1080/08830185.2022.2079642. [Epub ahead of print]

[100] Lauring AS, Hodcroft EB. Genetic variants of SARS-CoV-2—What do they mean? Journal of the American Medical Association. 2021;**325**(6):529-531. DOI: 10.1001/jama.2020.27124

Chapter 18

SARS-COV-2 Pandemic: How to Maintain a COVID-free Hospital

Marco Bassanello, Ugo Coli, Antonio Tegon, Maria Teresa Pasqualini, Aldo Farencena, Matteo Geretto and Maurizio D'Aquino

Abstract

The emergence of severe acute respiratory syndrome type 2 coronavirus (SARS-CoV-2) and its complications have demonstrated the devastating impact of a new infectious pathogen since the first months of 2020, especially on Health Systems. The work to maintain a COVID-free hospital in terms of reorganization of operational processes and surveillance against SARS-CoV-2 has allowed us to maintain the structure suitable for activities for non-positive patients. The commitment related to this reorganization (not only in terms of costs) is largely satisfied by the responses to the health needs of non-COVID patients. The results obtained during the First Pandemic phase at the Giovanni XXIII Hospital in Monastier di Treviso have allowed the maintenance of the status of a COVID-free hospital. These results are supported by multiple studies in other parts of the world.

Keywords: SARS CoV-2, COVID hospital, COVID- 19, coronavirus, pandemic, vaccines, immunity

1. Introduction

COVID-19 [1] (acronym of Coronavirus Disease 19), or Severe Acute Respiratory Syndrome from SARS-CoV-2 or more simply Coronavirus disease 2019, is an infectious respiratory disease caused by the virus SARS-CoV-2 belonging to the Coronavirus family. The first cases were found in China (Wuhan Province) during the COVID-19 pandemic of 2019–2020 [2]. Coronavirus mainly affects the lower respiratory tract with flu-like symptoms [3, 4], such as fever, cough, shortness of breath, muscle pain, fatigue and diarrhea [5]; up to pneumonia, ARDS, sepsis and septic shock, and death of the patient. More studies indicate the endothelium as the virus site of the attack, therefore the involvement is systemic. A mass vaccination campaign is underway with two types of vaccines: mRNA and protein vaccines. Currently, treatment consists of isolating the patient and managing clinical symptoms [3]. An infected person may present symptoms after an incubation period that can vary between 2 and 14 days approximately (although there have been cases of 29 days), during which they can still be contagious [6, 7]. To limit its transmission,

IntechOpen

precautions must be taken, such as adopting careful personal hygiene, washing hands frequently and wearing Personal Protective Equipment (PPE) [8]. Those who believe they are infected must remain in quarantine, wear a surgical mask and call a doctor immediately in order to receive appropriate guidance [4, 9]. Today monoclonal antibodies and antivirals prevent serious complications when taken in the first days of infection [10]. But the only weapon in our possession is the isolation of infected communities. Due to its characteristics, a hospital is the structure with the greatest risk of transmission of pathogenic microorganisms, due to the high number of users, the permanence of many of them in the wards or common areas (emergency room, polyclinics), invasive diagnostic-therapeutic procedures to which patients are subjected and the immunosuppression state of many of them. The occurrence of epidemic clusters within hospitals can lead to such serious consequences that it is essential to take all necessary measures to prevent these. In the United Kingdom, during the second wave, some hospitals were defined as COVID-free Hospitals in order to guarantee the National Health Service (NHS) the possibility of treating cancer patients or other diseases, without suspending elective management as during the first pandemic wave. In fact, this approach was criticized by doctors and charities as it would increase the number of deaths and slow down millions of elective treatments in an unsustainable manner. The March closures allegedly denied vital care to non-COVID patients, with the exclusive treatment of COVID-positive patients. Planned treatments such as oncological surgery, joint prosthetic surgery, and ophthalmic surgery were discontinued. According to the NHS, a COVID-free Hospital should have been kept as free as possible from COVID-positive patients, unlike what happened during the first pandemic wave. This should also have reduced the risk of patients hospitalized for normal care being infected with COVID-19 while inwards. In north London, Whittington Hospital has designated a COVID-free site. It did not receive infected patients so that it could make time for planned non-urgent surgeries. COVID-19 patients would have been treated at University College London hospital or the nearby Royal Free hospital. Likewise, for hospitals in northwest London. In fact, millions of people have been denied NHS assistance after the fight against the coronavirus became a priority in the first wave. A record total of more than 2 million people - three times the figure from the same period last year - had to wait more than 18 weeks to begin hospital treatment in England, according to data from that period. Some hospitals, however, continued to provide COVID and non-COVID care in the same facility while maintaining strict infection control (by The Guardian of 21.09.2020 "Some hospitals in England to be kept COVID-free in second wave").

During the Italian pandemic of February–April 2020, the small hospital "Giovanni XXIII" in Monastier di Treviso, in the province of Treviso, was declared COVID-free by the local health authorities.

During this pandemic phase, SARS-CoV-2 circulated in this territory involving about 2.1% of the population [11].

This function has changed the management of hospitalized patients and the duties of health personnel working there.

2. The Health Organization in Veneto (Italy) during the first SARS-CoV-2 pandemic wave

Friday 21 February 2020 is a central date for the Italian situation linked to the new coronavirus (date of the first death from COVID in Italy, in Vò Euganeo in Veneto).

On that date, several cases of coronavirus emerged in Lombardy: these were people from outside China, a new outbreak whose extent was not yet known. Some of the affected villages (Codogno, Castiglione d'Adda, Casalpusterlengo and others) were in fact closed, a bit like it is now for Italian "protected areas". Outside China, the number of infected people is very high in Italy, Iran and South Korea, even if for the WHO, COVID-19 is not yet a pandemic. However, between the end of February and the first days of March 2020, after Italy, an increasing number of cases and an epidemic were also detected in other states (Europe and beyond). 4, 8 and 9 March: the three key dates of the measures in Italy. The infection spread in our country, especially in the north, but it was also starting in other regions. For this reason, on Wednesday 4 March the government gave the green light for the closure of schools and universities throughout Italy until 15 March. As of the 4th, according to data from the Civil Protection, the positives were about 2700 and there were already some cases (dozens or a few) in all regions. While on Sunday 8 March came the decree that provided for the isolation of Lombardy, by far the most affected, and of other 14 provinces, which became the "red zone". Although the still unofficial draft of the decree had already been published by some newspapers on the evening of the 7th. Finally, we arrive at the last (for now) important date for Italy: that of Monday 9 March. On that day, the government extended the measures already taken for Lombardy and the other 14 provinces to the whole country, so much so that all of Italy became a "protected area". The new rules were contained in the new decree Dpcm March 9, 2020, which came into force on 10 March. In fact, the rule is contained in the hashtag #iorestoacasa, you could only go out for proven reasons of necessity such as shopping, for work needs, for the purchase of medicines or other health reasons.

On 11 March 2020, Tedros Adhanom Ghebreyesus, World Health Organization (WHO) Director General, announced in the briefing from Geneva on the coronavirus epidemic that COVID-19 "can be characterized as a pandemic situation". The WHO's goal is to appeal to all nations to counter the spread of COVID-19. This condition remained valid until the gradual recovery with Phase 2 of the pandemic crisis.

The "Regional guidelines for the reopening of health activities - Phase 2 COVID 19 - interim document" of 28/04/2020, provided specific indications on the operation and organization of hospitals in Veneto, guided by criteria for maximum risk containment of the SARS-CoV-2 infection and to guarantee safe treatments to patients who have it, which can only be provided in this context, as well as to protect the health personnel who work there. In particular, it indicated the aspects of hospital management in Phase 2 COVID-19.

The main mission of the hospital, as a technical-functional structure dedicated to the treatment of acute and immediate post-acute conditions, is to provide appropriate, timely and excellent health services, emergency/urgent health services and highly complex programmed services, aimed at patients with a high level of vulnerability, also due to infectious diseases. It follows that, among the different types of health facilities, the hospital is the one at the greatest risk of transmission of pathogenic microorganisms, due to the number of users, the permanence of many of them in the wards, invasive procedures and diagnostic-therapeutic treatments to which they are subjected and the immunosuppressive state of many of them. The eventuality that epidemic clusters may arise within hospitals entails such serious consequences that it is essential to implement all the necessary measures to prevent their occurrence. Therefore, the hospitals of the Veneto Region should have permanently adopted access procedures in compliance with the guidelines contained in this document which represented, for the hospitals, a tool to be used, not only in this epidemic phase, to prepare specific operational processes and paths of access but also aimed at the prevention and management of infections from different pathogens. This task was carried out by the Medical Departments of the Presidium which, for this purpose, would have collaborated with the corporate Risk Management Services.

This document, therefore, had the purpose of:

- returning the hospital to its main management function emergency/urgency and health services based on the provisions of the "Hub and Spoke" model, reaffirmed within the Veneto Regional Social-Health Plan of 2019–2023;
- reducing all the low-complexity functions that can be performed in other health facilities, in order to drastically reduce the flows of users who access them, with a view to preventing infectious diseases with particular reference to SARS-CoV-2 infection;
- further strengthening the pathways aimed at containing hospital infections, with particular reference to SARS-CoV-2, for patients, in particular the most fragile ones, who need treatment for other pathologies;
- ensuring the safety of personnel working within hospitals.

This document was aimed at all regional health authorities and accredited public and private hospitals, in order to provide the necessary and appropriate directives with respect to the access of hospitals to:

- the users/patients who came for treatment.
- the health, technical and administrative personnel operating there.
- the staff of external companies that provided services to the hospital (cleaners, employees of service cooperatives, etc.)
- workers in internal utility services.
- visitors.
- providers.
- volunteers.

This document was divided into the following operational lines:

1. General criteria for user access to hospital facilities.
2. Criteria for access to the emergency room.
3. Criteria for managing admissions activities.
4. Criteria for carrying out the surgical activity.

5. Criteria for carrying out outpatient activities.

6. Healthcare services in private practice.

7. Internal support services.

8. Relations with users.

9. Rules for employees.

10. Personnel related to service, work and supply companies.

11. Hygiene of the environments.

12. Morgue.

The general criteria for user access to hospital facilities are divided into prevention and compartmentalization measures for the containment/zeroing of the risk of contagion and can only be obtained by rethinking and radically redefining the organizational and care processes, the operational and connection spaces and separation of the different activities that take place within the hospital. The principle must be emphasized that every access to the hospital must have an adequate reason and, outside of urgent/emergency situations, it must, as a rule, be booked. The fronts to consider in defining these measures are:

- the methods of access for people to the health facility, depending on the purpose, the activities/services to be used and their conditions at the time of access;

- the precautionary, preventive and protective measures of the various subjects;

- the definition of suitable routes to convey, as neatly as possible, the flows of people, separating, as far as possible, the areas and routes for admissions, clinics and services;

- the need to guarantee the safe use of health services for people who need them;

- the need to consider the logistical and organizational characteristics of each individual structure, respecting the freedom of each managerial figure to adapt the prevention and protection measures to their own contexts;

- the definition of the sanitary and hygienic measures of prevention in the environments.

In order for anyone to access the hospital in safe health and hygiene conditions, minimizing the risk of transmission of pathogenic microorganisms, it is necessary to scrupulously observe the principle that only people who must access the hospital.

- to benefit from health services such as: urgent or planned admission, PS services, outpatient services (urgent or planned) or services related to a previous admission, etc.

- take advantage of other services that cannot be provided remotely (e.g. picking up of drugs for exclusive hospital distribution, administrative services that cannot be accessed from home due to lack of IT means, etc.)
- visit a relative, assist a minor or a disabled person.
- work there, in any capacity.

This principle implies the regulation of access and the maintenance of the set of hygiene and public health measures aimed at limiting the risk of transmission of microorganisms through the circulation of people in the hospital environment; these measures include:

1. the limitation of access to cases of real need;
2. the definition of differentiated paths;
3. social distancing;
4. the prevention of transmission through droplets;
5. hand hygiene.

The application of these preventive measures was also referred to in the Ordinance of the President of the Regional Council no. 40 of 13 April 2020 and would have been maintained, in order to prevent the transmission of SARS-CoV-2 infection, even after the end of the ongoing pandemic.

3. Results

3.1 Organization of the activity in our hospital

The end of the lockdown corresponded to a gradual relaxation of the restrictive measures put in place for the purpose of the containment determined by the coronavirus pandemic SARS-CoV-2 (COVID-19), which hit the health and economic system of our country in the spring 2020 and in a particular way our Region.

This moment coincided with the start of Phase 2 of the COVID-19 which also involved the Monastier Hospital with a significant commitment of human and economic resources, in order to guarantee the status of COVID-free Hospital, already been in place since the beginning of the pandemic itself.

In fact, during Phase 1, the Hospital remained operational at all times, with a central role in the organizational and health management chessboard of the eastern Treviso area.

From the end of February 2020, the strategic management of ULSS 2 decided to confer on the Monastier Hospital on the maintenance of urgent activities in a COVID-free context (i.e. free from coronavirus), in order to guarantee all medical emergencies and surgical-orthopedic "safe treatments" to safeguard the integrity of the patient, often elderly, who was admitted and treated there.

To this end, the Nursing Home management has put in place a "very tight mesh network" of controls based on evidence and reasonableness, adapting them to the inevitable changes that medical science has brought, allowing us to move from a critical Phase 1 to the current state.

During Phase 1, the Hospital management adopted the following progressive measures to maintain the status of a COVID-free Hospital:

- It has always adapted to all national and regional regulations and standards in force.
- All the material and instrumentation (respirators, monitors, infusion pumps, etc.) of the first aid and reanimation have been sold to the intensive care unit (ICU) of the reference area hospital (hub centre of reference), in that moment in a great state of the managerial shortfall.
- Health personnel have been made available to the hub centre of reference for any needs or critical issues that cannot be overcome.
- The organization of the structure has been transformed: from a hospital with a programmed elective activity of excellence to a hospital with emergency activities (although it does not yet have its own operational emergency room), creating shifts for the availability of health personnel that has allowed hundreds of patients (especially elderly at risk) to receive urgent specialist care, keeping them "protected and safe".

All this was possible thanks to the establishment of an Operational Crisis Unit h24 / 7on7 until the end of Phase 1.

- The staff (health and non-medical) who accessed the Nursing Home have been checked through the access gates to the Nursing Home, which allows temperature control and daily medical history of the subject who accessed the facility, producing a daily report for the purpose of epidemiological surveillance.
- All subjects with body temperatures higher than 37.5°C were entrusted to the caregiver. All patients entering the admissions regime were subjected to a throat swab for specific RNA-COVID-19 research, and COVID-19 negative patients admitted exclusively in single rooms (in the medical department, more at risk, with negative air pressure).
- All the staff operating in the Nursing Home were subjected to active surveillance in order to preserve their integrity and of the frail hospitalized patients, placing the subjects at risk in quarantine until their negativity to the tampon and subsequent serological tests were determined qualitatively.
- The use of PPE has been arranged systematically to healthcare personnel and patients, in order to ensure safety towards potentially infected patients and fragile subjects who are certainly not infected and the healthcare staff themselves.
- In all cases of admission, a device (tablet for video calls) has been made available to the patient during the hospital stay for communication with the family, preventing access to accompanying persons/relatives (except in special cases).

- Social distancing measures have been guaranteed at the time of access, during waiting, in the departments and admission areas.
- Antibody screening has been done with the qualitative determination of COVID-19-specific antibodies (IgM and IgG) in subjects (patients or staff) with clinical doubt when these procedures have become accessible and reliable.

3.2 COVID-free hospital organization

Phase 2, therefore, began after having guaranteed the status of COVID-free Hospital to the Monastier Hospital and the safety of the subjects who up to now have passed through it.

In this new phase, the difficulty in eliminating the risk of contagion (which, however, will increase) has led to further restrictive decisions, in order to maintain a closer and therefore more effective control network.

The management of the Nursing Home has therefore decided to create a "lean" structure to direct these operations coordinated by a COVID manager.

This structure will make use of all the best technical-scientific and specialist skills in order to further safeguard the integrity of the Hospital's COVID-free status and to make access to it still safe for patients, staff (and therefore their families) and all those who want to take advantage of the excellences that are available to a territory and a population that at this moment needs "Safe Care".

To this end, it was decided to reorganize the resumption of services as follows:

- Arrangement of 5 filter zones for the entrance to the Nursing Home (**Table 1**).
- Arrangement of 5 gates in the filter areas equipped with turnstiles to determine the access flows of subjects to the Nursing Home (**Table 2**).
- Arrangement of four check-in areas for patient registration.
- Preparation of routes for patients who must access treatments and clinics by appointment (**Tables 3, 4, 6–9, 11–13**).

A (WHITE)	Access for patients destined for outpatient clinics, cardiology, admission, symptomatic patients, patients in an ambulance, others	Tensile structure in front of the entrance above the access ramp to the Nursing Home
B (BLUE)	Access for patients destined for pre-admission, dentistry, post-operative check-up, swabs	External entrance to the ambulatory-cardiology reception area
C (YELLOW)	Access for patients destined for physiotherapy	External entrance to the physiotherapy reception area
D (NO COLOR)	Access for employees, specialists, suppliers, technicians or others	Rear access tunnel
E (RED)	Access to laboratory, radiology, handicapped people, minors	Hot room of the accident and emergency department
F (BLACK)	COVID Point	Tensile structure for tampons

Table 1.
Filter areas A-B-C-D-E.

Waiting room with entrance gate
Seats with a minimum distance of one and a half metres
Turnstiles with fever measurement and PPE control
Entrance gates and infrared thermo-scanner
Diversified path for symptomatic or febrile (sub-febrile) patients through filter area A
Check-in for booked patients
It is desirable to reach 100% of online or telephone bookings (CUP) as soon as possible
Check-in for unbooked patients (It is desirable to reach 0% of accesses without booking as soon as possible)
Presence of a room assistant
Water-drink-coffee dispenser
Mask and gloves dispenser

Table 2.
Gate features.

Seats with a minimum distance of 1-m
Certain tensile structure at Gate A, no tensile structure at Gate B, no tensile structure at Gate C, tunnel already present at Gate D, hot room of the accident and emergency department already present at Gate E
Summer air conditioning with a negative air pressure circuit in the tensile structure or natural air recycling
Doors/windows that can be opened to allow air to be recycled in the tensile structure or in the waiting rooms
Seating with fixed chairs spaced one and a half metres apart
Monitor skip queue (Filter Zone B-C)
TV monitor (Zone B-C)
Totem for booking at Gates A and B
Disinfectant dispenser
The turnstiles with fever measurement and device control allow control of access and exit flows (with data centralization and remote access control) for patient access at presentation time with a thermo-scanner and alarm if: • TC ≥ 37°C • no PPE (Mask)

Table 3.
Management of outpatient areas – waiting room with entrance gate.

If the patient is febrile (TC ≥ 37.5°C), he/she is sent to the entrance to the Emergency Department (ramp side) upon communication of the room assistant from the Gate sending the room assistant of Gate E
If a patient with 37°C ≤ TC <37.5°C, re-evaluation of the temperature by the Room Assistant with the tympanic or axillary thermometer. If confirmed, sent as in the previous point
If a patient is without PPE (mask and gloves), he/she is asked to purchase them
The Room Assistant must provide for patients who are unable to purchase surgical masks and gloves
The patient must enter and exit (if possible) the Nursing Home through the same turnstile

Each turnstile must be "controlled and governed" by the Room Assistant
The Room Assistants must be equipped with manual thermo-scanners (even in the case of turnstiles with thermo-scanners)
The filter area E can be controlled by a volumetric thermo-scanner
Infrared thermo-scanners are turnstile devices
The temperature check is guaranteed by the Room Assistant
The Gate and waiting area for symptomatic or febrile (sub-febrile) patients are located in the waiting room of the emergency department

Table 4.
Various events.

If the reason for accessing the Nursing Home is the symptom or fever he/she presents, the procedure already established at the time of booking will be followed
If the reason for access is different and there is no urgent need for access to the Nursing Home, he/she will be sent to the care provider for territorial care
If the reason for access is different and there is an urgent need for access to the Nursing Home, the referral specialist will be contacted
If the referral specialist is not reachable or is unable to define the problem or urgent management, the patient will be placed in safety and sent to the referral emergency room with 118
If the symptomatic or febrile (sub-febrile) subject is the carer, he/she will be sent to the care provider for territorial care
Surveillance protocol applications already in place

Table 5.
Diversified path for symptomatic or febrile (sub-febrile) patient through Gate A – the symptomatic or febrile (sub-febrile) patient, sent to the waiting room of the emergency department, is taken in charge by the assistant of Gate E and accommodated there.

The booking is made via CUP or online
The booking must be detailed and also include an information check (no interview) of the patient's health status (information report attached to the booking)
The patient must be present in the Filter Zone indicated 20 minutes before the time indicated for the visit
The passage from the turnstile to go to check-in: Gate A - Central Cashier Area Gate E - Central Cashier Area, Emergency Triage, Radiology Cashier area Gate B - Outpatient Reception Area Gate C - Physiotherapy Reception Area
The arrival of the patient at the outpatient clinic dedicated to the time of examination
Check-in filter totem at Gate A-B

Table 6.
Check-in for booked patients - it is desirable to reach 100% of online or telephone bookings as soon as possible.

Such patients should be referred to Gate A
Non-booked patients must ask the Room Assistant for a manual booking
These patients will be able to book their examination by entering with a report, one for every five patients already booked (1/5) at check-in

Table 7.
Check-in for non-booked patients – it is desirable to reach 0% of accesses without booking as soon as possible.

The presence of a Room Assistant is foreseen, positioned at each gate
This person will refer to the user
He/she will act as an intermediary with the check-in
He/she will control the body temperature or provide PPE if not available
He/she (at Gate A-E) will be the liaison with the switchboard for the search for the specialist
He/she (at Gate A) must deliver the information form for registration at check-in to patients who show up without registration
He/she will verify the regularity of the procedures, will give information on the path to follow, will verify that all the safety protocols are adopted: maintaining distance between people, correct use of PPE, avoiding assemblies
He/she will have to use gentle, appropriate manners, avoiding any conflicts that can arise in waiting situations
He/she will end his/her function with the Gate closed
He/she will write a report of the most significant events that emerged during his/her function

Table 8.
Presence of a waiting room.

Patients (and carers) who will pass through filter zones A and B can access the parking in front of the Nursing Home (PARK A-B)
Patients (and carers) who cross the filter area C can access the rear parking (access to physiotherapy) at the Nursing Home (PARK C)
Patients (and carers) who will cross the filter area E can access the rear-lateral parking (after the roundabout) at the Nursing Home (PARK E).
At the rear and side parking (after the roundabout) at the Nursing Home (PARK D) all the personnel (medical, technical and support) will be able to access the filter area D

Table 9.
Parking - the distribution and indications for the parking areas will be given by the civil protection volunteers.

This paper information form will be delivered to the patient who shows up without a booking and delivered to the assistant in Gate A (who will access him with a 1/5 ratio)
Questions to ask when booking: • Name • Surname • Date of birth • Address • Telephone number • Name and surname of accompanying person (only 1 per patient) • Reason for booking

• Access gate • Presentation day • Presentation at the Filter Area 20 minutes before the time of the examination (with absolute prohibition to arrive earlier) • Time of examination • Inform the patient about the path to follow • Exit after max 15 minutes of the end of the procedure • Exit from the access gate • Fever • Symptoms (cough, rhinitis or respiratory symptoms, pharyngitis, diarrhea, anosmia, other) • Quarantine • Previous contagion and / or positivity to COVID-19 • Call booking number if 15-16-17-18 on the day of the booking • For those accompanying: if 15-16-17-18 on the day of booking, it is useful to change the accompanying person • Carry masks (surgical or other valveless) and vinyl / latex gloves • Front Park (Park A-B) for Gate A-B - Rear Park (Park C-E) for Gate C-E • Inform about probable delays due to checks and filter • Inform if handicapped or non-self-sufficient people (input Filter Zone E) • Inform if a minor (Filter E Zone input)

Table 10.
Booking information form - it is desirable to reach 100% of online or telephone bookings as soon as possible.

After check-in, the patient must follow the path indicated at the time of booking and confirmed at check-in
The patient will arrive at the waiting room at the appointed time and he/she will receive the examination or service booked
Along the routes there will be stewards/hostesses who will check the regularity of the procedures, give information on the path to follow and verify that all safety protocols are adopted (maintaining distance between people, correct use of PPE also by personnel, avoiding assemblies)
Once the examination has been completed, the patient can go to the cashier, the bar and try to limit the stay in the Nursing Home to a maximum of 15 minutes
elf-sufficient patients must have individual access to the visiting areas
In any case, the access of a companion of non-self-sufficient patients or minors is allowed
The exit from the facility will take place through the entry gate (if possible)
Surveillance protocol application already in place
In the clinic, the operator must present himself with the following PPE: • FFP2 or FFP3 mask without valve • Vinyl or latex gloves • Overshirt if invasive maneuvers on the airways or other invasive maneuvers are foreseen: • Visor • Shoe covers • Change of PPE after each patient with these characteristics

Table 11.
Outpatient clinics – service areas to be provided.

After check-in, the patient must follow the path indicated in the instructions given for admission and confirmed at check-in
The patient will arrive at the waiting room of the reference ward at the established time where he/she will prepare for admission

In this circumstance, the temperature will be re-measured and the Head of the Department informed by the reception nurse
Along the routes there will be stewards/hostesses who will verify the regularity of the procedures, give information on the path to follow and verify that all safety protocols are adopted (maintaining distance between people, correct use of PPE also by personnel, avoiding assemblies)
Self-sufficient patients will have to access the admission areas individually
In any case, the access of a companion of non-self-sufficient patients or minors is allowed
In all cases, a device (tablet for video calls) will be made available during the hospital stay for communication with the family
Surveillance protocol applications already in place

Table 12.
Departments – hospital areas.

Sanitation
Basic Medical Information
External Information
IT Procedures

Table 13
Connections.

- Preparation of a path for patients who must access treatments and clinics by appointment, but with critical issues (**Table 5**).
- Preparation of a personal report during telephone booking at the CUP of the structure (**Table 10**).
- Preparation of guidelines for administrative and health care.
- Updates of the organizational status, in case the needs and/or priorities of access to treatment, should change.

The strategic combination of operating procedures (as represented by the tables) and sequencing of Reverse Transcriptase-Polymerase Chain Reaction (RT-PCR) tests have proved successful, allowing uninterrupted system operativity.

All patients admitted to our hospital (DH-DS included) will be subjected to RT-PCR tests (T0) performed the day before hospitalization at Gate F – COVID Point (7.00–9.00), in order to promptly intercept any positive cases before hospitalization. Patients will continue with molecular swabs from hospitalization, following the scheme:

- T1: at the entrance of the patient in the ward (Day Hospital – Day Surgery included).
- T2: every 48 h after T1.
- T3: in the case of active or passive surveillance.
- T4 (RAPID MOLECULAR SWAB from 2021): to patients transferred from other hospitals who have not performed the molecular swab at that site (**Table 14**).

T0	Before hospitalization
T1	At the entrance of the patient in the ward
T2	Every 48 h after T1
T3	In the case of active or passive surveillance
T4 (from 2021)	To patients transferred from other hospitals who have not performed the molecular swab at that site

Table 14.
Sequential swabs.

The surveillance with sequential molecular swabs for the health and non-health personnel operating at the facility has also made it possible to avoid the formation of clusters within the structure and propagate the infections. The temporal variability of these swabs for staff will change depending on the course of the epidemic outside the hospital and will diversify into active or passive surveillance [12, 13]. These RT-PCR tests were performed on hospital staff up to once per day.

During the First Pandemic Phase of Coronavirus in Veneto in Spring 2020, we can distinguish three periods of activity at our hospital. An initial block Phase from 22 February to 9 March, a Phase 1 (total block) from 10 March to 3 May and a Phase 2 from 4 May to today (data collection deadline 18 June 2020).

The admissions activity at our hospital was referable only to urgent patients with admissions to the Departments of Orthopedics, Physiotherapy and Medicine. The outpatient activity was only possible on patients of various specialties of an urgent nature or with priority evaluation within 7 days.

In the initial phase, 85% of outpatient visits were carried out and 98.5% of patients were seen compared to the same period in 2019, and there were 102% admissions compared to 2019.

In Phase 1, 21% of outpatient visits were made and 18% of patients were seen compared to the same period in 2019 and there were 26.4% of admissions compared to 2019.

In Phase 2, 94.7% of outpatient visits were carried out and 101.6% of patients were seen compared to the same period in 2019 and there were 81.3% of admissions compared to 2019.

During the Initial Phase and Phase 2, the recovery of activity highlighted by the numbers above led to an optimization of the Health Organization according to the still present and important external circulation of SARS-CoV-2.

All while continuing to maintain the structure of a COVID-free hospital.

4. Discussion

When community cases of COVID-19 increase:

1. Emergency departments immediately enact new pathways and protocols for triage, evaluation and admission [14].

2. Hospitals begin to assess and enhance inpatient capacity, often by opening units not traditionally used for general medical care (for example, postoperative care units) as COVID-19–designated areas [15].

3. Hospitals reduce elective surgical activity, merge specialized ICUs, and increase costs due to the need to have more staff available for the care of critical patients. The monitoring of patient flows between departments is optimized and the communication of news about patients' conditions to family members is simplified [16].

In addition to the macro-processes, the micro-processes are completely revised, involving all the Operational Units of the Hospital. New equipment such as beds and mechanical fans is provided in specific areas. PPE and reagents for laboratory tests are purchased. Medical, nursing and paramedical personnel, even newly recruited, are diverted to critical departments and trained for emergencies. Common areas such as canteen, laundry and sanitation are organized with access scheduling. Suppliers are diverted to different areas of the building. In addition, monitoring and critical patient management guidelines are introduced. [17]. Kadri and colleagues present findings from a nationally representative cohort of 144,116 hospitalized patients cared for in 558 hospitals to understand the effect of COVID-19 surges on patient outcomes. Nearly 1 in every 4 deaths and almost 6000 total deaths may have been attributable to hospital strain due to COVID-19 [18]. However, Kadri and colleagues' analyses may not capture the tightrope that many of us walk today as we balance COVID-19 and non– COVID-19 care. Shared learning platforms to understand how hospitals are managing COVID-19 care could be launched [17].

An interesting programme was the Mi-COVID-19 initiative in Michigan, where Blue Cross Blue Shield of Michigan and Blue Care Network, the Michigan Health & Hospital Association, the Society of Critical Care Medicine, and 40 hospital systems came together to improve COVID-19 care [19]. The Mi-COVID-19 initiative served as an amalgam for clinicians and hospital leaders across the state to tackle important questions ranging from therapeutic strategies and excess antibiotic use to provider wellbeing and long-term outcomes of COVID-19 survivors [20, 21].

Besides patients, there are other victims when COVID-19 strikes hospitals: health care workers. And although some have raised their voices asking for change [22], surveys suggest that many are considering leaving the field after being battered by wave after wave of COVID-19 [23].

Measures to control SARS-CoV-2 infections include active surveillance for early identification of the positive subject, with his/her isolation in dedicated rooms and the systematic use of PPE; and passive surveillance for the tracking of potential secondary cases (perhaps asymptomatic) [24–27].

Effective infection control measures against SARS in 2003 were less successful against SARS-CoV-2 [28], due to the greater number of asymptomatic (but infectious) cases, and the presence of a peak of viral load with the presentation of symptoms. Therefore, the systematic screening of patients and healthcare staff by RT-PCR reduces the risk of outbreaks in hospitals [29]. The risk of hospital transmission increases if asymptomatic COVID-19 patients are placed in non-AIRI rooms, and/or in high-flow oxygen or non-invasive ventilation [30]. Therefore, the use of PPE by healthcare personnel and inpatients should be applied to reduce the risk of SARS-CoV-2 droplet transmission [31]. Universal masking in the community also reduced the incidence of COVID-19 in the general population [32]. Also, appropriate use of PPE is associated with a decreased risk of COVID-19 [33]. The huge number of patients admitted to the COVID-19 Hospital also greatly increases the risk of expansion of the nosocomial epidemic. In China (Singapore), Hong Kong, UK, USA, temporary hospitals have been built (using tents or existing buildings such as conference or exhibition halls) to cope with a sudden increase in COVID-19 cases [34–36]. During the SARS-CoV-2 pandemic in Italy, some hospitals became fully COVID-Hospitals, while in most others, parts of the hospital were converted or created to treat COVID-19 patients. In the latter cases, other parts of the hospital, "no-Covid-19" departments, treated COVID-negative patients. Bo et al. reported their experience within a COVID-free department, with asymptomatic patients or with negative RT-PCR tests. During the study, a proportional increase in surveillance tests against SARS-CoV-2 was adopted based on the increase in the community spread of COVID-19, together with the use of PPE. Their findings demonstrate that there is a not negligible risk of "hospital-acquired" SARS-CoV-2 infection, both for patients and hospital staff, particularly within overcrowded supposed no-COVID-19 wards [37].

In our hospital, the winning strategy was to avoid the spread of SARS-CoV-2 infection with modular surveillance models on the course of the pandemic: increased surveillance tests (RT-PCR tests) with the worsening of the pandemic curve. Also important were the systematic adoption of PPE, the use of passive surveillance tests (with contact tracing, both for patients and healthcare personnel) in the face of an alleged case of COVID-19 or contact [38] and, where possible, patient isolation and safe distancing.

5. Conclusions

During Phases 1 and 2 of the SARS-CoV-2 pandemic that struck Italy in the months from February to April 2020, the re-organization of the hospital structure with strict containment rules and surveillance with RT-PCR tests allowed it to remain a hospital free of SARS-CoV-2, with zero infections.

The admissions activity at our hospital was referable only to urgent patients with admissions to the Departments of Orthopedics, Physiotherapy and Medicine. The outpatient activity was only possible for patients with various specialties of an urgent nature or with priority evaluation within 7 days.

The subsequent pandemic waves, faced with the same methodological approach, have allowed the Giovanni XXIII Hospital to remain a COVID-free Hospital.

Acknowledgements

We thank all the staff working at the Microbiology Laboratory and Service of the Giovanni XXIII Hospital in Monastier di Treviso for their unwavering commitment to the fight against COVID-19. We also thank Gabriele Geretto and Massimo Calvani (respectively CEO and President of our Hospital) for the commendable organizational support during the pandemic.

Conflict of interest

The authors declare no conflict of interest.

Author details

Marco Bassanello*, Ugo Coli, Antonio Tegon, Maria Teresa Pasqualini, Aldo Farencena, Matteo Geretto and Maurizio D'Aquino
Casa di Cura Giovanni XXIII Monastier di Treviso, Treviso, Italy

*Address all correspondence to: bassanellomarco@hotmail.com

References

[1] Zhun ZD, Wang W et al. China novel Coronavirus investigating and research team. A novel coronavirus from patients with pneumonia in China. The New England Journal of Medicine. 2020; **382**(8):727-733

[2] Munster VJ, KoopMans M, Van DoreMalen N, Van Riel D. A novel coronavirus emerging in China - key questions for impact assessment. The New England Journal of Medicine. 2020; **383**(8):692-694

[3] Q&A on COVID-19, ecdc.europa.eu

[4] Australian Government Department of Health, Novel Coronavirus. 2019. Available from: https://www.health.gov.au/diseases/covid-19- COVID-19

[5] Jinyang G, Bing H, Jian W. COVID-19: Gastrointestinal manifestations and potential fecal-oral transmission. Gastroenterology. 2020;**158**(6): 1518-1519

[6] Harapan H, Itoh N, Yufika A, Winardi W, Keam S, Te H, et al. Coronavirus disease 2019 (COVID-19): A literature review. Journal of Infection and Public Health. 2020;**13**(5):667-673

[7] Expert reaction to news reports that the China coronavirus may spread before symptoms show | Science Media Center. sciencemediacentre.org. [Accessed on: February 11, 2020]

[8] Sequence for Putting on Personal Protective Equipment (PPE). Available from: https://www.cdc.gov

[9] MOH Updates on 2019 Novel Coronavirus (2019-nCoV) Local Situation www.moh.gov.sg

[10] Bartoletti M, Azap O, Barac A, Bussini L, Ergonul O, Krause R, et al. ESCMID COVID-19 living guidelines: Drug treatment and clinical management. Clinical Microbiology and Infection. 2022;**28**(2):222-238

[11] Bassanello M et al. Epidemiological study in a small rural area of Veneto (Italian region) during Sars-Cov-2 Pandemia. Scientific Reports. 2021;**11**: 23247

[12] Vandenberg O, Martiny D, Rochas O, van Belkum A, Kozlakidis Z. Considerations for diagnostic COVID-19 tests. Nature Reviews. Microbiology. 2021;**19**(3):171-183

[13] Lai CKC, Lam W. Laboratory testing for the diagnosis of COVID-19. Bioche mical and Biophysical Research Communications. 2021;**538**:226-230

[14] Whitwell K, Maynard R, Barry N, et al. Strategic planning and response to COVID-19 in a London emergency department. Emergency Medicine Journal. 2020;**37**:567-570

[15] Griffin KM, Karas MG, Ivascu NS, et al. Hospital preparedness for COVID-19: A practical guide from a critical care perspective. American Journal of Respiratory and Critical Care Medicine. 2020;**201**:1337-1344

[16] Chopra V, Toner E, Waldhorn R, et al. How should U.S. hospitals prepare for coronavirus disease, COVID-19. Annals of Internal Medicine. 2019; **2020**(172):621-622

[17] Chopra V. When COVID-19 strikes your hospital. Annals of Internal Medicine. 2021;**174**(9):1319-1320

[18] Kadri SS, Sun J, Lawandi A, et al. Association between caseload surge and COVID-19 survival in 558 U.S. hospitals.

Annals of Internal Medicine. 2021;**174**: 1240-1251

[19] University of Michigan Institute for Healthcare Policy and Innovation. COVID-19 Hospital Network Shares Key Lessons to Improve Care. 2021. Accessed at https://ihpi.umich.edu/news/covid-19-hospital-network-shares-key-lessons-improve-care [Accessed on: June 20, 2021]

[20] Vaughn VM, Gandhi TN, Petty LA, et al. Empiric antibacterial therapy and community-onset bacterial coinfection in patients hospitalized with coronavirus disease 2019 (COVID-19): A multi-hospital cohort study. Clinical Infectious Diseases. 2021;**72**:e533-e541

[21] Chopra V, Flanders SA, O'Malley M, et al. Sixty-day outcomes among patients hospitalized with COVID-19 [letter]. Annals of Internal Medicine. 2021;**174**: 576-578

[22] Essex R, Weldon SM. Health care worker strikes and the Covid pandemic. The New England Journal of Medicine. 2021;**384**:e93

[23] Delaney RK, Locke A, Pershing ML, et al. Experiences of a health system's faculty, staff, and trainees' career development, work culture, and childcare needs during the COVID-19 pandemic. JAMA Network Open. 2021;**4**: e213997

[24] Cheng VCC, Wong SC, Chuang VWM, et al. Absence of nosocomial transmission of coronavirus disease 2019 (COVID-19) due to SARS-CoV-2 in the prepandemic phase in Hong Kong. American Journal of Infection Control. 2020;**48**:890-896

[25] Cheng VCC, Wong SC, Wong SCY, et al. Directly observed hand hygiene - from healthcare workers to patients. The Journal of Hospital Infection. 2019; **101**:380-382

[26] Wong SC, AuYeung CH, Lam GK, et al. Is it possible to achieve 100 percent hand hygiene compliance during the coronavirus disease 2019 (COVID-19) pandemic? The Journal of Hospital Infection. 2020;**105**:779-781

[27] Cheng VCC, Wong SC, Chen JHK, et al. Escalating infection control response to the rapidly evolving epidemiology of the coronavirus disease 2019 (COVID-19) due to SARS-CoV-2 in Hong Kong. Infection Control and Hospital Epidemiology. 2020;**41**:493-498

[28] Cheng VC, Chan JF, To KK, et al. Clinical management and infection control of SARS: Lessons learned. Antiviral Research. 2013;**100**:407-419

[29] Kai K et al. Lessons learned 1 year after SARS-CoV-2 emergence leading to COVID-19 pandemic. Emerging Microbe s Infection. 2021;**10**:507-535

[30] Haymet A, Bassi GL, Fraser JF. Airborne spread of SARS-CoV-2 while using high-flow nasal cannula oxygen therapy: Myth or reality? Intensive Care Medicine. 2020;**46**:2248-2251

[31] Klompas M, Morris CA, Sinclair J, et al. Universal masking in hospitals in the covid-19 era. The New England Journal of Medicine. 2020;**382**:e63

[32] Cheng VC, Wong SC, Chuang VW, et al. The role of community-wide wearing of face mask for control of coronavirus disease 2019 (COVID-19) epidemic due to SARS-CoV-2. The Journal of Infection. 2020;**81**:107-114

[33] Liu M, Cheng SZ, Xu KW, et al. Use of personal protective equipment against coronavirus disease 2019 by healthcare professionals in Wuhan, China: Cross

sectional study. British Medical Journal. 2020;**369**:m2195

[34] Chen S, Zhang Z, Yang J, et al. Fangcang shelter hospitals: A novel concept for responding to public health emergencies. Lancet. 2020;**395**: 1305-1314

[35] Wong SC, Leung M, Tong DW, et al. Infection control challenges in setting up community isolation and treatment facilities for patients with coronavirus disease 2019 (COVID-19): Implementation of directly-observed environmental disinfection. InfectionControl and Hospital Epidemiology. 2021;**42**(9):1037-1045

[36] Chia ML, Him Chau DH, Lim KS, et al. Managing COVID-19 in a novel, rapidly deployable community isolation quarantine facility. Annals of Internal Medicine. 2021;**174**(2):247-251

[37] Bo M, Brunetti E, Presta R, Rota M, Dutto F, Cortese A, et al. To keep a COVID-19-free hospital ward: Mission possible? Aging Clinical and Experimental Research. 2020;**32**(8): 1627-1628

[38] Black JRM, Bailey C, Przewrocka J, et al. COVID-19: The case for health-care worker screening to prevent hospital transmission. Lancet. 2020;**395**: 1418-1420